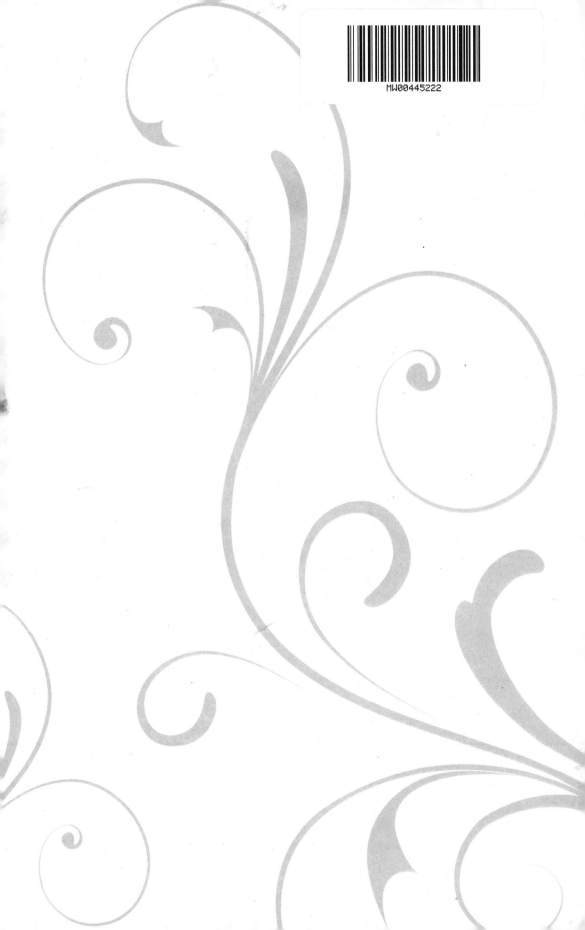

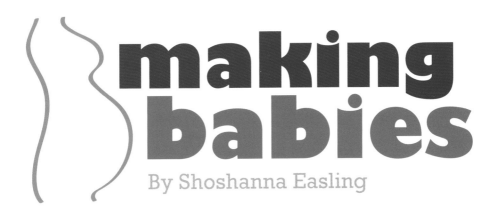

making babies

By Shoshanna Easling

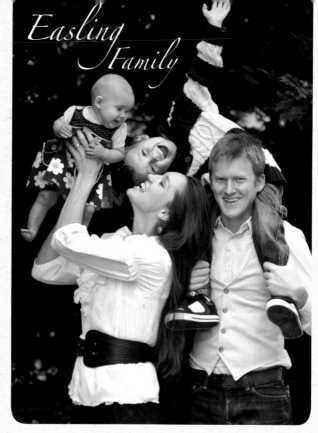

Easling Family

James and Shoshanna Easling and their two children, Jeremiah James, 6 years, and Penelope Jane, 1 year, live life together happily. They are passionate about keeping their family first and enjoying life, friends, and community involvement. Together the Easlings love working in their family business, Bulk Herb Store. Even though the Easling family is always busy working, they do not have a day without play. They love swimming, volleyball, peek-a-boo, wrestling, and so much more.

Live · Laugh · Love

MAKING BABIES

Editor in Chief: Shoshanna Easling

Design & Layout: Audrey Madill

Photography: Laura Newman Photography
See page 480 for Patricia Cohen
photo credits Lauren Brandt
Nate Crouch Photography
Clint Cearly
Alicia Easling
Hannah Stoll
Erin Harrison

First Edition October 2011
First Reprint March 2012
ISBN: 978-1-937478-04-9

Food staging and styling: Lauren Brandt
Patricia Cohen
Shoshanna Easling
Audrey Madill

Copy Editors: Michael Aprile
Steve Bailey
Jennifer Brooks
Patricia Cohen
Lisa Joyner
Laura Newman
Talitha Snow

Baby Diary Illustrations: James Easling

Contents

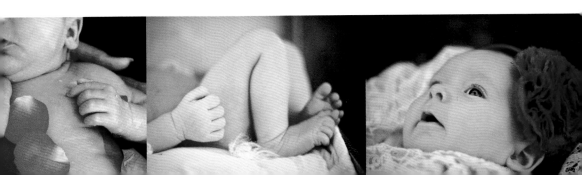

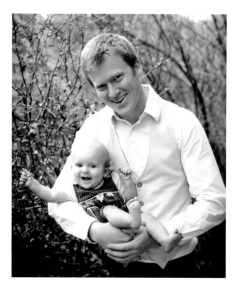
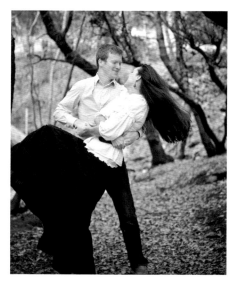
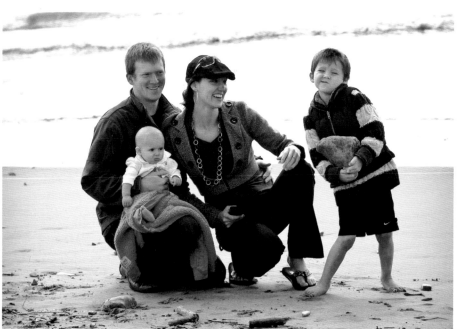
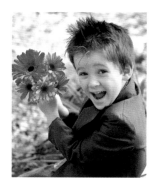
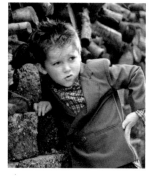
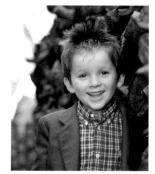

I dedicate this book to my wonderful husband (James) and amazing family (Jeremiah and Penelope). James supported me and helped with the kids every day of this project. I could never have done this without him. He was the rock that kept me going. Jeremiah James and Penelope Jane were my inspiration and my giggles along the way. They are the best kids in the world!!!! I love all of you guys and can't wait to live the rest of my life with you. Everything is better when we are together.

Love,
Mama (Shoshanna Easling)

Introduction

I got my inspiration for the *Making Babies* series from the pregnancy and birth of my first child. I loved every stage of my pregnancy and birth! I enjoyed learning and researching when I had morning sickness and when I got indigestion. Every time I was faced with another bridge, I would research, study, learn, apply, and rise to new heights of excitement. I knew everything I did, and did not do, would make a difference with me and my growing baby. It is not always easy finding good food to eat, knowing what exercises to do, and asking the right questions to the right people, but I researched it step by step and enjoyed a healthy pregnancy and birth.

I grew up in an Amish community. Talk about making babies--whoa, they make a lot! No, I am not Amish, but I am a blood-bought child of God. Twenty-five years ago my parents were artists living in Memphis, Tennessee. They wanted to raise us five children in the country so we could learn the dying art of homemaking and the skills of country living. Hard work, herbal remedies, nutritional health, home births, and common sense were all part of the lifestyle in the Amish community. In November 2004, my husband James and I found out we were pregnant with our first child. I knew I wanted to have my baby in the soothing warmth of my own home, so I went to talk to a midwife. I had assisted in two births before I got married, and knew I wanted my children's births to be better. With good food, the right exercises, and relaxation, the birth of Jeremiah James was WONDERFUL! The midwife that attended had been to over 350 births and said it was the best she had ever attended. Since my firstborn, I never stopped researching the wonderful world of making babies.

I have been asked many questions about healthy foods, recipes, exercises, and herbal remedies from family, friends, and customers at Bulk Herb Store. In November 2009, we got pregnant with our second child. I was so excited about my pregnancy journey. I was going to have another baby! I thought about all the horrible births I had heard about, and wanted to show women across the world how beautiful pregnancy and birth can be, so I started the *Making Babies* series.

Making Babies is a fresh, organic look at the simplistic beauty of pregnancy and birth. From delectable recipes, superb remedies, must-have tips, birthing exercises, and resources, to relaxing techniques, this is a fun, energetic video and book series. Follow me through my pregnancy and the birth of Penelope Jane Easling.

-Shoshanna Easling

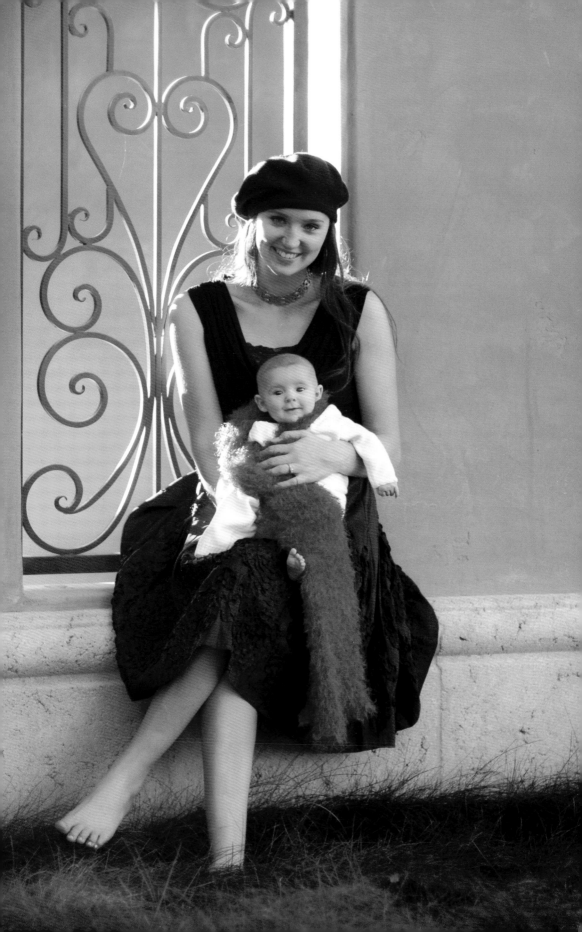

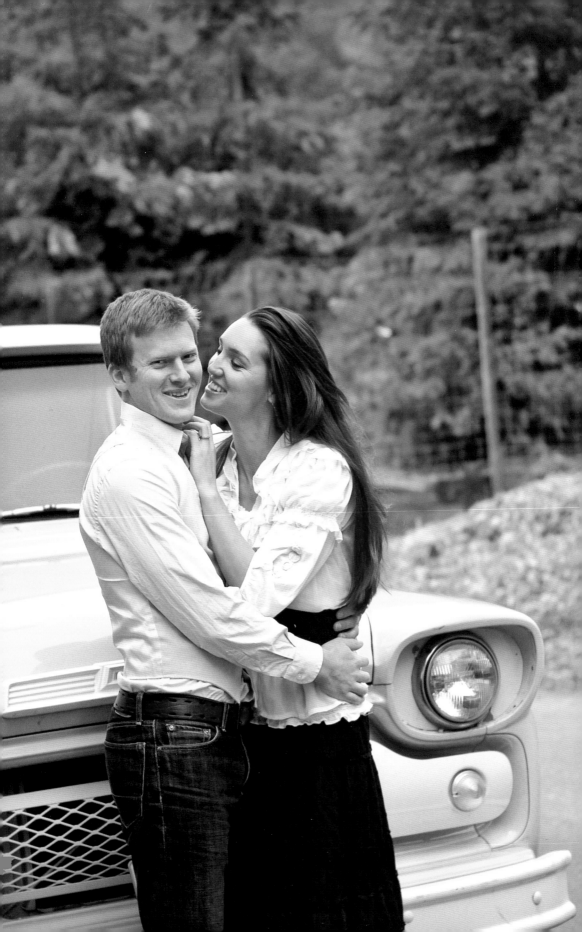

making babies
Conception Through the First Trimester

Look for this symbol throughout the book to find gluten-free/ low casein or casein-free food recipes. *

* *Recipes are provided as recommendations for preparing allergen-free dishes. It is the responsibility of the reader to make sure all recipe ingredients are gluten- or casein-free.*

Making babies is a miracle! It is a spectacular event when the sperm and egg meet and make a life inside of you. A tiny living heartbeat. A tiny living soul. A baby that is a part of you, living inside your body. You are its very life. You nourish it and help it grow. You introduce it to food, sound, movement, feelings, and so much more. You are a mother.

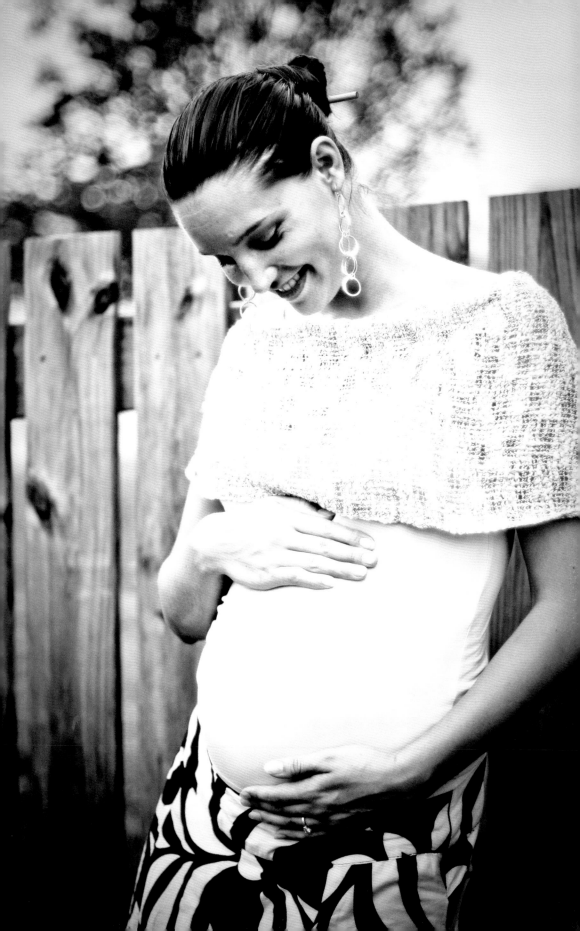

Berry Herbal Brew

Grandma's Brew and Remedy for Fertility

1 cup Berry Herbal Brew Mix

3 cups water, warm, not hot

2 cups Concord grapes, fresh or thawed

1 cup blueberries, fresh or thawed

1½ cups raw sugar (turbinado) or 2½ cups of honey

1. Add Berry Herbal Brew Mix to a glass gallon jar.

2. Pour water over brew mix. With a clean hand, combine thoroughly.

3. Cover jar with a cloth, secure with a rubber band, and let sit until dried herbs are hydrated (3 to 5 hours).

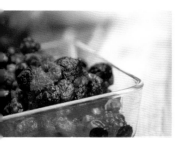
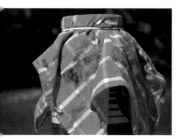
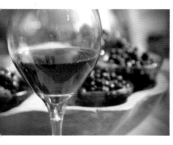
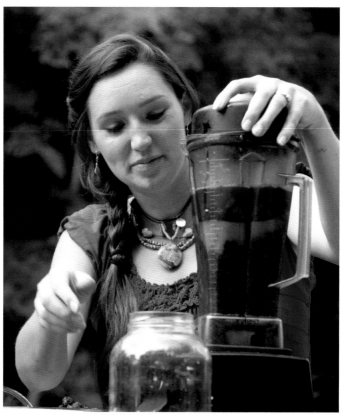

For more info, see *Making Babies DVD - Vol. 1*

4. Place Concord grapes with seeds, blueberries, and sugar in a food processor or blender. Add Berry Herbal Brew liquid mixture to the berries and sugar. Blend for about 1 minute. Put blended mixture in gallon jug, cover with a clean cloth that can breathe, and put a rubber band around the mouth of the jar to keep out fruit flies.

5. Near the end of the first week, mix Berry Herbal Brew once with clean hands for about 2 minutes. Make sure you have a towel over the opening to keep out fruit flies. After mixing, cover with a tight cloth and rubber band over the mouth of the jar. Set jar in cool, dark place for 3 weeks (can be months).

6. LATER (after 3 weeks or longer), in a clean glass gallon jug, drape a thin cloth (cheesecloth works great) down in mouth of jar. Use a rubber band to firmly secure cloth around jar mouth. Slowly pour brew through cloth to strain into clean jar. It might take awhile, so use another cloth to keep any pesky flies away!

7. When it stops straining, use clean hands to twist the cloth together (keeping herbs inside) to squeeze out as much liquid as possible. Discard the remaining herb mixture. You can then pour the strained liquid into an old wine bottle or whatever you choose. I like using wine bottles because they have small openings, colored glass, and the cork fits tightly, keeping the brew well protected.

Whatever glass container you use, remember that the Brew will keep fermenting, so you will want to use something like a cork to seal it. This will keep it from exploding in the container you are storing it in or when you open it. If you do decide to use a regular lid, you will want to open it every once in a while to release the pressure.

Keep Berry Herbal Brew in a cool, dark place - a cabinet works great.

Tip From Shoshanna:

You can use the strained herbs as an additional starter for your next batch.

Mama's Red Raspberry Brew

Prepare Your Body for the Workout of Your Life.

"This tea blend is so tasty! I drank red raspberry leaf during my first pregnancy. I had a very fast and smooth labor/natural birth." -Elizabeth

Red raspberry strengthens the uterus, but use caution when taking it. Some studies have shown it to cause miscarriages when it is started during the first trimester. Also, avoid alfalfa if you have a family history of lupus.

For a Cup of Hot Tea

1 to 2 tsp. of Mama's Red Raspberry Brew herb mix

1 cup water

Raw honey, to taste (*optional*)

For a Pitcher of Tea

10 tsp. of Mama's Red Raspberry Brew herb mix

8 cups water

Raw honey, to taste, (*optional*)

Never miss a chance to dance.

Prep: 5 min.   Steep: 5-10 min.   Yield: 1 cup or 1 pitcher

1. Boil water.

2. Add Mama's Red Raspbery Brew.

3. Let steep for 5 to 10 minutes, strain, and add honey to taste.

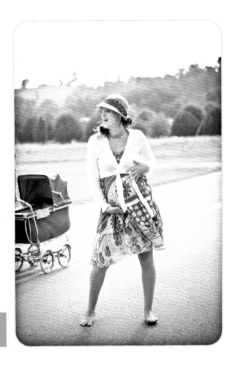

For more info, see *Making Babies DVD - Vol. 1*

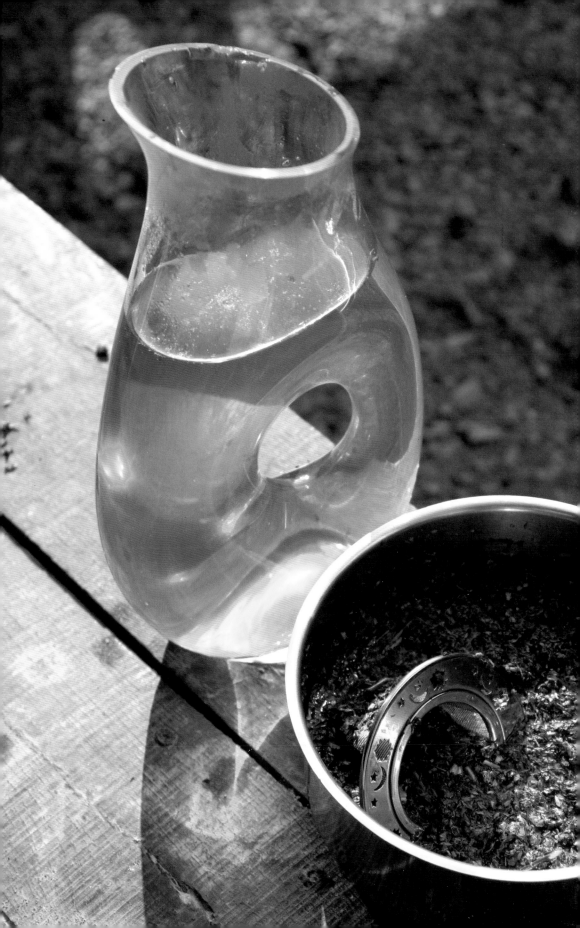

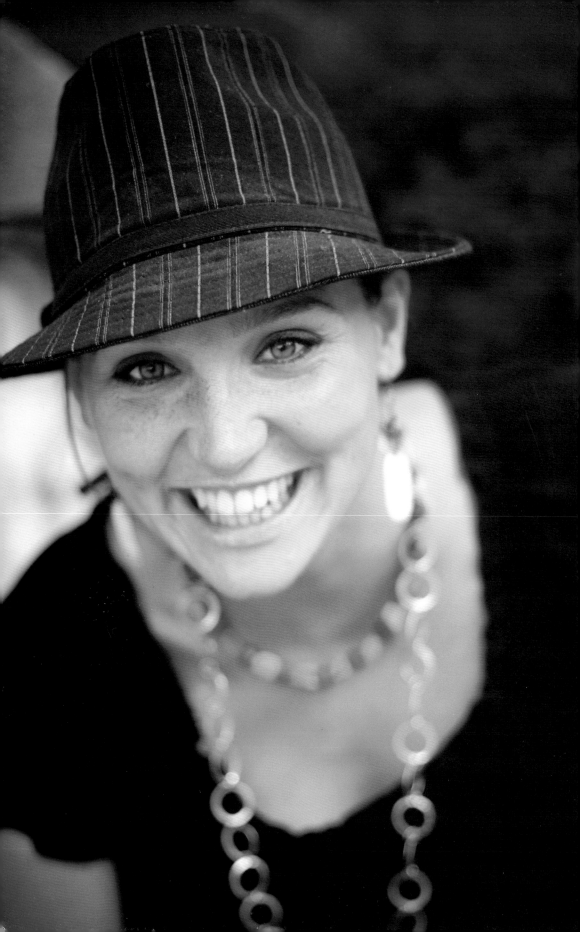

Energy Balls

Raw Protein and High Energy - Yummy!

Almonds are full of folate. Folate is the natural form of folic acid (see page 349) and is great for you and baby. Check out page 382 to read about good fat versus bad fat.

2½-3 cups shredded coconut, unsweetened

1 cup almond butter

½ cup raw honey or maple syrup

1 cup raisins

2 tsp. cinnamon

1½ cups pecans or your favorite nut, chopped

Shredded coconut, unsweetened, for coating balls.

Prep: 5 min.   Yield: 18 balls

1. Place first 6 ingredients in a mixing bowl.

2. Mix on low for 3 minutes and blend until ingredients look combined. Dough will be a little crumbly-looking.

3. Pinch a small, palm-size handful of dough (Approx. ⅛ cup) and roll between hands to form into a ball.

4. Roll ball in shredded coconut to cover. Repeat steps 3 and 4 until you have used all of the dough.

5. Lay balls out on a plate, cover, and refrigerate until cold.

6. Enjoy the delicious taste of energy! These will store very nicely for up to 10 days.

For more info, see Making Babies DVD

Liver Cleanse Tincture

Clean Your Filters and Strengthen Your Body.

"Wow, this combination of herbs really works. I made the liver cleanse tincture and immediately started using it; two weeks later I noticed that my energy level had gone up." -Alex

3 T. dandelion leaf, cut

2 T. hawthorn berries, whole

2 T. eleuthero root (commonly known as Siberian ginseng) cut

2 T. astragalus root, cut

2 T. ginger root, cut

3 T. turmeric, powder

4 T. Amalaki berry, powder

2 T. wurdock, cut

4 T. St. John's wort, cut

5 T. milk thistle, whole

1 ½ T. licorice root, cut

Vodka *(Any vodka works and does not need to be expensive. You can also substitute with glycerin if you prefer. See page 22 for an example of how to make a glycerin tincture).*

Herbs can be fresh or dried.

Prep: 5 min.   Total Time: 2 to 6 weeks

1. Place all herbs in a quart jar with just enough hot water to dampen them.

2. Fill jar with vodka (leaving a space of 1-2 inches from lid), close tightly, and store for 2-6 weeks in a dry, cool place, shaking the jar daily.

3. After 3 weeks, strain and discard the herbs; bottle the liquid and label it.

I like to start with a dropper a day for a week. (1 dropper equals about ¼ tsp.) Then 2 droppers a day, working my way to 3 droppers a day for 1 to 3 months or until pregnant. I stop if I become pregnant, because you do not want to be doing cleanses while your body is trying to build a baby.

If you want to evaporate the alcohol, place your dose in a hot liquid, such as tea or hot water before taking.

The herb mix for this tincture can be purchased at Bulk Herb Store.

For more info, see *Making Babies DVD - Vol. 1*

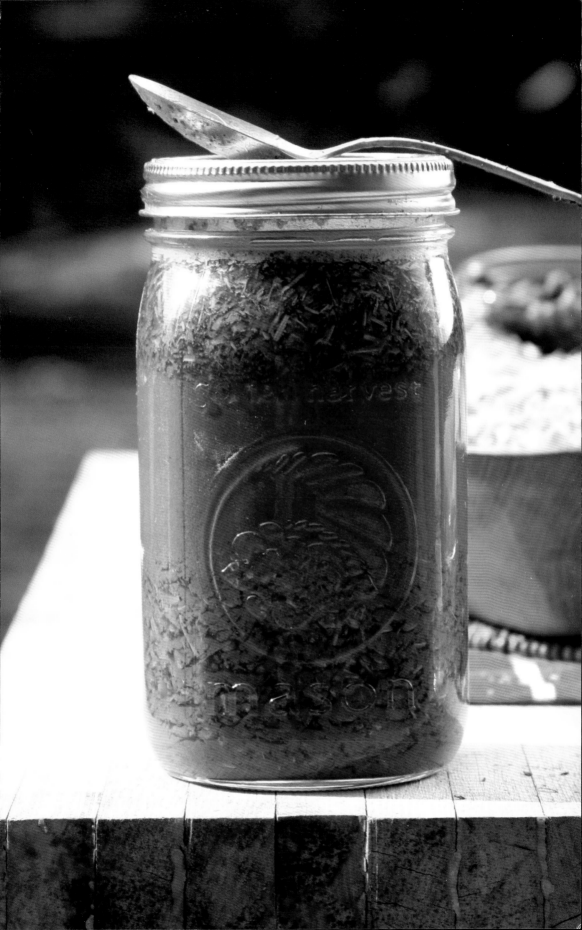

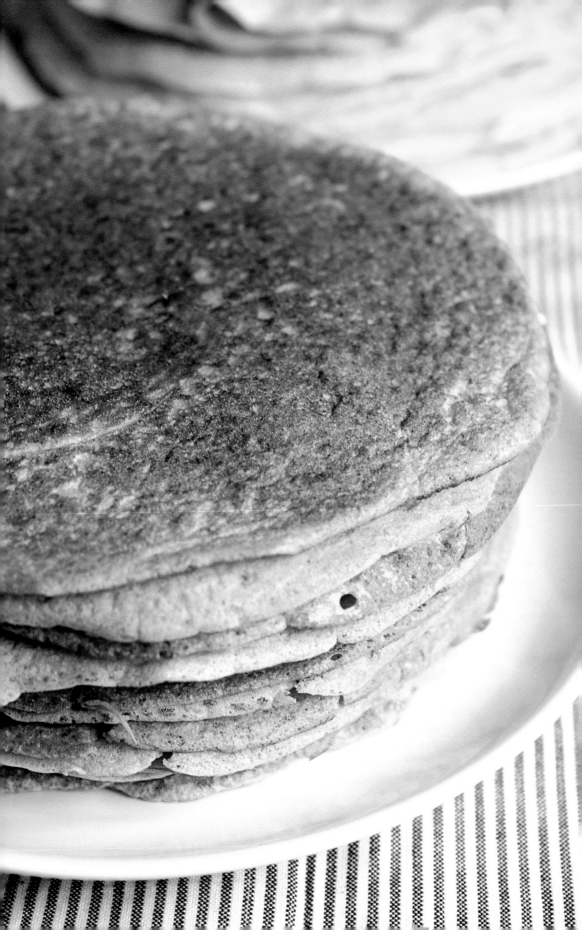

Buckwheat Pancakes & Berry Syrup

Pancakes This Morning and a Date Tonight

Pancakes

1 cup buckwheat flour

½ cup whole wheat flour

2½ tsp. baking powder

½ tsp. baking soda

1 tsp. sea salt (See page 464.)

1-2 T. butter or coconut oil

2 eggs

4 T. butter, melted

¾ cup yogurt

1 cup water

2 tsp. raw honey

1 tsp. vanilla

Berry Syrup

4 cups mixed berries, frozen

2 T. water

2 T. arrowroot powder

⅛ cup water

¼ cup raw honey

½ tsp. vanilla

Prep: 5 min. Cook: 20 min. Yield: 12-18 pancakes

Pancakes

1. In a medium-size bowl, whisk together all dry ingredients until thoroughly combined.

2. In a separate bowl, crack and beat eggs and add all liquid ingredients. Whisk together.

3. Add liquid ingredients to dry ingredients, and mix until just combined.

4. Oil griddle or frying pan with butter or coconut oil and heat pan to medium-high heat or about 350° F.

5. Using a ¼ measuring cup, pour batter onto the hot griddle.

6. When tiny holes appear all over the top of the uncooked pancake side, flip and cook until browned on both sides.

Berry Syrup

1. In a small bowl, combine water and arrowroot. Stir until arrowroot dissolves.

2. Place berries and water in a small saucepan and bring to a low boil, stirring occasionally.

3. Immediately bring to a simmer and add arrowroot mixture. Stir constantly until thickened into a syrup.

4. Stir in honey and serve over hot pancakes.

Pre-Pregnancy Healthy Tincture

Get Your Insides in Shape!

3 T. alfalfa, cut

1 T. eleuthero root (commonly known as Siberian ginseng) cut

2 T. dandelion root, cut

2 T. blessed thistle, cut

2 T. nettle leaf, cut

2 T. chamomile flowers, whole

2 T. ginger root, cut

1 T. garlic, powder

2 T. ginkgo, cut

1 cup red raspberry leaf, cut

2 T. mustard seed, powder or whole

2 T. horsetail/shavegrass, cut

Water

Glycerin

Herbs can be fresh or dried.

Prep: 8 min. Cook: 3 days Yield: about 3 cups

1. Place herbs inside a quart jar.

2. Fill jar with 40% hot water and 60% glycerin, leaving 1-2 inches of space from the top.

3. Close jar lid tightly and place it in a Crock-Pot with a small towel underneath to keep the jar from breaking.

4. Fill the Crock-Pot with water up to the top of the jar (not touching the lid), and turn it on the warm setting for 3 days, keeping the glycerin hot, but not boiling. Add water to the Crock-Pot as necessary.

5. Strain out herb solids and place liquid in a tincture bottle.

6. I take 1 dropperful every morning and evening, or more as needed.

Warning: If your Crock-Pot gets too hot and water has boiled down, turn it off and do not touch until cool. Never pour water over a hot glass jar, as it can explode or crack.

For more info, see *Making Babies DVD - Vol. 1*

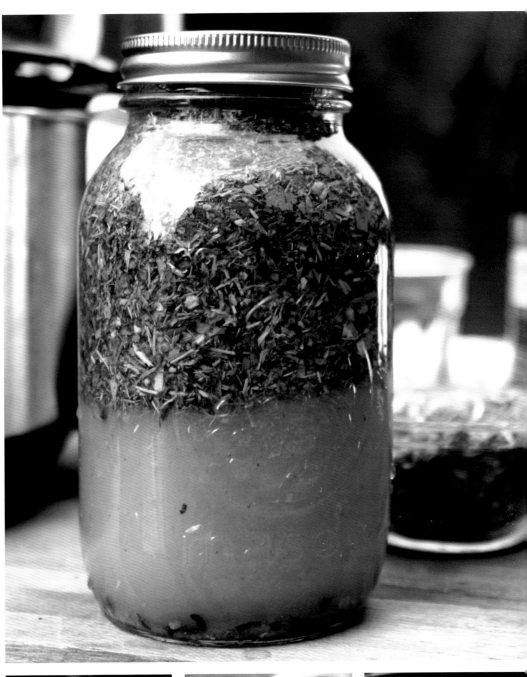

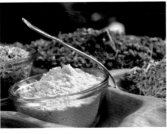
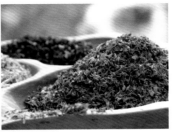
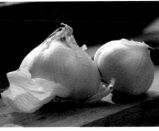

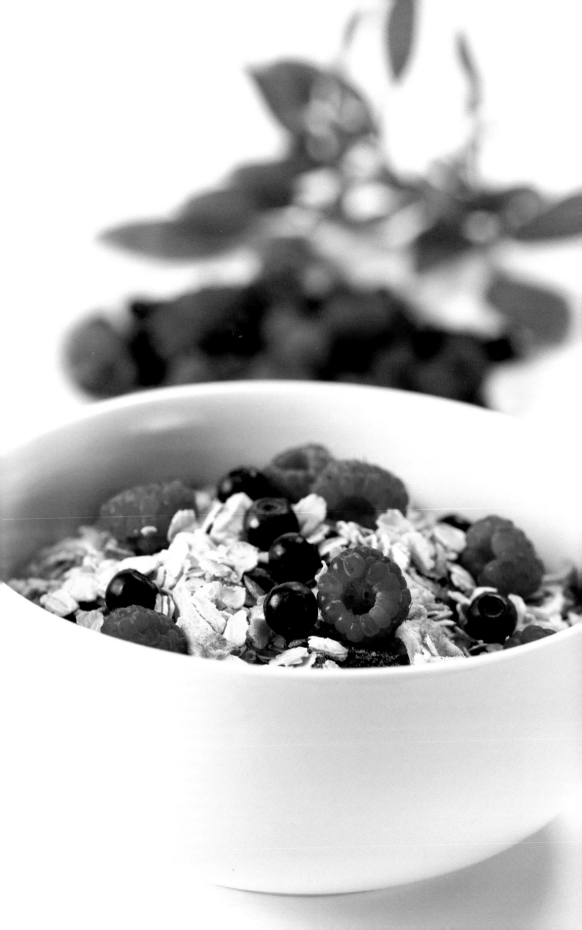

Simply Granola
Granola That Keeps You Moving

4 cups rolled oats, gluten-free

½ cup pecans

½ cup shredded coconut or coconut flakes, unsweetened

1-5 tsp. cinnamon, to taste

1 tsp. sea salt

½ cup raw honey

½ cup flax

½ cup butter, melted

Butter or coconut oil, for oiling pan

Prep: 10 min. Cook: 1 hour Yield: 5 cups

1. Butter a 9-inch pan and preheat oven to 200° F.

2. In a large mixing bowl, combine all ingredients until thoroughly combined.

3. Pour granola mixture into pan and spread around evenly.

4. Bake for 1 hour, stirring every 15 to 20 minutes.

For more info, see *Making Babies DVD*

Egg Shell Water

Passed Down from Grandma

This is great for bone pain. Egg shell water has been used for strengthening bones and bone inflammation. It is high in calcium, magnesium, and more.

8 egg shells, rinsed

4 cups water, hot

Prep: 5 min. Yield: 4 cups

1. Crush egg shells in a quart jar.

2. Pour water over egg shells. Cover and let cool.

3. Strain the liquid into another clean glass jar. Screw lid on and refrigerate.

4. I take a sip of the liquid one to two times a day. One recipe lasts for 3 or 4 days, after which I like to make it fresh again.

Tip From Shoshanna:

Choose free-range, organic eggs straight from the farm if you have access to them. They are richer in nutrients than the eggs from the supermarket.

For more info, see Making Babies DVD - Vol. I

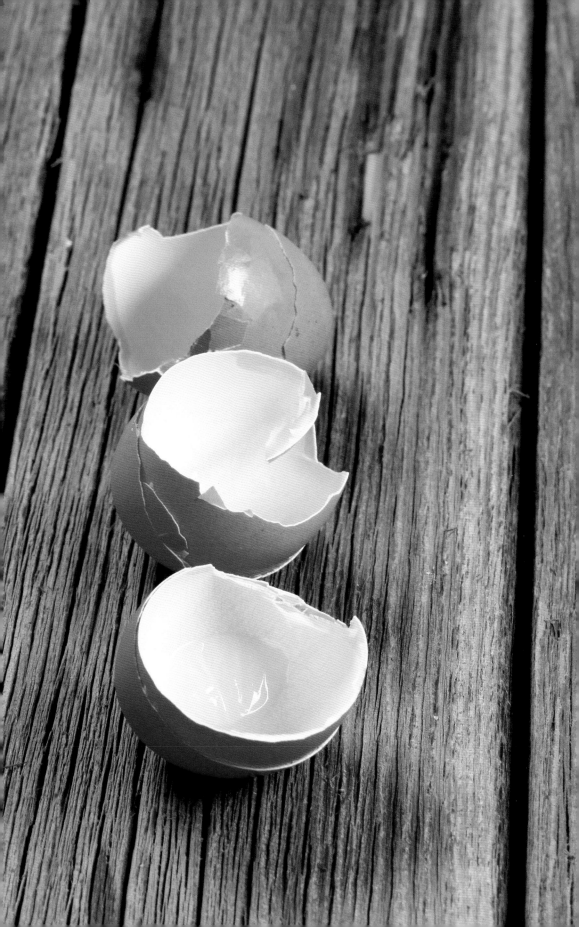

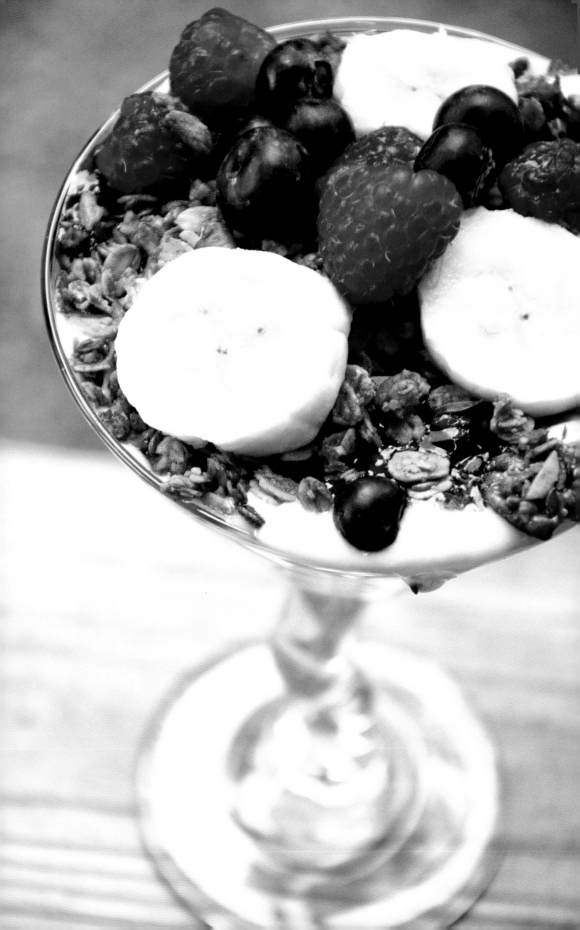

Yogurt Parfait

Breakfast Awesomeness – That's What I'm Talking About!

⅛ cup raspberries

⅛ cup blueberries

⅛ cup strawberries

⅛ cup kiwi, sliced

⅛ cup banana, sliced

¼ cup yogurt

3 T. **Berry Syrup** (page 21)

⅛ cup **Simply Granola** (page 25)

Fruit, to garnish

Prep: 5 min.   Serves: 1

1. Wash fruit, then layer it in a glass parfait cup.

2. Pour yogurt over fruit.

3. Drizzle berry syrup over and sprinkle with granola.

4. Garnish with fruit of choice. Yumm!

Tip From Shoshanna:

This is great for morning sickness! Also, B6 has been scientifically proven to help with morning sickness. For more about morning sickness, see page 354.

For more info, see Making Babies DVD

Tilapia on a Bed of Herban Rice
Flaky Fish That Feeds Your Brain

Herban Rice

2 cups *Simple and Basic Brown Rice*, cooked, still hot (page 339)

1 T. butter

½ tsp. peppercorns, freshly ground

1 lime, juiced

¼ cup chives

¼ cup cilantro

½ cup tomatoes, chopped

Salt, to taste

Baked fish

6 tilapia fillets

2 T. butter, softened

1 T. onion powder

1 tsp. sea salt

2 garlic cloves, crushed

1 pepper, thinly sliced *(Red Marconi peppers are my favorite. You can grow them during the summer or get them at Costco during the winter.)*

1 T. cilantro or parsley

Prep: 15 min. Cook: 15 min. Serves: 4-6

Herban Rice

1. Mix all rice ingredients together.

Baked Fish

2. Preheat oven to 400° F.

3. Rub butter on tilapia fillets and place in a large baking dish.

4. Sprinkle onion powder, salt, and crushed garlic cloves over fillets.

5. Place pepper slices over fillets. Sprinkle cilantro or parsley on top.

6. Bake fillets in preheated oven for 15 minutes or until flaky.

For more info, see Making Babies DVD - Vol. 1

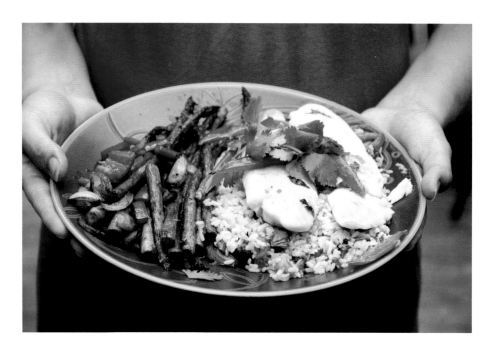

 # Asparagus
Brain Food! Good Food!

1 bunch of asparagus, ends cut off 1 inch from asparagus base

1 tsp. sea salt

½ tsp. onion powder

½ onion, wedged and layers separated

⅛ cup red peppers, sliced

Prep: 5 min. Cook: 8 min. Serves: 4-6

1. Place asparagus and onions in a large skillet and sprinkle with sea salt and onion powder.

2. Sauté on medium-high for 5 to 8 minutes.

3. Remove asparagus from heat and place on a platter.

4. Sprinkle red peppers over and enjoy.

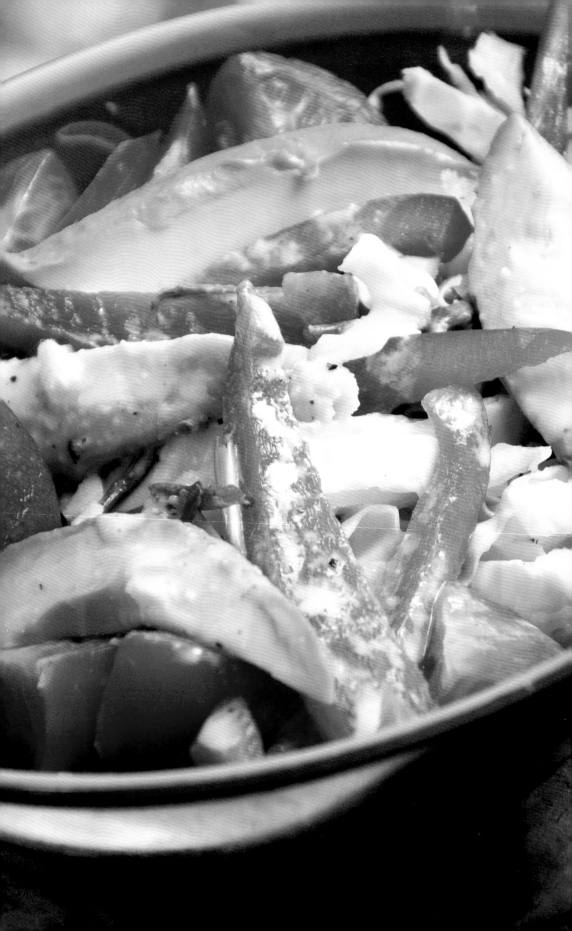

Cabbage Salad
Get Your Man Going! Wow!

Salad

1 cup cabbage, thinly sliced

⅛ cup tomato, chopped

1 T. chives, chopped

3 slices red pepper

⅓ cup avocado, chopped

1 lime, juiced

Dressing

2-3 garlic cloves

½ cup virgin olive oil

1 tsp. peppercorns, freshly ground

½ cup apple cider vinegar

1 tsp. onion powder

1 tsp. sea salt

1 tsp. raw honey

Prep: 8 min.   Serves: 1

Salad

1. In a salad bowl, combine the first five ingredients.

2. Drizzle dressing over salad, and garnish with lime wedges. Yummy!

Dressing

1. Crush garlic cloves.

2. Mix all ingredients well.

Tip From Shoshanna:

Cabbage is high in boron which makes it good for a man's testosterone.

Iron Infusion

Herban! Iron Your Body Can Digest

½ cup nettle leaf

½ cup dandelion root

½ cup alfalfa

½ cup yellow dock

½ cup red raspberry leaf

Water, simmering

Herbs can be fresh or dried.

Prep: 24 min.   Yield: 3 cups

1. Place all herbs in a quart glass jar and pour simmering, hot water over herbs until jar is full.

2. Screw lid on jar and let sit until cool. Strain off herbs.

3. Refrigerate liquid. I like to sip throughout the day for a dose of iron infusion.

Keeps in refrigerator 3-4 days.

You can also make this into a tincture. (See page 18 to see an example of how to make a vodka tincture, or page 22 for a glycerin tincture.)

For more info, see *Making Babies DVD - Vol. I*

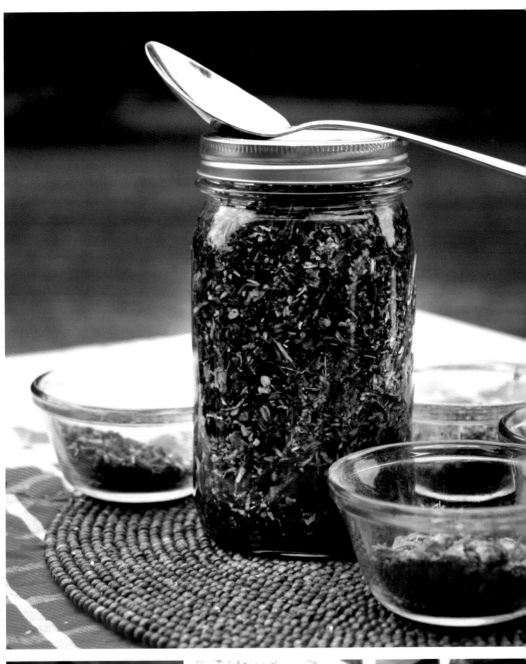

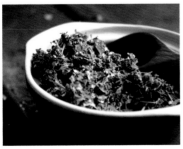

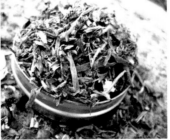

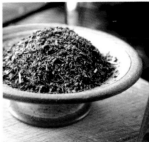

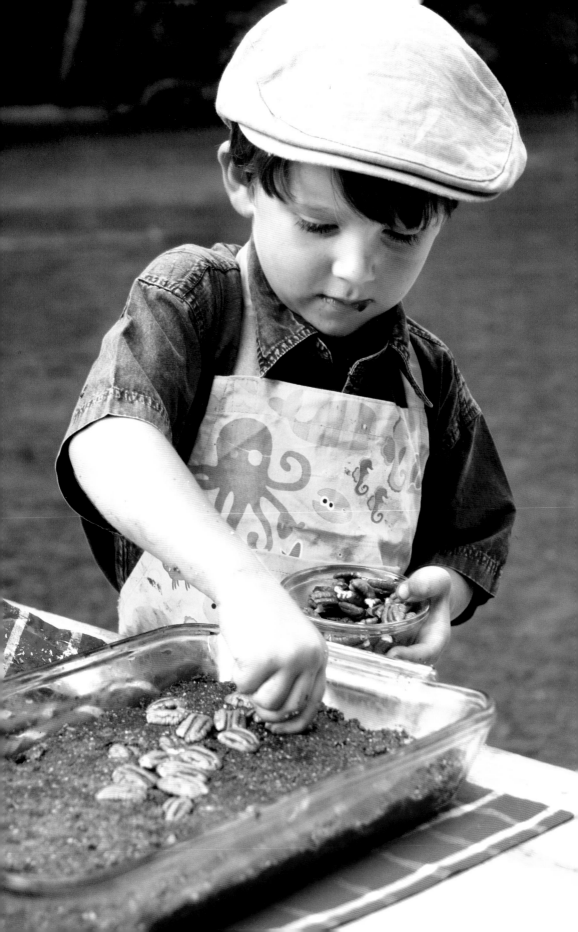

Chewy Chocolate Bars
Life's Motto: Add More Chocolate

1 cup almond butter

3 cups coconut flakes, unsweetened

⅔ cup cocoa powder

⅔ cup raw honey

1 tsp. sea salt

½ tsp. vanilla

½ cup almond flour (*optional*)

Prep: 5 min.   Yield: 12 bars

1. Place all ingredients in a food processor or bread machine and blend until combined.

2. In a shallow baking dish, spread mixture evenly to desired thickness.

3. Refrigerate until chocolate is firm.

4. Cut into bars and serve. Enjoy!

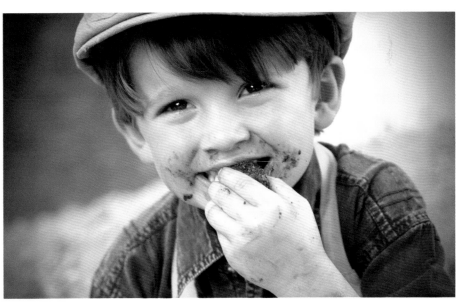

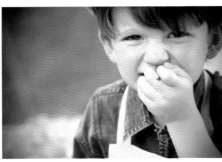

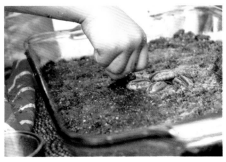

Chicken Broth

Drink Your Broth; Grandma Knows Best.

1 chicken, whole, organic

2 carrots, roughly chopped

4-5 garlic cloves, crushed

5 parsley sprigs

1 tsp. peppercorns, freshly ground

6 egg shells

1 rosemary sprig

1½ tsp. sea salt

3 celery stalks

4 T. vinegar, with the mother

6 or 8 cups water, depending on how strong you want the broth

1 onion, cut in wedges

Prep: 10 min. Cook: 3 hours Yield: 8 cups

1. Wash veggies and rinse meat. Place all ingredients in a large pot.

2. Bring to a boil, then reduce heat to low; cover.

3. Lightly simmer for 2 to 3 hours, covered.

4. Turn off heat and let stand 45 minutes or until cool enough to remove chicken, or to make a more nutrient-rich broth, remove cooked chicken and let bones, fat, and vegatables simmer for 24-48 hours. Reserve meat for a meal.

5. Allow broth to cool; then, using a strainer, strain broth into a container.

6. Use broth as desired.

For more info, see *Making Babies DVD - Vol. 1*

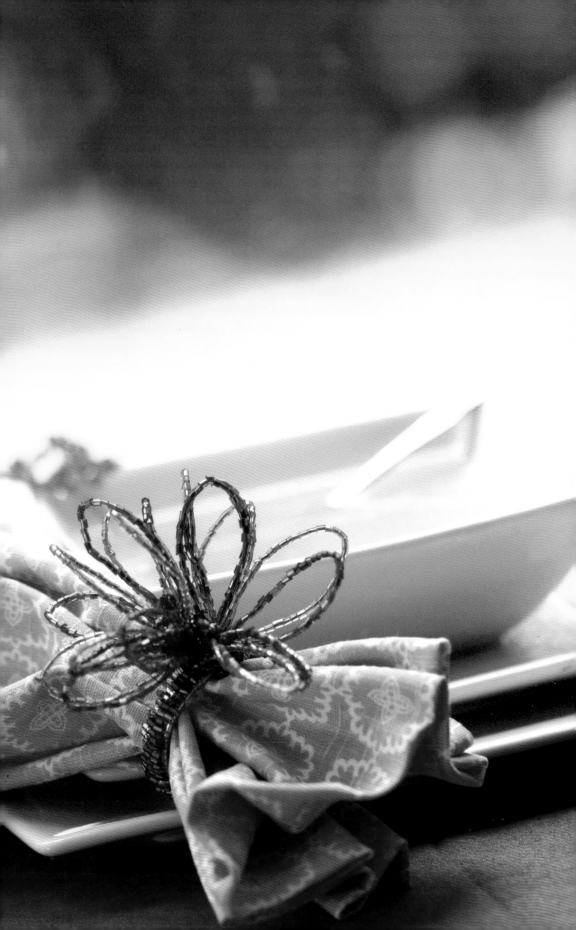

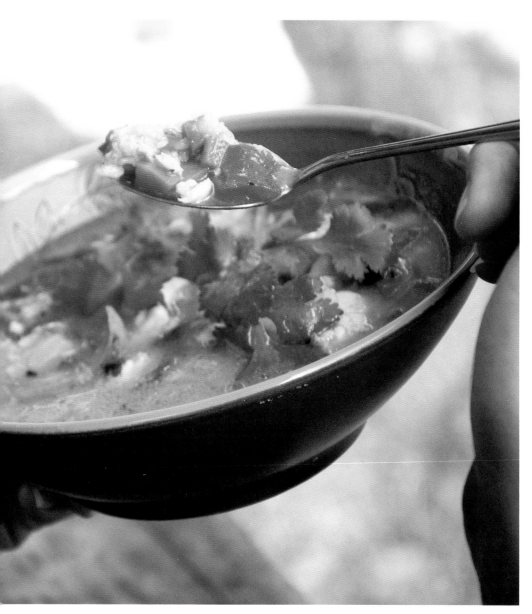

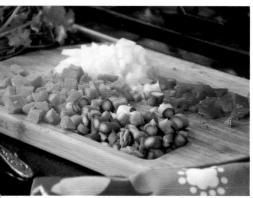

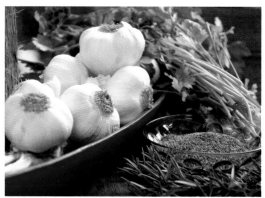

Soooo Good Fish Soup
Easy to Digest; Makes You Feel Great!

½ cup onions, chopped small

½ cup carrots, chopped small

1 T. olive oil

½ cup asparagus, chopped

½ cup red peppers, chopped

4 fillets of tilapia

4 cups **Chicken Broth** (page 38) or **Vegetable Broth** (page 320)

½ cup **Herban Rice** (page 30)

½ tsp. pepper

2 tsp. onion powder

¼ cup cilantro

1 lime, juiced

1 T. butter

Prep: 5 min. Cook: 28 min. Serves: 4-6

1. Wash and chop veggies.

2. In a large sauce pan, sauté first five ingredients on medium-high for 3 minutes. Add tilapia. Cook 5 minutes.

3. Chop fish into large bite-sized pieces while it is cooking. Add the rest of ingredients and cook for 20 more minutes. Garnish with cilantro.

4. Serve hot. This soup is sooo good!!

For more info, see Making Babies DVD

Making a Pretty Necklace

Beautiful and Fashionable All Nine Months

I string

I bead, button, or stone

1. Cut your preferred string about 2 to 3 feet long, depending on how long you want your necklace. Fold string in half.

2. Thread the string's loop side through a bead, button, or stone. Open loop, and thread other end of string through loop.

3. Pull until tight around bead. Tie necklace around neck. You are looking fabulous!!!

4. At least one day every week of your and your baby's nine months, wake up and dress fabulously. Show the world how beautiful God made pregnancy.

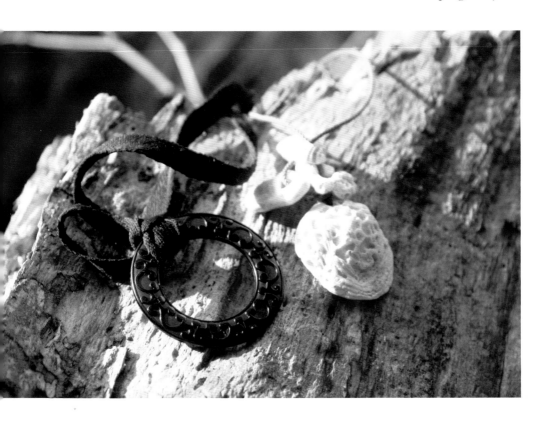

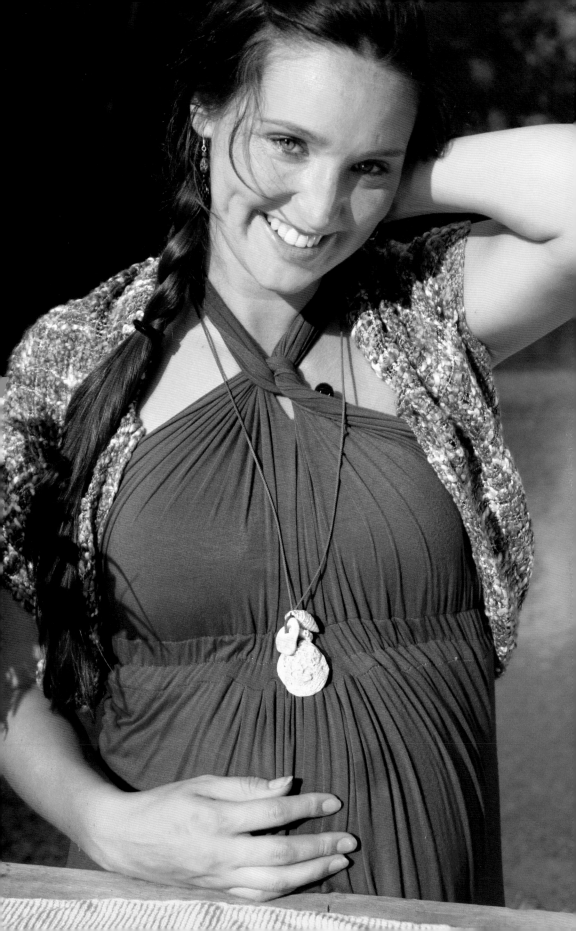

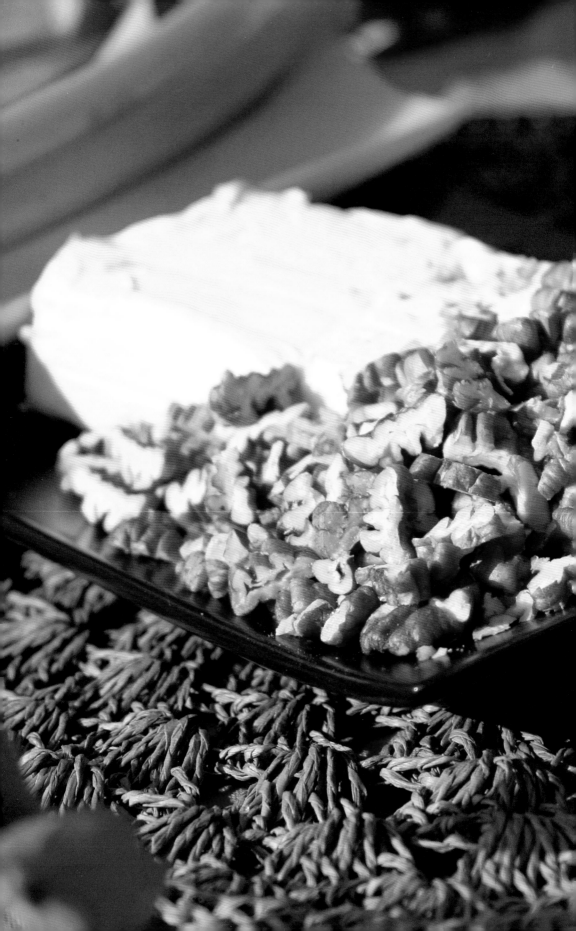

Celery and Pecans

I Love This Even Though I Don't Like Celery.

This one is great for scaring away morning sickness, and it tastes good too.

¼ cup cream cheese

½ cup pecans or walnuts, toasted and chopped

2 sticks celery, washed and ends removed

Prep: 3 min.   Serves: 2

1. In a small bowl, mix cream cheese and pecans.

2. Simply fill a celery stalk with cream cheese mixture.

3. Take a bite and enjoy!

For more info, see *Making Babies DVD*

Ginger Tincture

This Made a Big Difference for Me!

2 lightly packed cups ginger, freshly grated

About 2½ cups vodka

Prep: 5 min. Brew: 2-6 weeks Yield: 2½ cups

1. Place ginger in a pint canning jar.

2. Fill jar up to one inch from the top with vodka.

3. Store in cabinet for 2-6 weeks.

4. Strain ginger off with an old T-shirt or cheesecloth. Pour liquid into a tincture bottle. Seal and label.

5. I like to take this tincture for nausea, morning sickness, and indigestion as I need it.

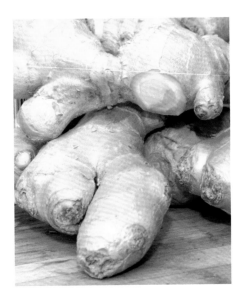
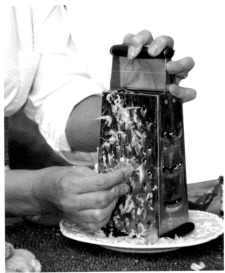

For more info, see *Making Babies DVD - Vol. I*

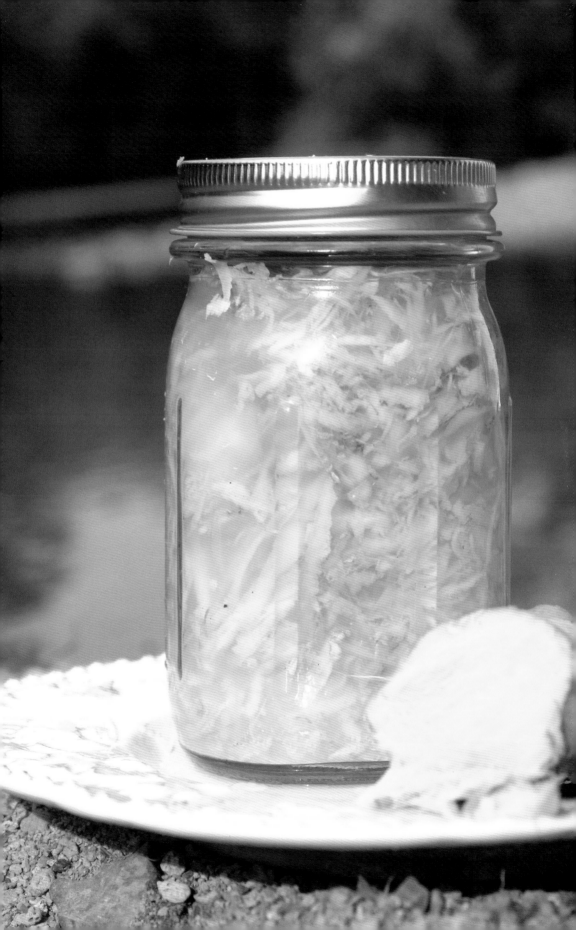

Pregnancy
TIPS

Constipation

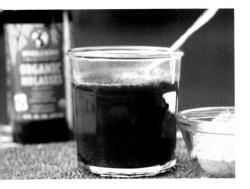

Prep: 2 min. Serves: 1

1 T. psyllium seed powder
2 T. blackstrap molasses
1 ½ cup water

1. Place all ingredients in a cup and stir quickly until thoroughly combined.

2. Drink immediately.

I drink this 1 to 3 times a day.

Immune Booster

If you are feeling under the weather and need a boost or just don't want to catch the neighbor's cold, here is a great thing to take.

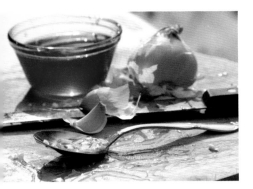

Prep: 2 min. Serves: 1

2 garlic cloves, minced
1 T. raw honey

1. In a small bowl, combine minced garlic and honey.

2. Scoop mixture onto a spoon and eat or swallow it down with water. Jeremiah does it with a smile!

For more info, see *Making Babies DVD - Vol. 1*

Peppermint Tea

Prep: 2 min. Steep: 10 min. Serves: 1

2 tsp. peppermint

2 cups hot water

Raw honey, to taste

Cream or coconut cream, to taste

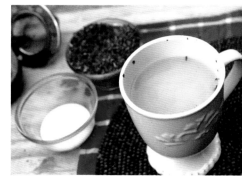

1. Pour hot water over peppermint. Let steep for 5 to 10 minutes.

2. Strain out herbs.

3. Mix in honey, until dissolved.

4. Add cream to taste.

At Bulk Herb Store we sell peppermint tea and tea strainers. I love them!!

Deodorant

We have glands under our arms. Every time we rub a deodorant stick under there, we are filling our bodies with chemicals that are bad for us and our babies. Here are some healthy alternatives that work great and keep you fresh:

1. When you are showering daily, make sure you wash under your arms well. Powder your underarms with baking soda, which is natural and fresh!!

2. This is one of my favorites! It is a salt rock/mineral rock. You can get it at almost any health store (JimBo's, Whole Foods). When you are showering daily, make sure you wash under your arms well. Get the rock wet and rub all over under your arms. It is healthy, fresh, and feels like nothing is there.

Recommended Books

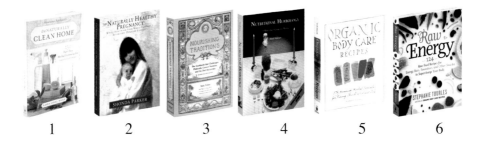

1 2 3 4 5 6

The Naturally Clean Home by Karyn Siegel-Maier
This book contains many great, earthy recipes to keep your home clean without all the chemicals.

Naturally Healthy Pregnancy by Shonda Parker
This book is filled with good reading for your pregnancy and herbal education.

Nourishing Traditions by Sally Fallon
Full of great recipes, this book is loaded with a lot of good information.

Nutritional Herbology by Mark Pedersen
This is a great book for learning what herbs are good for, how to use them, and dosages.

Organic Body Care by Stephanie Tourles
This book has wonderful recipes to keep your body clean and natural for you and your baby.

Raw Energy by Stephanie Tourles
Full of information, this book has fun recipes that are loaded with nutrients.

With every book there is always stuff I do not agree with, but why discard the good because of some bad? It is like a peach. You still eat it if it has a rotten spot. You eat the good and just don't eat the rotten spot. Like I always say, "Learn and live well!!!"

For more info, see *Making Babies DVD - Vol. I*

Five Essentials

Cranberries
Juice, concentrate, frozen, fresh - any way you like them, just not in sugar. Cranberries are great to take for urinary tract infections, including bladder and kidney infections.

Eden Salve has many great uses, from a lubricant to an herbal antibiotic cream. I use it every day!!

Digestive Enzymes help you digest your food. Having a baby squashing your gut sometimes makes digestion difficult. Enzymes work great!!!

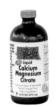

Liquid Cal-Mag really helps if you are cramping. Our babies are needing so many vitamins and minerals that sometimes they take them from our bodies' store. Then we get cramps, arthritis pain, and stuff. That is why our vitamins are so important. Cal-Mag can be used to help keep those pains away.

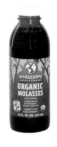

Blackstrap Molasses is great for a dose of iron or for giving your colon a helping hand. It is important to not be constipated while you are pregnant, but because of your changing body it can happen easily. Blackstrap can be there when you need it.

Nature's Face Wash

2 T. oats

1 T. milk

Prep: 2 min. Yield: 3 Tablespoons

1. Place oats and milk in a small blender, and blend until the mixture has a gritty consistency.

2. Using upward circular motions, rub over face.

3. Rinse face with water.

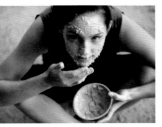 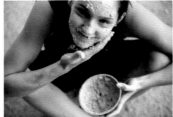 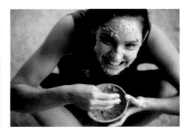

Lotion

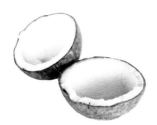

¼ to ½ tsp. coconut oil

1. With clean finger tip, lightly dab oil all over face. Allow five minutes for oil to soak in, then pat face with dry, clean rag.

Kegel Exercise

A strong Kegel muscle is important for a great birth. It also makes "making babies" more fun. I exercise mine at red lights, in bed at night, and…well lets just say, I have a strong one! Your body can be in shape and you can still have a weak Kegel muscle. For at least five minutes a day, take the time to work it out. It will be worth it!

Tighten up, starting at your anus and moving all the way to your clitoris, hold it as long as you can, and then do it again.

Sugar Scrub

This is great for your skin. You know what is in it, and making it is a fraction of the cost of buying it.

Prep: 5 min. Yield: 3 cups

2 cups raw sugar

2 cups olive oil or coconut oil

20-30 drops orange essential oil

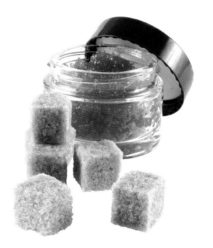

1. In a large bowl, combine all ingredients.

2. Store in a glass jar with lid. I keep mine by the bath. Love it!!!

Berry Beautiful Smoothie

Prep: 5 min. Serves: 1

1 kiwi

¾ cup berries, frozen

1 T. coconut oil

1 T. flax oil

1 dropper *Horsetail Tincture* (page 395)

½ cup pomegranate juice or seeds

¼ or ⅛ cup raw honey or maple syrup (*optional*)

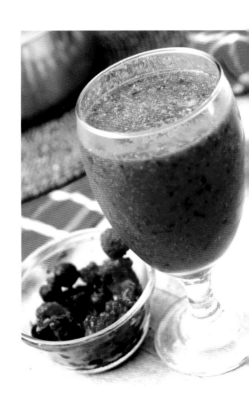

1. Place all ingredients in a blender.

2. Blend thoroughly and enjoy!

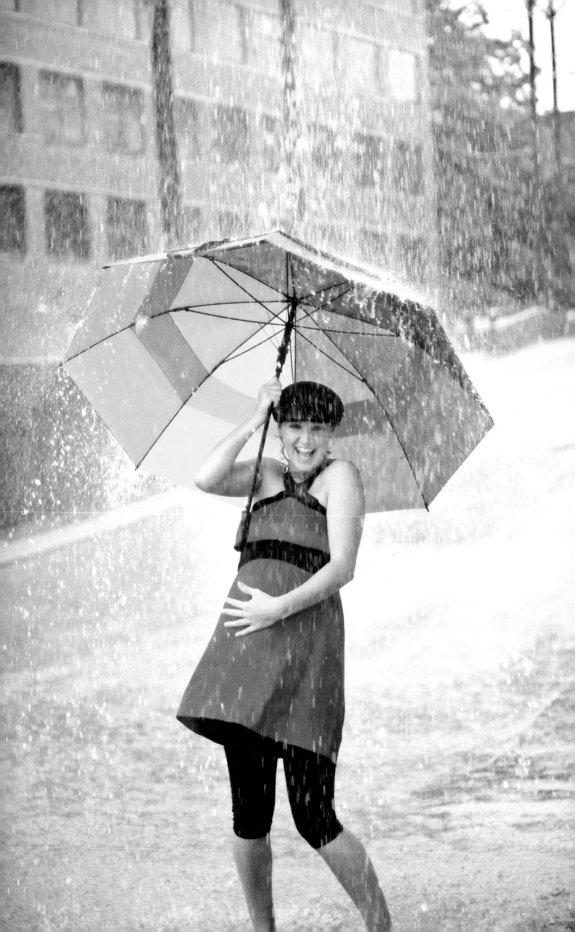

Second & Third Trimesters

Making babies is such a beautiful thing. It is truly amazing how we can mold our babies' bodies, touch their souls, and pave a way for them to grow. Your baby feels your heart beat. He knows your voice. She knows your emotions and feels them with you. He eats your food and drinks what you do. She is a part of you.

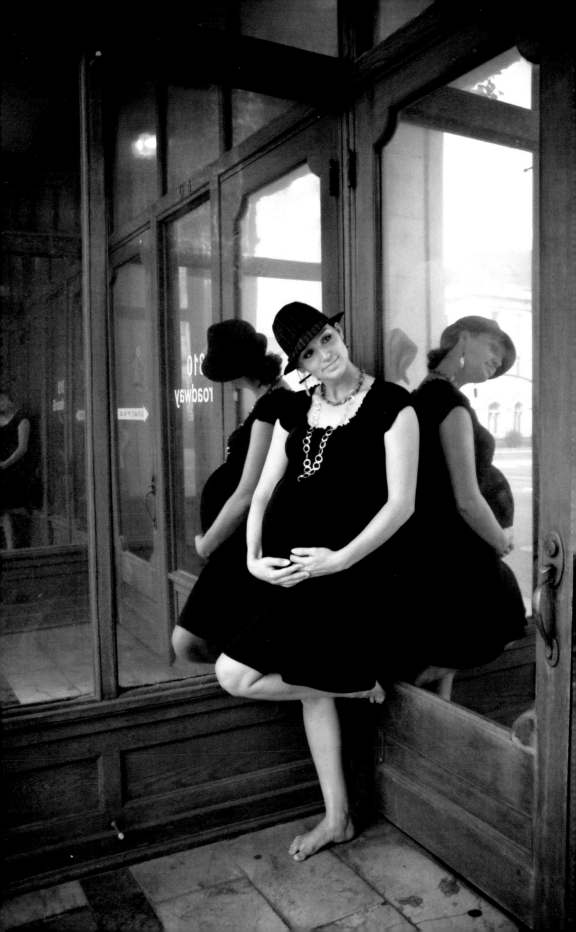

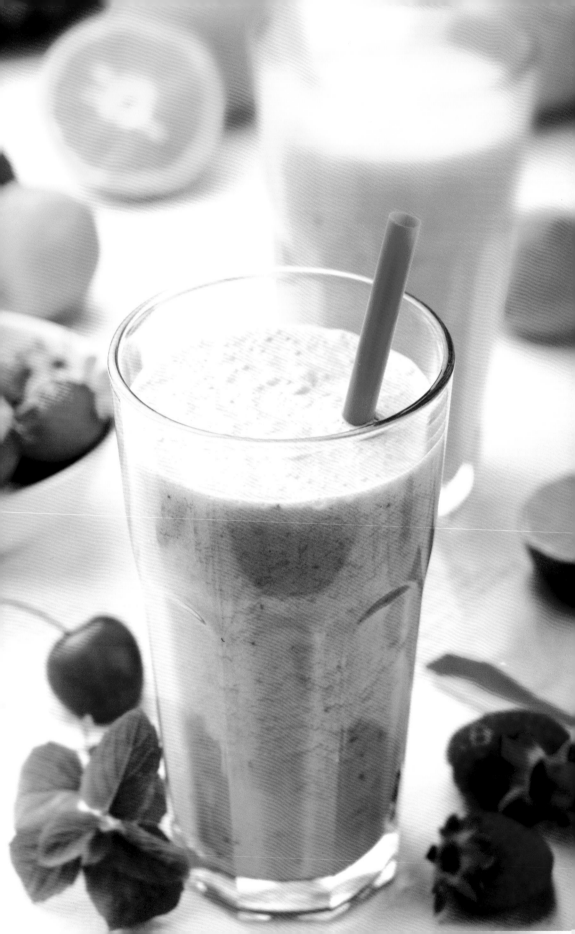

Enzyme Smoothie
Energy in a Glass

Smoothies are a great way to take care of a lot of different problems during pregnancy, from acne to cellulite, indigestion to a lack of energy. Smoothies taste great and make you feel better.

Enzymes are mostly protein molecules that are responsible for digesting, transporting, metabolizing, and more. Enzymes are catalysts that help the chemicals of your body work better together.

2 T. orange juice concentrate

⅛ cup banana (about 3 pieces)

¼ cup papaya, cubed

¼ cup mango, cubed

½ cup blueberries

¾ cup coconut water

½ cup ice

1 kale leaf

5 strawberries (*optional*)

½ tsp. Herba-Smoothie mix, found at Bulk Herb Store (*optional*)

Fruit can be frozen or fresh.

Prep: 5 min.   Serves: 1-2

1. In a blender combine all ingredients. Blend until smooth. Enjoy!

If fruit is frozen you can omit the ice and add more coconut water.

Mix and match your fruits and vegetables. Try making a different smoothie every time.

For more info, see *Making Babies DVD* - Vol. 2

Probiotic Smoothie

Feeling Great All Day Long

Fruits are full of enzymes, and kefir and yogurt are full of probiotics. Probiotics are specific bacteria that are necessary components of the digestive tract. They make up a living colony that lines our digestive tract, aiding in our digestion, nutrient intake, and immune support. Fruits, kefir, and yogurt make up a great healthy gut combination in this smoothie.

⅓ cup kefir, plain

⅓ cup yogurt, plain

4 T. orange juice concentrate

⅔ cup blueberries, fresh or frozen

½ of a kiwi, peeled; fresh or frozen

½ banana, frozen (*optional*)

½ cup ice

½ tsp. Herba-Smoothie mix, found at Bulk Herb Store. (*optional*)

Prep: 5 min.   Serves: 1-2

Fruit can be frozen or fresh. In a blender combine all ingredients. Blend until smooth. Enjoy!

Don't stop here! You can make all kinds of smoothies. Use your favorite fruit, nuts, oils, greens, veggies, and more.

For more info, see *Making Babies DVD - Vol. 2*

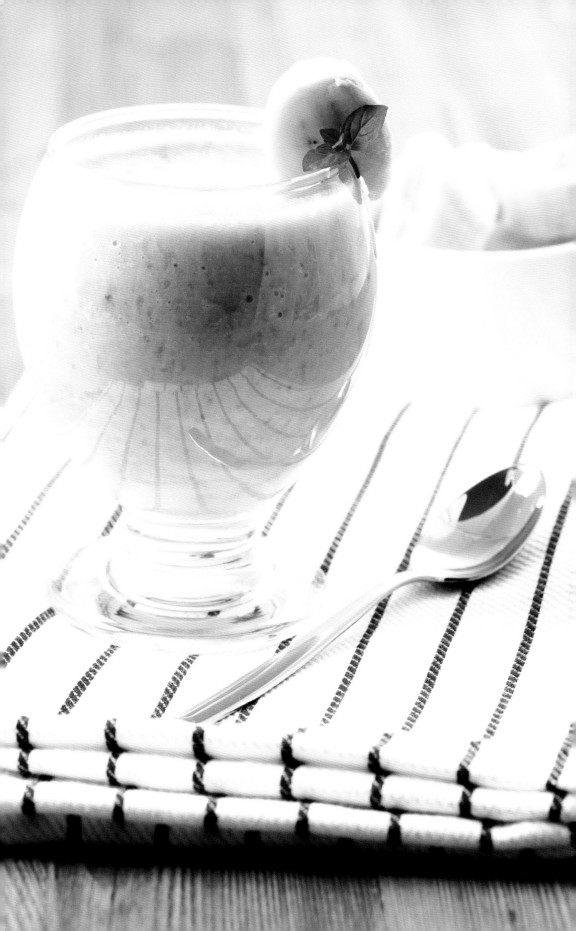

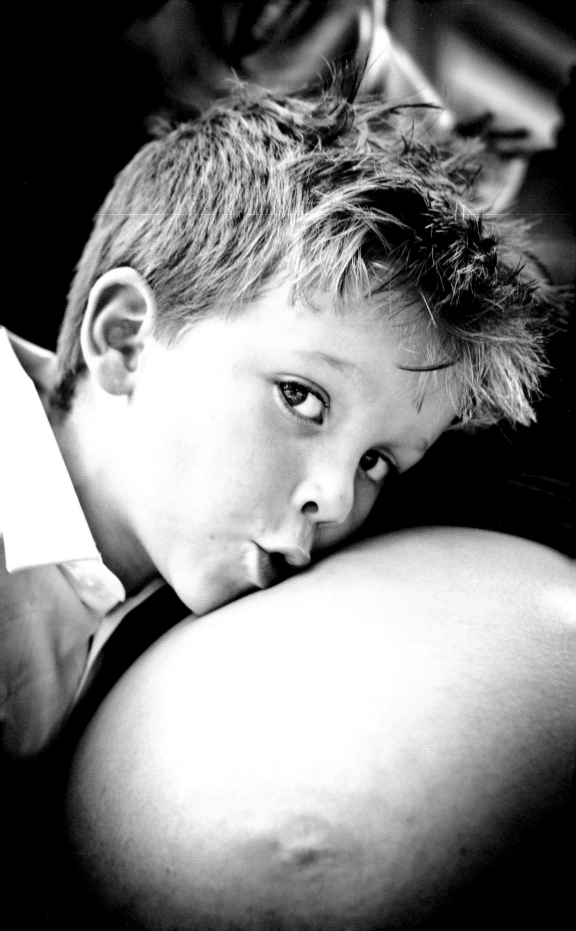

Belly Butter

Baby Your Belly With Your Belly Butter.

Pregnancy skin can get itchy. Here are a few things you should know: itchy skin is a sign of toxins as well as stretch marks trying to get you. You need to eat good oils – avocados, fish, and raw nuts. Take your omega fish oil. Stay hydrated by drinking 8 glasses of water a day. Keep your skin moisturized with quality oils. Here is a great recipe for preventing stretch marks.

2½ cups horsetail/shave-grass, cut

3½ cups oil of choice (Coconut is my favorite.)

½ cup beeswax

1½ to 2½ cups aloe vera juice

2 T. vitamin E oil

These are optional but I think they make a big difference:

1 cup jojoba oil

½ cup shea butter

1 T. vitamin K oil

10 drops myrrh essential oil

10 drops lavender essential oil

10 drops rose essential oil

½ tsp. grapefruit seed extract

Prep: 5 min. Cook: 72 hours Yield: about 6 cups

1. Fill a quart-size glass canning jar ⅓ full with herbs. Add coconut oil or olive oil. Make sure you leave at least one inch between mixture and top of jar. Screw lid on tightly and place jar in a Crock-Pot with a small towel underneath to keep the jar from breaking. Fill the Crock-Pot with water up to level of tincture in jar, but not over lid. Turn Crock-Pot on lowest setting, and leave it on for 3 days. Add more water to Crock-Pot as necessary.

2. After about 72 hours, remove from heat and let cool. Strain the oil through a cheesecloth into a glass container, squeezing the herbs to release the finished oil. Throw the used herbs away. Pour oil in a sauce pan and heat on low. Add beeswax. Stir until wax is melted. Pour mixture into a glass cake pan to cool, making it a salve.

3. In a blender add your salve and the rest of the ingredients. Blend and stir until white and creamy. You can blend in ½ cup water if you want a lighter cream. Pour into a clean glass jar with lid; date and label. Keep in the cabinet out of heat and light. Will keep through pregnancy.

Chiller for UTIs

Stay Hydrated. No Sugar. Eat Green.

1 cup ice

2-4 T. blueberry concentrate

1 T. pomegranate concentrate

1 cup 100% cranberry juice (no sugar added)

Prep: 5 min. Serves: 1

1. In a blender, blend all ingredients.

2. Enjoy the delicious chill!

Tip From Shoshanna:

A **urinary tract infection** (UTI) is a bacterial infection in your urinary tract.

Symptoms include:
- Frequent need to urinate.
- Pain during urination.
- Cloudy or strong smelling urine or urine that contains blood.
- Discomfort, pressure, or bloating in the lower abdomen or pain in the pelvic area or back.
- Fever.

This is what I do when I think I have a UTI:
- Drink 8-10 glasses of water or herbal tea a day.
- Take 1000 mg of Vitamin C every day.
- Drink 12-24 ounces of cranberry juice a day.
- Avoid sugar.
- Drink 1 tablespoon of apple cider vinegar "with the mother" with eight ounces of water 1-3 times a day.

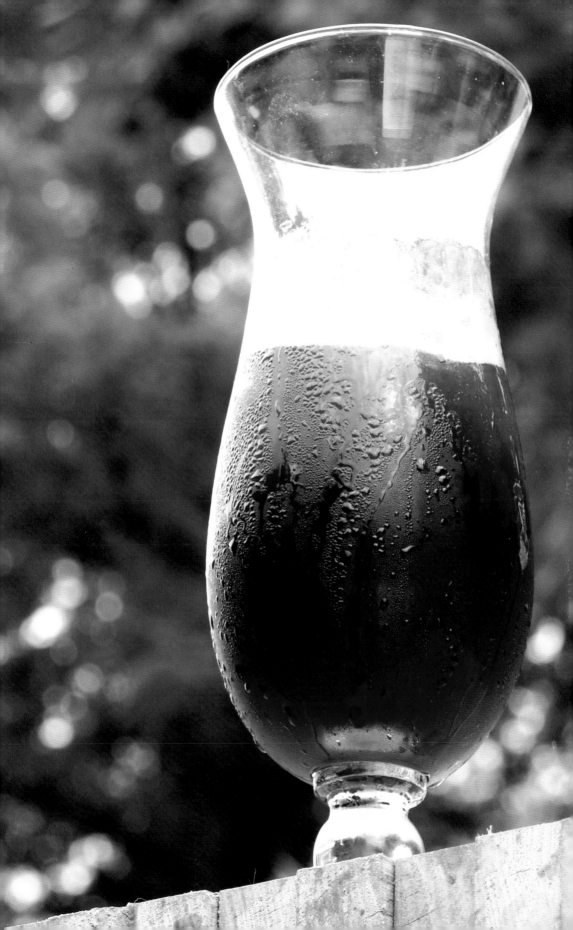

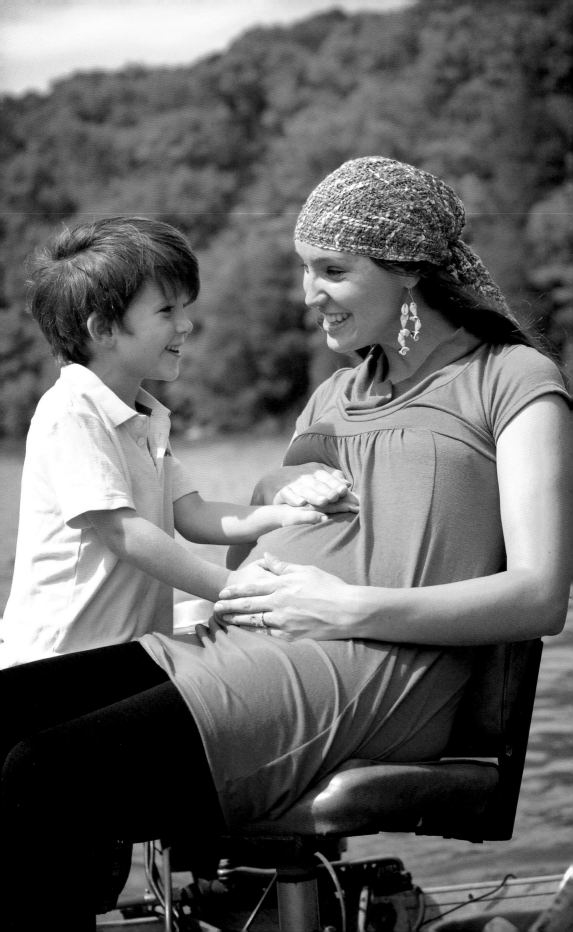

Tea with Minerals

Refreshingly Healthy

Your baby is growing faster than ever! That means he is using more vitamins and minerals too. His bones are hardening up and he needs a lot of calcium and magnesium, as well as many other minerals and vitamins. If you are not ingesting enough vitamins and minerals, then they are pulled from your bones and muscles. Your muscles need calcium and magnesium and many other vitamins just like your bones do. If your muscles do not get enough, then you get leg cramps and charley horses. Pain!! This is a great and refreshing tea that can help replenish your body. I love drinking 2 to 4 glasses of this tea a day.

Tea Mix

¼ cup alfalfa

⅓ cup oatstraw

⅛ cup peppermint

Honey or stevia to taste

Tea

1 cup water

1-2 tsp. tea mix

Prep: 5 min. Steep: 5-10 min. Yield: about 3/4 cup

Tea Mix

1. Mix all herbs

Tea

1. Add herbs to boiling water.

2. Let steep for 5 to 10 minutes, strain, and add honey or stevia to taste.

Warning: Do not use alfalfa if you have a family history of lupus.

Tip From Shoshanna:

Cal-mag is great to keep on hand. If you get charley horses at night, then take some liquid cal-mag before you go to bed. It helps you sleep and keeps you from getting those painful cramps.

Baked Turkey
Deliciously Lean Protein

Whole turkey, thawed

4 cups leeks, washed and chopped

1 large onion, chopped

6 celery stalks, chopped

1 stick butter, melted

Prep: 10 min.   Cook: 6 hours Yield: 1 Turkey

1. Wash turkey and pat it dry with a paper towel. Place in a large casserole dish or turkey pan.

2. Wash and chop vegetables. Stuff turkey with vegetables and butter; place extra veggies around turkey.

3. Bake turkey at 200° F for 6 hours or overnight, or until thickest part of turkey reaches a temperature of 165° F.

Nanny was the best grandma ever!!! I think of her often, up in heaven, looking down on me. I can still see her making that big Thanksgiving turkey. Yummy! She was always in the kitchen or the garden. I miss my Nanny!

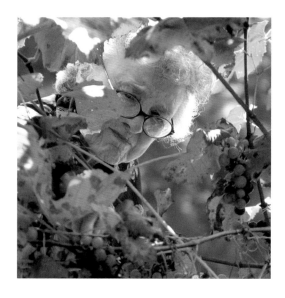

For more info, see *Making Babies DVD - Vol. 2*

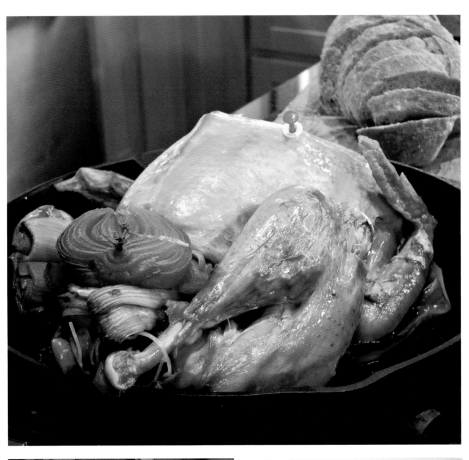

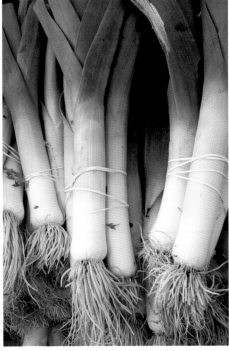

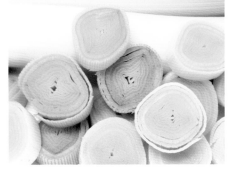

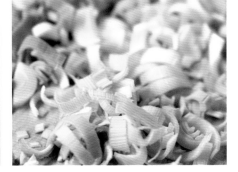

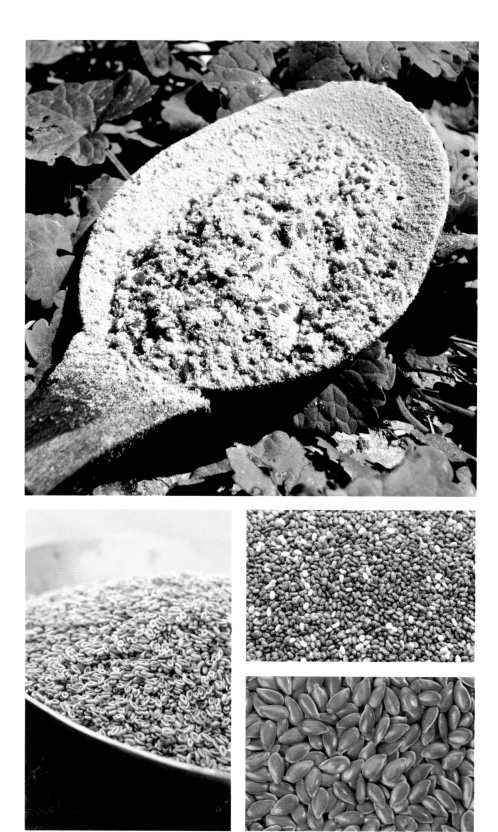

Nutritional Fiber
Giving You Energy and Good Health

Fiber Mixture

½ cup flax seeds

½ cup apple pectin

½ cup chia seeds

1 cup psyllium seed powder

Drink

2 T. fiber mixture

2 T. blackstrap molasses

2 cups water

Prep: 4 min.   Yield: 2½ cups mixture, 1 drink

Fiber Mixture

1. Thoroughly mix together dry ingredients.

Drink

2. In a large cup, mix together 2 T. of fiber mixture, blackstrap molasses, and water.

3. Stir quickly. I drink it immediately.

For more info, see *Making Babies DVD - Vol. 2*

Pizza Perfect
Gourmet at Home

1 T. butter

2 cups spinach

1 tomato, washed, patted dry, and sliced

8 basil leaves

1-2 garlic cloves, crushed

½ cup mozzarella, grated

Sea salt, to taste

Red pepper, sliced

Onions, thinly sliced

Turkey, cooked and chopped

1 slice pita bread

Prep: 10 min. Cook: 5 min. Serves: 2

1. Wash and chop veggies.

2. Melt butter in a saucepan.

3. Add spinach and sauté until spinach is wilted and becomes dark green. Season spinach with sea salt to taste.

4. Toast pita bread in an oven set to broil.

5. Drizzle olive oil over tomatoes and lay them on the pita bread along with spinach, turkey, basil leaves, crushed garlic, mozzarella, onions, and peppers.

6. Broil pita pizza for five minutes or until hot and golden. Wow!!! That is good!

For more info, see Making Babies DVD - Vol. 2

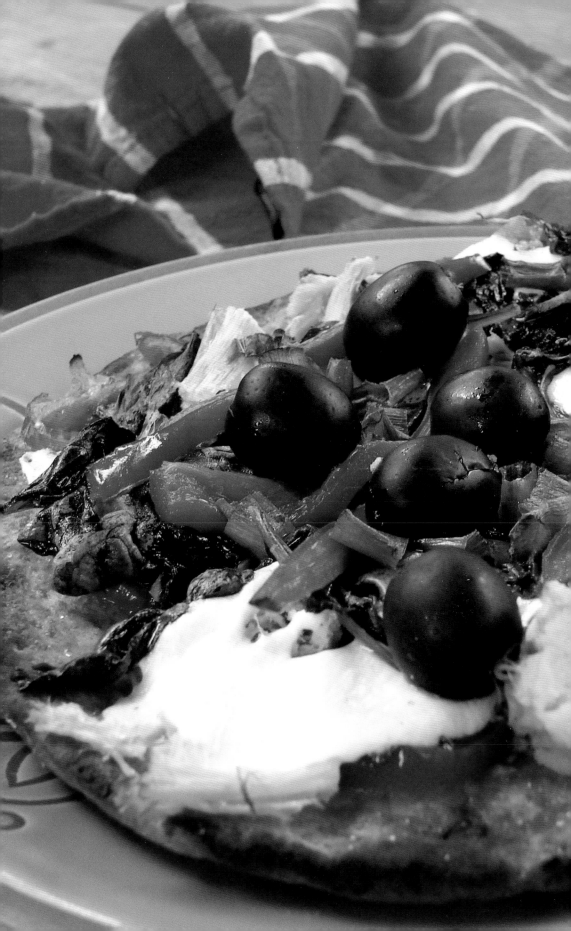

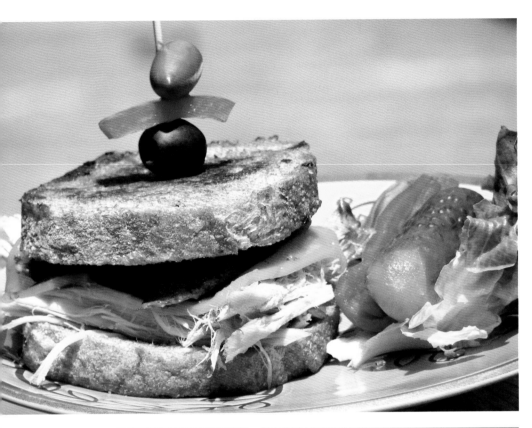

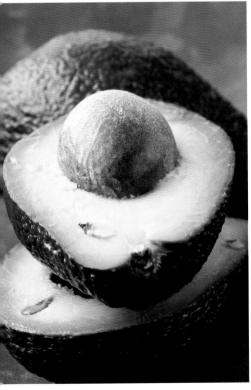

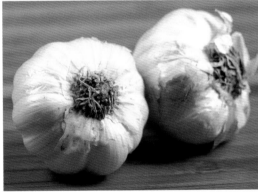

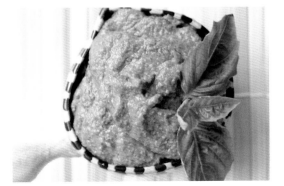

Turkey Melt
Toasty, Juicy, and Just Right

1 T. butter

2 slices bread

½ cup turkey

1 slice cheddar cheese

2 slices of avocado

1 garlic clove, crushed

1-2 T. **Original Pesto** (Page 316)

Prep: 5 min. Cook: 8 min. Yield: 1 sandwich

1. Rub butter on bread and place on a skillet, butter-side down, on medium heat.

2. Place all the ingredients on top of bread, and place second slice on top of sandwich.

3. Cook each side until golden brown (about 4 minutes on each side) and allow the cheese to melt.

For more info, see Making Babies DVD - Vol. 2

Turkey Salad

I Love This!!! Snack, Lunch, or Dinner

2 cups turkey, cooked and chopped

¼ cup red grapes, halved

¼ cup apple, chopped

¼ cup pecans, chopped

2 T. Vegenaise

½ tsp. sea salt

⅛ cup Craisins (*optional*)

Prep: 7 min. Yield: 2¾ cups

1. Wash and chop fruit.

2. Stir together all ingredients.

3. Place turkey salad in a lettuce wrap, tortilla, or on bread.

For more info, see *Making Babies DVD - Vol. 2*

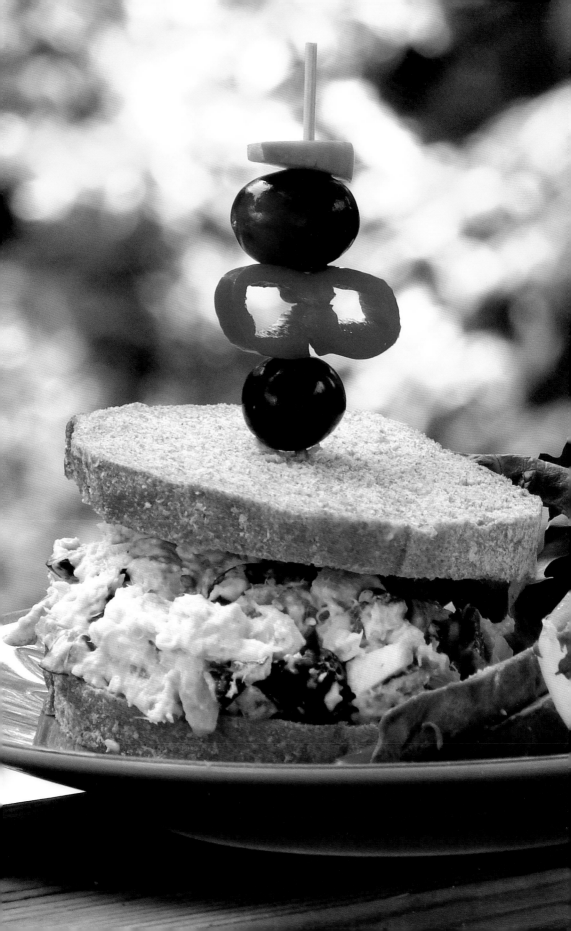

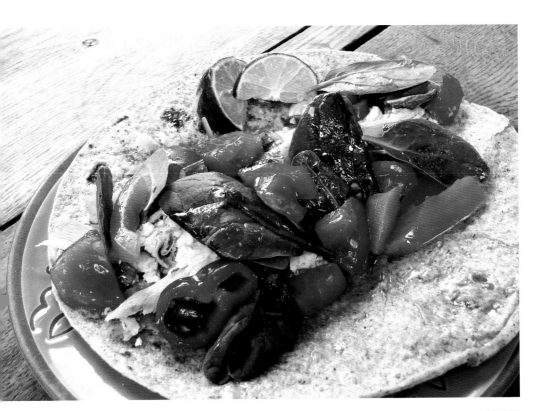

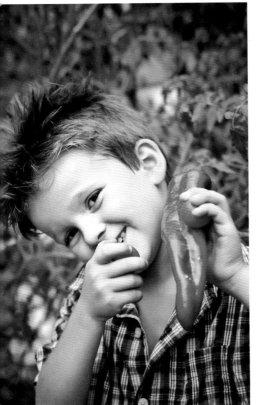

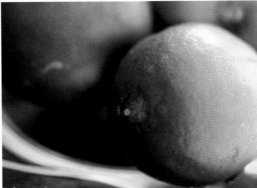

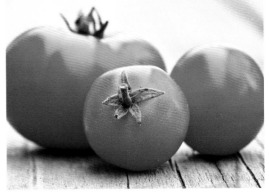

Turkey Wrap

Full of Fresh Flavor and Antioxidants

1 tortilla

1 garlic clove, crushed

½ cup turkey

⅛ cup red pepper, such as Marconi, chopped

⅛ cup green onions

½ cup spinach, fresh

¼ cup tomatoes, chopped

1 or 2 lime wedges

2 T. olive oil

¼ tsp. sea salt

4 Mediterranean olives

Prep: 8 min. Serves: 1

1. Rub garlic on inside of tortilla.

2. Lay next 5 ingredients vertically in center of tortilla.

3. Squeeze lime juice, sprinkle salt, and drizzle olive oil on tortilla and wrap.

4. Serve with olives on the side.

For more info, see *Making Babies DVD - Vol. 2*

Tincture for Inflammation

This is Great to Keep on Hand.

In your third trimester, your hips are separating. It can cause pain and inflammation. Your body is preparing for your baby to come through the birth canal. Your feet can also cause you pain during your third trimester. After standing or walking, your feet might be so painful you can barely stand. Did you know you can set yourself up for arthritis for the rest of your life? Your baby needs vitamins and minerals to build her body. If you are not ingesting enough, then the vitamins and minerals are pulled from your bones and muscles, giving you achy bones and sore muscles. This is a tincture to help reduce inflammation and to strenghten your body with vitamins and minerals. Also see: Egg Shell Water (page 26), Cal-Mag (page 369), and Flat-Footed Squat (page 108).

1 ½ cups oat straw

2 cups nettle leaf

Hot water

Glycerin

Herbs can be fresh or dried.

Prep: 5 min. Cook: 3 days Yield: 2-3 cups

1. Place herbs in a clean, glass, quart jar with lid.

2. Fill jar 40% with hot water and 60% with glycerin, leaving 1-2 inches from top of the jar.

3. Close jar tightly, place in a Crock-Pot with a small towel underneath to keep the jar from breaking.

4. Fill the Crock-Pot with water up to the top of the jar (not touching the lid), and leave it on the lowest setting for 3 days, keeping the glycerin hot, but not boiling; add water as necessary.

5. Strain out herb solids and place liquid in a tincture bottle.

This tincture is made with nutritious herbs, like whole foods. That is why I feel comfortable taking a lot more of this tincture. I take up to 1 tablespoon 3 times a day depending on how I feel.

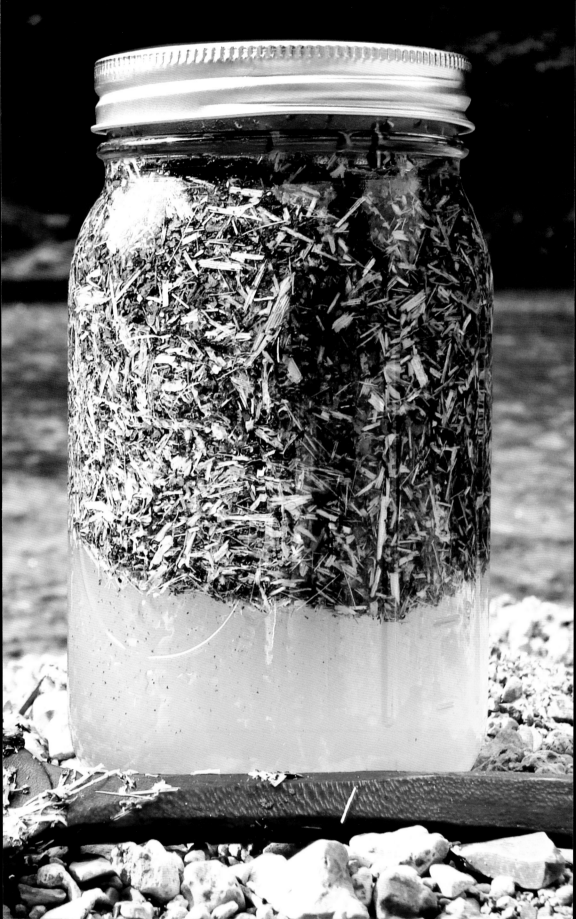

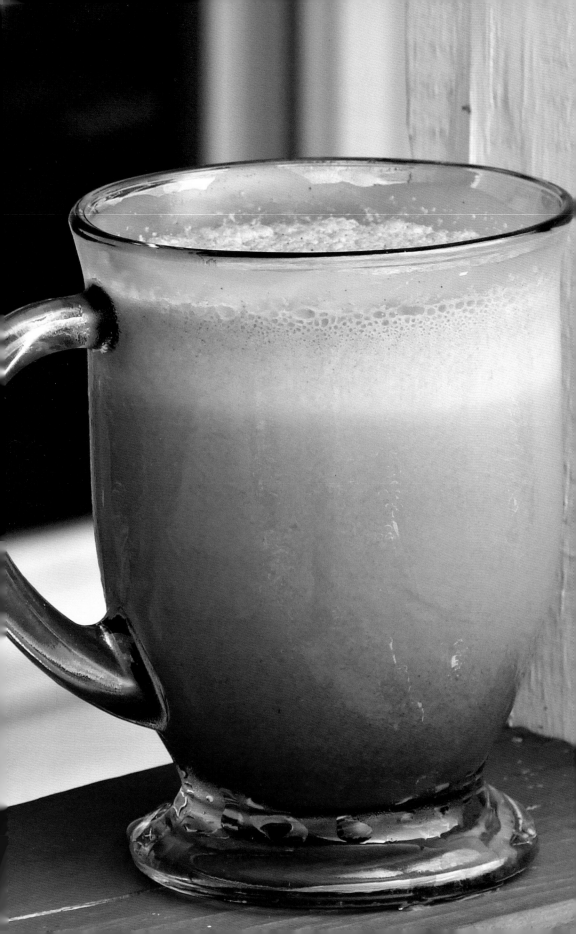

Chocolate Milkshake
Shake It Up With a Healthy Shake!

Sometimes you just need a deliciously chocolate milkshake. This is it!!

½-¾ cup plain yogurt

2-4 T. cocoa powder, organic

⅛ cup cream or coconut cream

⅛ tsp. sea salt

¼ tsp. vanilla

3 T. raw sugar or maple syrup

½ cup milk or coconut milk

Prep: 5 min. Yield: 1 shake

1. Make yogurt into 5 cubes by freezing it in an ice tray about 2 hours or overnight.

2. In a blender, blend all ingredients until smooth.

3. Drink and enjoy.

For more info, see *Making Babies DVD - Vol. 2*

Rhubarb Crisp

The Richer the Red, the Better.

4 cups rhubarb

2 cups green apple

1 T. lemon zest

1 T. lemon juice

1 tsp. vanilla

1½ cups raw sugar
(turbinado)

2 T. arrowroot powder

1 T. whole wheat flour

¼ tsp. nutmeg

1 tsp. cinnamon

1 tsp. sea salt

3 T. butter

Topping

3 cups oats

½ cup whole wheat flour

1 cup brown sugar or raw
sugar

¼ tsp. nutmeg

1 tsp. cinnamon

1 cup pecans, chopped

½ cup butter, cold

Prep: 10 min. Cook: 45 min. Serves: 8

1. Preheat oven to 350° F.

2. Wash rhubarb and apples and chop in ¾-inch cube pieces.

3. Toss rhubarb and apples with lemon juice, zest, and vanilla.

4. Mix next seven ingredients together and toss with rhubarb mixture, then pour mix into a 9½ x 11 dish.

Topping

1. Combine all topping ingredients except butter.

2. Cut in butter using a pastry cutter or 2 knives until butter looks like little pearls covered with flour.

3. Sprinkle evenly over rhubarb mix. Do not press topping mix on rhubarb – allow to rest on top.

4. Bake in oven for 45 minutes.

Tip From Shoshanna:

Rhubarb strengthens your uterus and prepares it for conception.

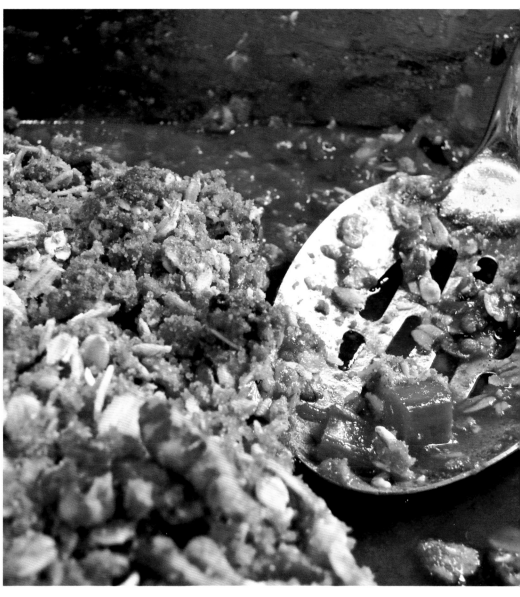

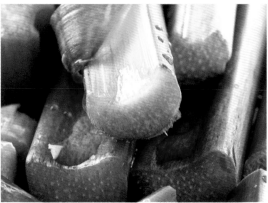

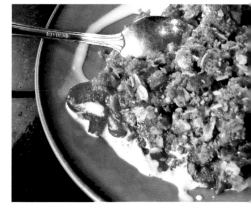

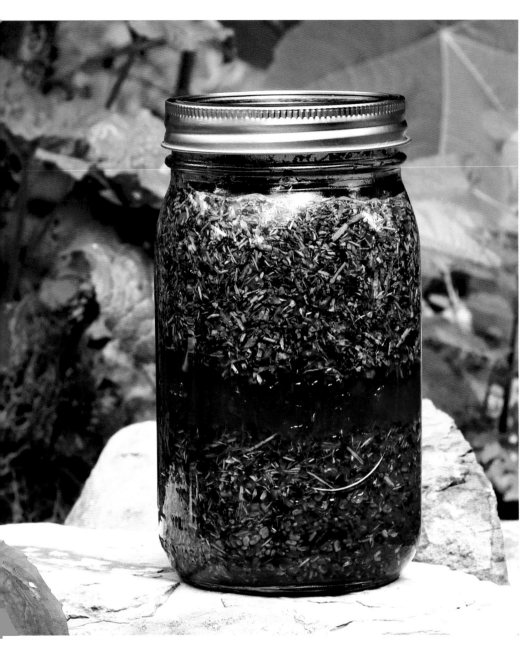

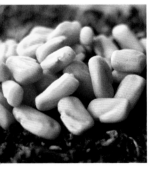
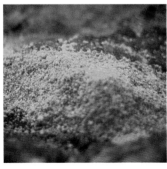
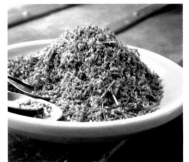

Vitamin B Tincture

Bs Are Very Important. Happy Vitamins!

Prep: 8 min. Soak: 6 weeks   Yield: 3 cups

4 T. alfalfa, cut

4 T. fenugreek, whole

5 T. burdock, cut

2 T. nettle, cut

3 T. catnip, cut

1 T. dandelion leaf, cut

3 T. chamomile flowers

4 T. eleuthero root (commonly known as Siberian ginseng), cut

1 T. cayenne, garlic, or onions

3 T. gingko leaf, cut (*optional*)

Vodka

Any vodka works. It does not need to be expensive. You can also make it with glycerine if you prefer. See page 22 for an example of how to make a glycerin tincture.

Herbs can be fresh or dried.

1. Place all herbs in a quart jar.

2. Fill jar with vodka up to 1-2 inches from the lid, close tightly and store for 2-6 weeks in a dry, cool place, shaking the jar daily.

3. After 3 weeks, strain and discard the herbs. Bottle the liquid and label it.

4. If you want to evaporate the alcohol, place your dose in a hot liquid, such as tea or water before taking.

5. I like to take 3 to 6 droppers a day with food. (1 dropper is equivalent to about ¼ teaspoon.)

For more info, see *Making Babies DVD - Vol. 2*

Chicken and Rice

Turmeric Is Great With Soup, Fish, and More.

6 cups turkey broth

3 cups brown rice

1 tsp. sea salt

6 T. turmeric powder

8 garlic cloves

½ cup leeks

½ cup cilantro

3 lbs. chicken

Prep: 5 min. Cook: 45 min. Yield: 10-12 cups

1. Wash and chop cilantro.

2. Chop and separate leek rings, then wash leeks.

3. Remove skin from garlic.

4. Chop chicken into about 2 by 3 inch pieces.

5. Combine all ingredients in a large saucepan.

6. Cook on stove top, with lid, for 45 minutes or until it stops steaming, holes appear on top of rice, and rice is tender.

7. Eat garnished with cilantro and green onions.

Tip From Shoshanna:

Turmeric is blood purifying, giving you more energy and keeping your body running better.

For more info, see *Making Babies DVD - Vol. 2*

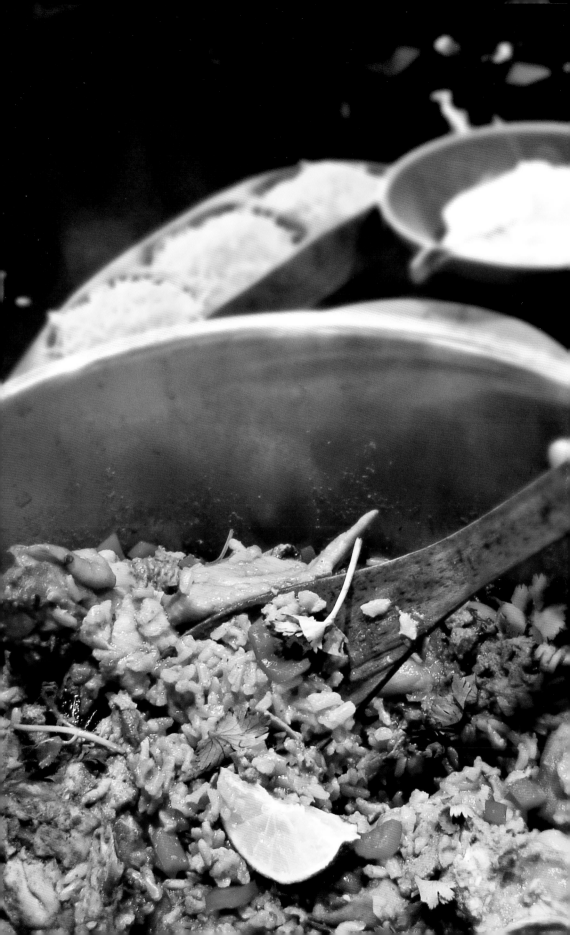

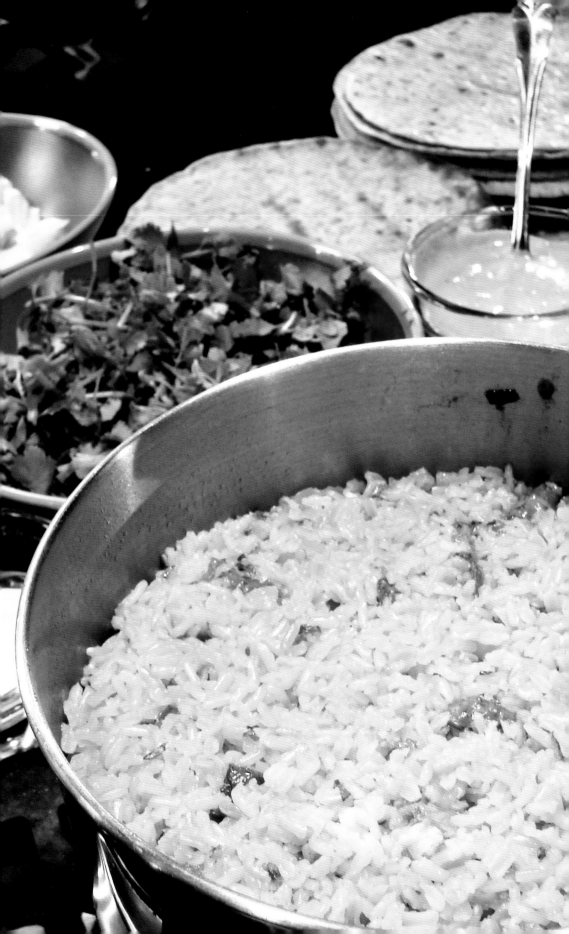

Beans and Rice

Beans Are Great to Eat Every Day.

I recipe **Simple and Basic Brown Rice**, cooked according to page 339 (with broth)

2 cups black beans, dried

9 cups water

2 tsp. garlic powder

I tsp. sea salt

¼ cup cilantro, washed and chopped

½ cup leeks, chopped, separated and washed

½ tsp. cumin, *optional*

Prep: 6 hours Cook: 45 min. Serves: 4-6

1. Soak beans in 5 cups of water for 6 hours.

2. Strain and rinse soaked beans.

3. Place beans, garlic powder, sea salt, and cumin (if using) into a medium-size pot with the remaining 4 cups of water.

4. Cook beans until soft (about 45 minutes).

5. Top with cilantro and leeks. Serve beans over bed of rice. Enjoy!

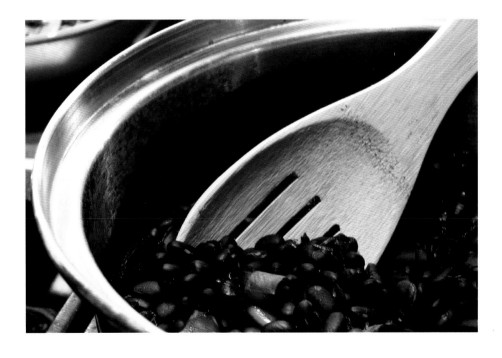

Mexican Pizza

Simply Delicious

1 pita, toasted

½ cup **Rice**, (page 91)

½ cup **Black Beans**, (page 91)

¼ cup green onions

¼ cup tomatoes

½ avocado, sliced

¼ cup cheddar cheese, grated (optional)

Sea salt, to taste

Mexican Sauce

1 T. sour cream

Pinch pepper, freshly ground

1-2 garlic cloves, crushed

1 tsp. taco seasoning

Prep: 5 min. Cook: 5-7 min. Serves: 1-2

Pizza

1. Preheat oven to broil.

2. Lightly toast pita on each side.

3. Sprinkle each topping, one at a time, on pita.

4. Broil pizza for 5 to 7 min.

5. Drizzle sauce over pizza and enjoy!

Mexican Sauce

1. Mix all ingredients together.

Indian Pizza

Leftovers Into Gourmet

1 cup **Chicken and Rice** (page 88)

¼ cup green onions

¼ cup green chilies

¼ cup cheese of your choice

¼ cup red pepper

Sea salt to taste

Prep: 5 min. Cook: 5-7 min. Serves: 1-2

1. Preheat oven to broil.

2. Wash and chop onions and peppers.

3. Lightly toast pita on each side.

4. Sprinkle each topping, one at a time, on pita.

5. Broil pizza for 5 to 7 min.

6. Enjoy!!

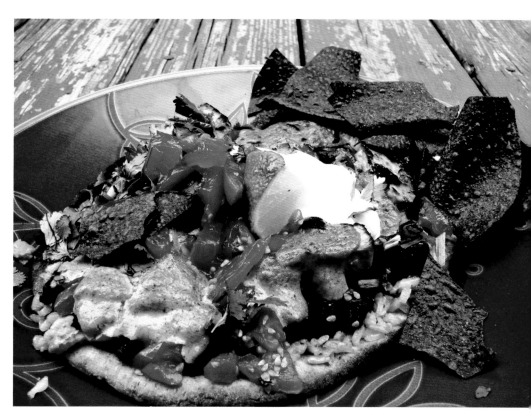

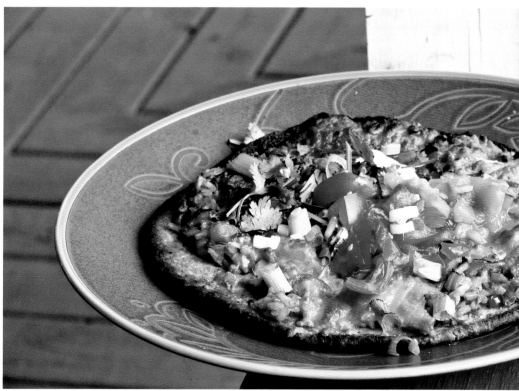

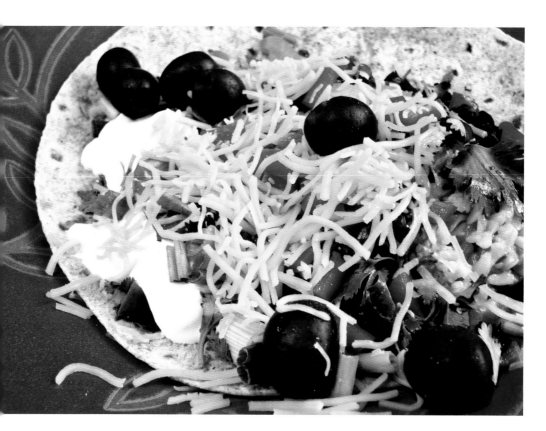

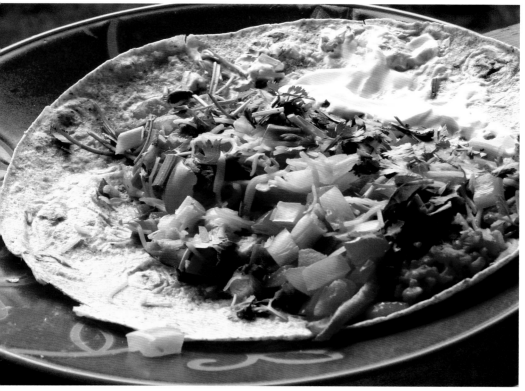

Mexican Burrito
Leftovers in Disguise

1 tortilla

½ cup **Black Beans** (page 91)

⅓ cup **Rice** (page 91)

⅓ cup chicken, cooked and chopped

½ cup cilantro

¼ cup green onions

¼ cup peppers

¼ cup green chilies

2 T. sour cream

¼ cup cheddar cheese

Olives (*optional*)

Prep: 7 min. Serves: 1

1. Lay ingredients elongated in center of tortilla.

2. Fold 3 sides of the tortilla over and you have it!!

Burrito With a Twist
Indian Meets Mexican Cuisine

1 tortilla

1 cup **Chicken and Rice** (page 88)

⅓ cup cilantro

¼ cup tomatoes

¼ cup peppers

¼ cup green onions

¼ cup cheddar cheese

2 T. sour cream

2 lime wedges

Prep: 7 min. Serves: 1

1. Lay ingredients elongated in center of tortilla.

2. Fold 3 sides of the tortilla over and you have it!!

For more info, see Making Babies DVD - Vol. 2

Mexican Salad
Creating Something New With Old

2 cups mixed greens

¾ cup black beans

¼ cup cilantro, chopped

¼ cup cheddar cheese

½ avocado, sliced

¼ cup peppers

¼ cup tomatoes

½ cup **Rice** (page 91)

2 lime wedges

2 T. **Mexican Sauce** (see **Mexican Pizza**, page 92)

Green chiles (*optional*)

Blue corn chips

Prep: 7 min. Serves: 1-2

1. Wash and chop all veggies.

2. In a bowl add greens and layer all ingredients, other than chips, on top.

3. Serve with blue corn chips on side.

Curry Salad
Keeping It Fresh

2 cups mixed greens

½ cup **Chicken and Rice** (page 88)

2 T. sour cream

¼ cup tomato

¼ cup peppers, chopped

¼ cup green onions

Corn chips (*optional*)

Prep: 7 min. Serves: 1-2

1. Wash and chop all your veggies.

2. In a bowl add your greens and then layer all ingredients on top.

Eat with corn chips or a fork

For more info, see *Making Babies DVD - Vol. 2*

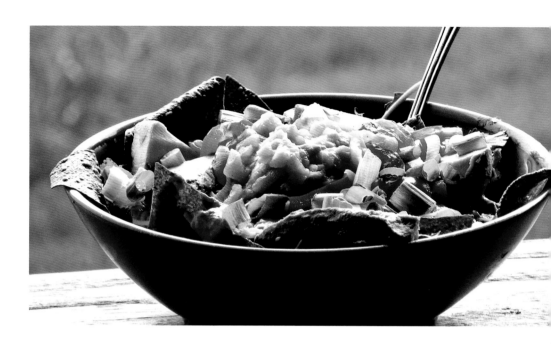

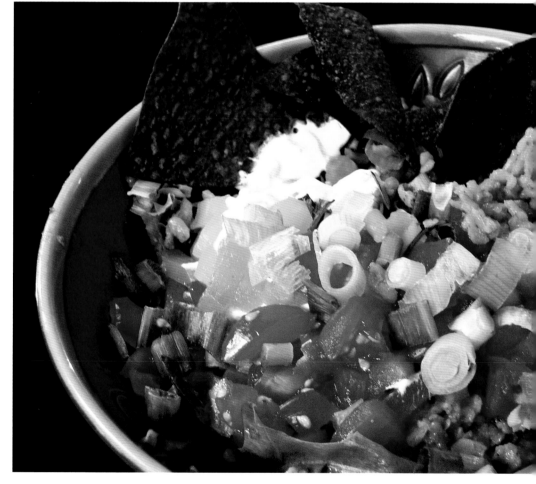

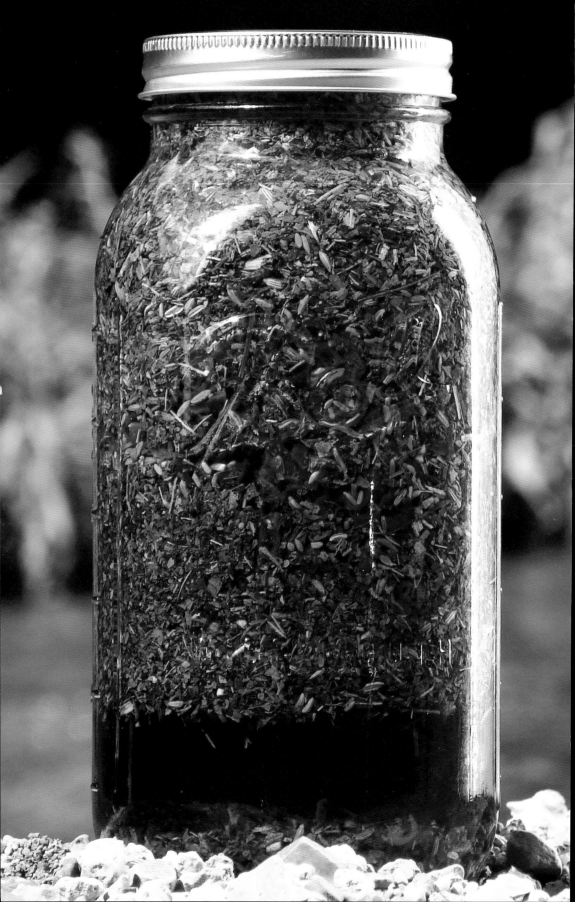

Iron Infusion

Keep Your Iron Up! Baby Needs It!

2½ cups nettle

1 cup rose hips

1 cup dandelion leaf

1 cup fennel

8 cups water, hot

Prep: 5 min. Steep: 12 hours Yield: 7½ - 8 cups

1. Place all herbs in a glass canning jar and cover herbs with hot water.

2. Cover and let sit overnight.

3. Strain out herbs.

4. I like to sip this throughout the day for an iron boost.

Keeps in the refrigerator for 3-4 days.

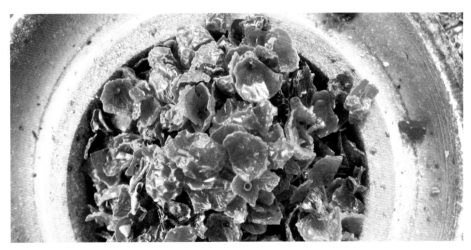

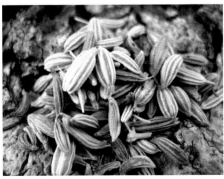
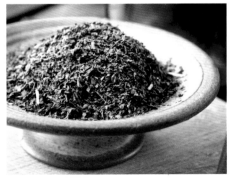

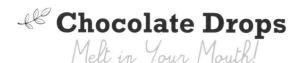 Chocolate Drops
Melt in Your Mouth!

1 cup coconut oil

½ cup raw honey

¼ cup cocoa powder

½ cup pecans or walnuts, chopped

½ cup coconut flakes, (*optional*)

Prep: 10 min.   Chill: 45 min.   Yield: 16

1. Place all ingredients in a food processor, and blend until combined.

2. Drop small spoonfuls of chocolate mixture onto wax paper. Chill in the refrigerator for 45 minutes.

3. Once chilled, enjoy a chocolate bite of heaven!

For more info, see *Making Babies DVD - Vol. 2*

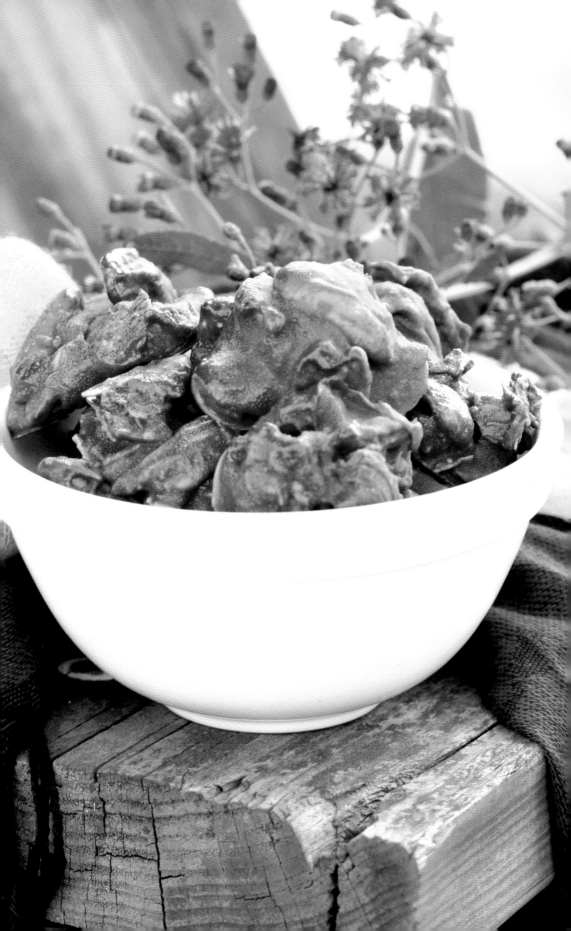

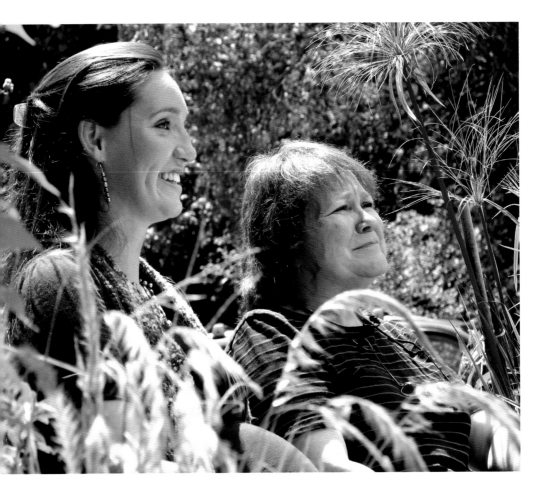

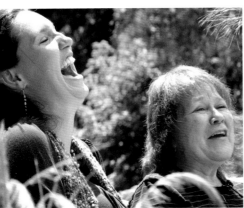

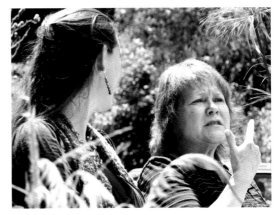

Interview With Elaine Wakeland

Learning From Those With Experience

In the Making Babies DVD series, we have some great interviews with different specialists. This interview is with Elaine Wakeland, one of the founders of Natchez Trace Maternity Center in Waynesboro, TN. She is a certified midwife and lactation specialist.

Question: What is the difference between hospital and midwife/maternity center?

Answer: In the hospital, the biggest difference is that 99% of the time you are going to be with an obstetrician. An obstetrician by nature is a surgeon, so they see birth differently compared to midwives. A midwife is trained specifically and exclusively to take care of women from birth control to postpartum, really through the rest of their lives.

Question: How does a woman choose whether to use a hospital, midwife at home, or maternity center for her birth experience?

Answer: That is what it is! Her birth experience! It is what she wants and thinks is safe for her baby.

Elaine and the other specialists, Johan C. Dinkelmann, DC, Dr. Nancy A. Armetta, MD, Elaine M. Wakeland, CNM, and Dr. Jay Gordon, MD, FAAP, have many great things to say. If you want to see the interviews, check out the Making Babies DVD series.

Check these out!! Here are some of Elaine's resources for you:

www.cappa.net
www.birthcenters.org
www.doula.com
www.midwife.org
www.dona.org

For more info, see *Making Babies DVD* - Vol. 2

Exercise Indian Style
Get Smart - Muscle Smart.

Going through labor and birth, you are using muscles you never used before. You need to prepare for the workout of your life. This exercise helps you stretch and get limber in the places you will need for your big day.

1. Sit Indian-style with knees bent and soles of feet facing and touching each other, or feet upside down, stretching foot out.

2. Using hands, push knees toward the ground, holding five minutes or more.

3. I do this throughout my pregnancy. By the third trimester, I'm doing this two to three times a day or more.

For more info, see *Making Babies DVD - Vol. 2*

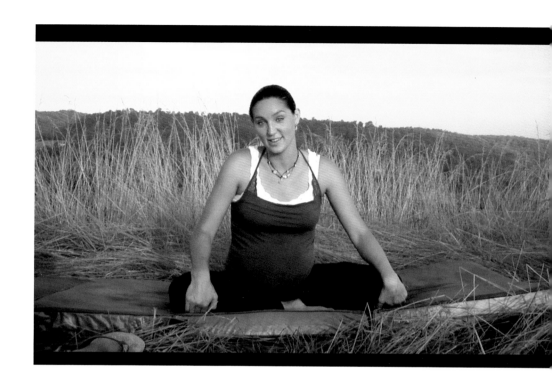

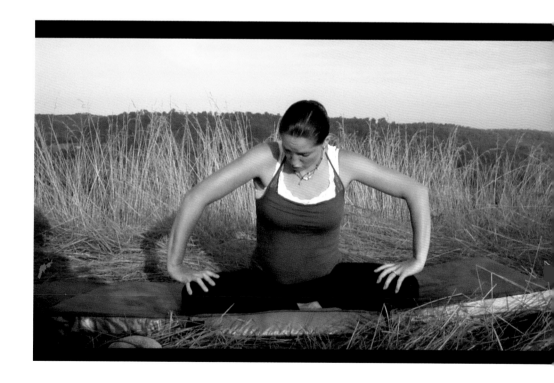

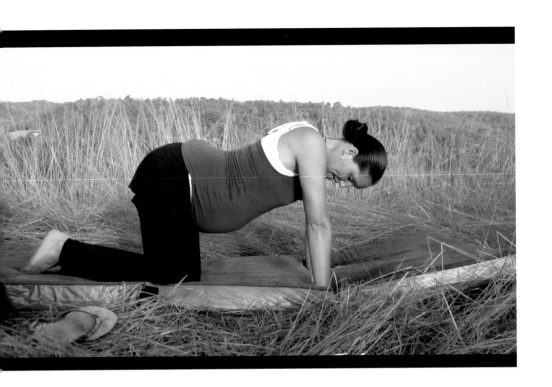

Cayenne, cinnamon, and garlic are all great herbs for increasing circulation.

Exercise and Circulation
More Than Relief; It's Prevention.

This is a great exercise for increasing circulation and relieving varicose veins and back pain. Your uterus is attached to your lower back. In your third trimester, it can cause some back pain. This exercise helps to relieve the vessels that are running down into your legs, as it moves the baby forward and relieves your back. This is not a race. Go slow and easy.

1. Get on your hands and knees. Your knees should be directly under your hips or slightly back. Make sure they are not in front of your hips. Your arms should be directly under your shoulders.

2. Tuck in your butt and tighten your abdomen. Try not to raise your shoulders.

3. I do this two or three times a day.

For more info, see Making Babies DVD - Vol. 2

Flat-Footed Squat

I Love This One!

Strengthening your kegel is very important!!!! This is a good exercise to keep up for the rest of your life. Not only is your kegel one of the most important muscles to strengthen for birth, it also makes the bedroom fun - out of this world! God blessed us girls with that one!!!!

1. Get your husband to help you until you are comfortable doing these exercises by yourself. Stand, facing each other. You both need to have a strong stance with your feet about a foot apart, flat on the ground.

2. Both you and your partner hold out your arms and hold onto each other. Start into a squat. Your goal is to be able to sit in a flat-footed squat, with your belly and arms between your legs, leaning forward a little.

3. This will help you prepare for birth. I do this one 30-45 minutes throughout the day.

For more info, see Making Babies DVD - Vol. 2

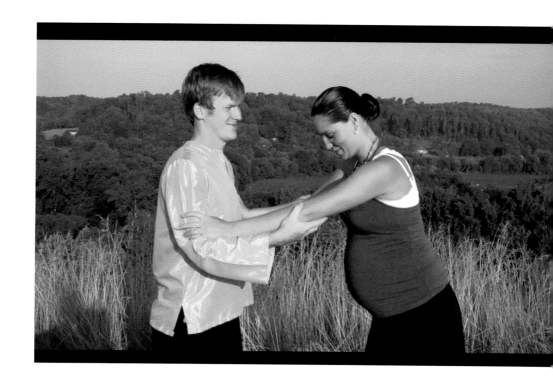

Tip From Shoshanna:

To learn more about the kegel muscle, see page 52.

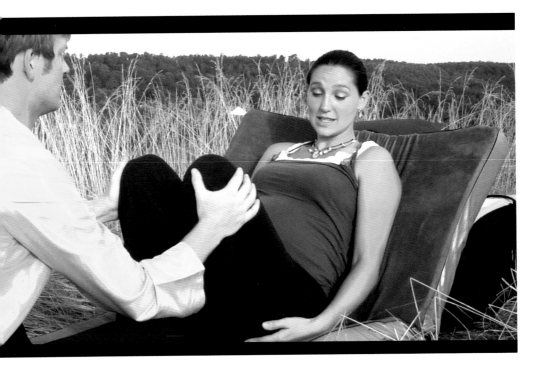

Practice, practice, practice! Exercise and relax. Your big day is coming - get ready for it!

Pillow Talk Exercise

Enjoy Some Time With Your Man.

My husband and I always had a great time doing this one, because it gave us a good reason to sit down and talk.

1. Sit on the bed with pillows propped against your back and lean back slightly.

2. Keep your knees bent and your feet flat and close to your butt.

3. Have your husband sit in front of you with his hands on your outer knees and apply enough pressure to give you some good resistance but not enough to cause you to strain.

4. Pull your knees apart as far as you can. Repeat ten to thirty times.

5. This is great to do 2 or 3 times a day!

For more info, see *Making Babies DVD - Vol. 2*

Relaxing Labor Exercise

On Your Mark! Get Set! Relax!

This is a position you should practice for labor. You don't want to have to teach your husband while you are having contractions, so both of you need to practice it now.

1. Sit on the bed with pillows propped against your back. You should be leaning back slightly.

2. Keep your knees bent and your feet flat and close to your butt.

3. Have your husband sit in front of you with his palms on either side of your stomach, slightly lower than your belly button, and rub in a circular motion.

4. You can also do this with him behind you and you leaning against him with his arms wrapped around you.

For more exercises and birth positions check out the Making Babies DVD Series.

For more info, see Making Babies DVD - Vol. 2

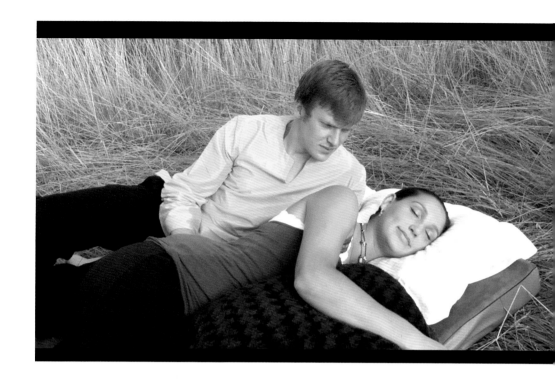

Tip From Shoshanna:

Don't wait for someone to help you relax. Learn to relax on your own and practice, practice, practice!

🌿 Trout
This Is an Awesome Fish! Healthy!

4 trout fillets

2 T. parsley

4 T. butter, softened

¼ cup leeks

½ tsp. lemon zest

2 T. lemon juice

1 tsp. garlic, minced

Peppercorns, freshly ground, to taste

Sea salt, to taste

Prep: 5 min. Cook: 15-18 min. Serves: 4

1. Preheat oven to 375° F.

2. Lightly butter a large glass baking dish.

3. Clean trout and pat dry. Rub with butter and layer evenly on baking dish.

4. Wash and chop veggies. Evenly sprinkle parsley, leeks, lemon zest, lemon juice, and garlic over fillets.

5. Sprinkle fresh ground peppercorns and salt over trout to taste.

6. Bake trout uncovered for 15-18 minutes, or until flaky.

🌿 Baked Tilapia
Tilapia Is One of My Favorites!

4 tilapia fillets

2 T. butter

1 T. lemon grass, chopped

¼ cup cilantro, chopped

¼ cup leeks

2 lemons, juiced

1 small clove garlic

Sea salt, to taste

1 tsp. lemon zest

1 tsp. ginger, freshly grated (*optional*)

Prep: 8 min. Cook: 18 min. Serves: 4

1. Preheat oven to 400° F.

2. Rub butter on tilapia fillets, and place them in a large baking dish.

3. Sprinkle lemon grass, cilantro, leeks, lemon juice, crushed garlic, salt, lemon zest, and ginger over fillets.

4. Bake fillets in preheated oven for 15-18 minutes or until flaky.

Carrots and Peas

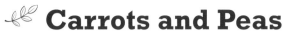
Eat Veggies With Every Meal.

2 cups carrots, chopped

2 T. butter

1 garlic clove

2 cups peas

1 ½ tsp. sea salt

Prep: 7 min. Cook: 7 min. Yield: 4 cups

1. Wash and chop carrots into ¾-inch pieces.

2. Wash peas.

3. Heat butter in pan, crush garlic, and add to pan.

4. Cook carrots in butter-garlic mixture for 4-5 minutes on medium-high to desired tenderness.

5. Add peas and cook, stirring often, for 3-4 minutes

6. Take off heat, salt, and serve.

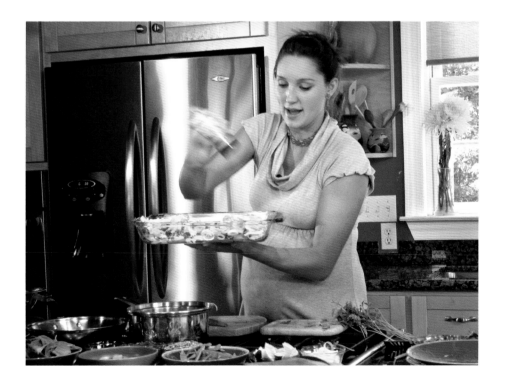

Artichokes

This Is a Great Superfood.

2 artichokes, large

4 quarts water, boiling

¼ cup virgin olive oil, for coating

3 cloves garlic, chopped

1 tsp. salt

½ tsp. black pepper, ground

1 lemon, quartered

¾ cup virgin olive oil, as dip

Prep: 5 min. Cook: 25 min. Serves: 4

1. Trim the tops from the artichokes, then cut in half lengthwise. Spoon out hairy center.

2. Add artichokes to boiling water, and cook for about 15 minutes.

3. Using tongs, place artichokes on a rack to drain for 5 minutes.

4. Preheat a pan or outdoor grill to medium-high heat.

5. Mix garlic, salt, pepper, and olive oil; coat cut side of artichokes with mix and place them face down in the preheated pan or grill.

6. Cook the artichokes for 5 to 10 minutes until a little toasted.

7. Serve immediately with lemon wedges; dip in virgin olive oil.

For more info, see *Making Babies DVD - Vol. 2*

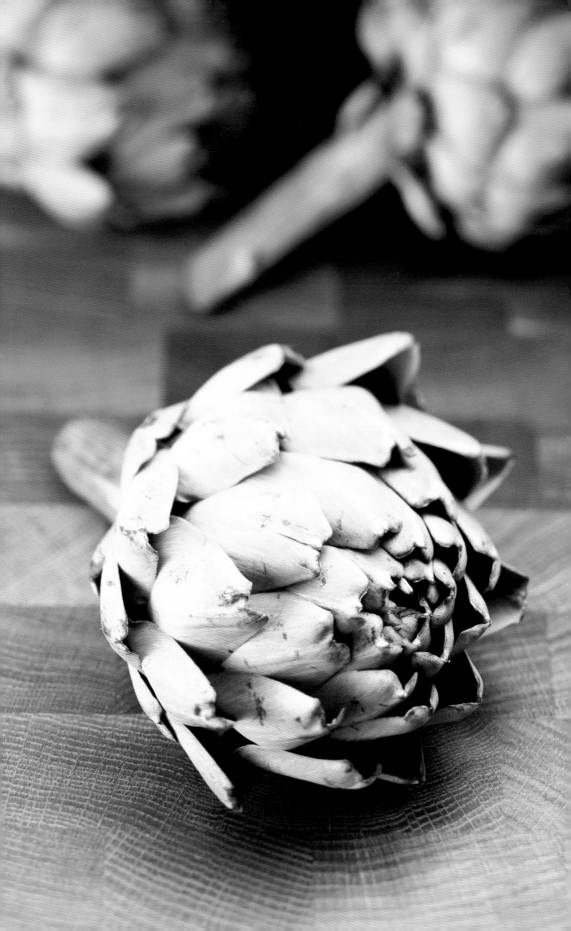

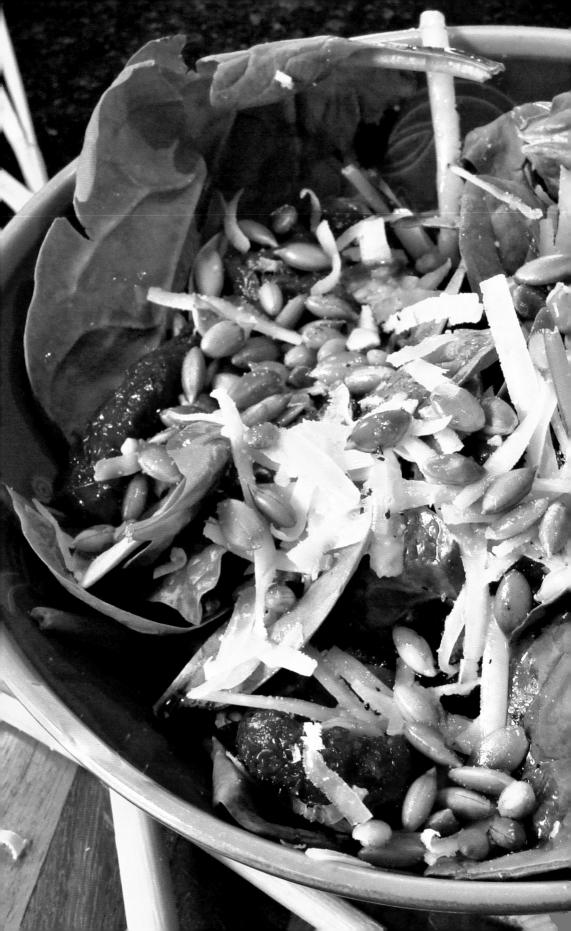

Spinach Salad

Mixing Citrus With Greens Helps Break Down Iron.

Salad

1 cup spinach

⅛ cup sun dried tomatoes

1 T. aged cheddar

1 T. pumpkin seeds

Dressing

1 T. lemon juice

1 T. olive oil

½ clove garlic

Pinch sea salt

Pinch pepper, freshly ground

½ tsp. raw honey

Prep: 5 min. Serves: 1

Salad

1. Wash spinach.

2. In a salad bowl, layer the salad ingredients.

Dressing

1. Crush garlic in another bowl.

2. Add other ingredients to dressing bowl, and mix.

3. Drizzle desired amount of dressing over salad and garnish with lime wedges. Yummy!

For more info, see *Making Babies DVD - Vol. 2*

Baby Powder
Going Organically Herbal for Baby

As a girl, I did a lot of babysitting. I remember the first time someone told me that store-bought baby powder can blind a baby. I thought, "Wow! We are still using it?" That is the way it is sold, so we buy it because we need it. When my babies came along, one of the first things I did was make a natural, herbal baby powder.

1 or 2 cups arrowroot powder

⅛ cup bentonite clay

¼ cup chamomile flower powder

⅛ cup lavender powder

Prep: 5 min.   Yield: 2½ cups

1. Mix ingredients together and put in a used (but clean) baby powder can.

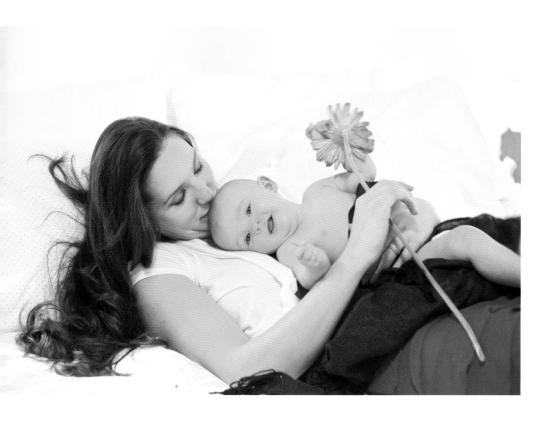

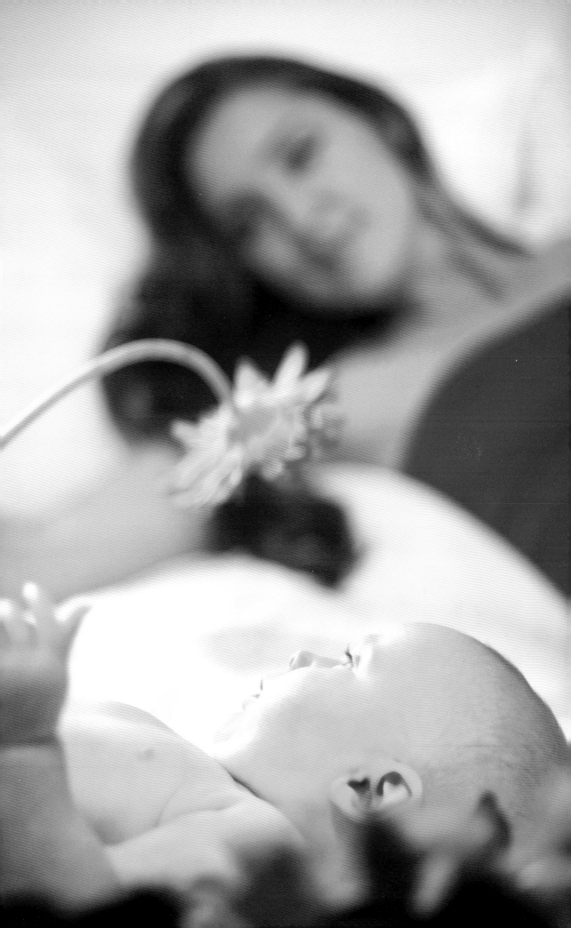

Pregnancy
TIPS

Cellulite

Use your homemade stretch mark cream or an organic lotion and rub, rub, rub! You need to get your circulation going. Upping your circulation helps to combat cellulite; so whether you are soaping up in the tub or moisturizing, rub, rub, rub!!!!

Acne

Your liver is working overtime when you are pregnant, taking care of you and your baby. Hormones, diet, or an overworked liver can cause acne. You need to make sure you are eating right, sleeping, exercising, and drinking water with a pinch of sea salt or a squeeze of lemon in it. Also, go organic in anything you can. Especially food, skin, and hair products.

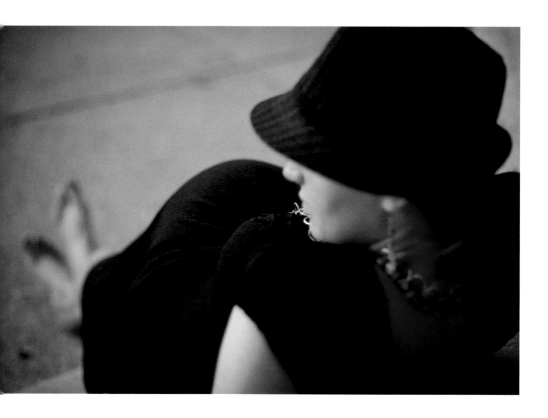

Pigment

Hormones change everything: your skin, hair, body, and the way you feel. Pregnancy hormones change a lot of women's pigment. Your nipples will darken, and some women might get more pigment with freckles, scars, or areas prone to friction, such as your underarms and inner thighs. This is normal and should fade within a few months after birth. The sun brings it out more. Wearing a hat to protect your face from the sun helps. Eating healthy, sleeping, and exercising help keep your hormones level.

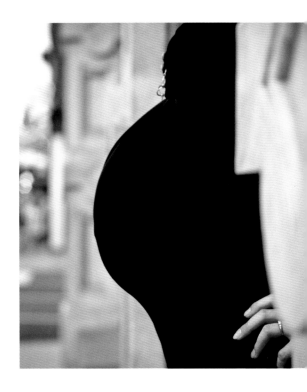

Natural Childbirth the Bradley Way
By Susan McCutcheon

The Bradley Method has been used and praised by women for more than thirty years. This is my favorite birthing book. It really teaches a woman how to feel her own body and know the birthing process. It teaches wonderful relaxing and exercise techniques that make such a difference in birth. Birth is the workout of your life. You need to be 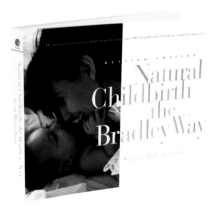 ready so you can enjoy it. My Amish midwife gave me this book when I was pregnant with my first child. I read it and practiced it throughout my pregnancy. My midwife had been to 350 births and said mine was the best she had ever seen. I know this book made the difference for me. We sell it at Bulk Herb Store. (www.bulkherbstore.com)

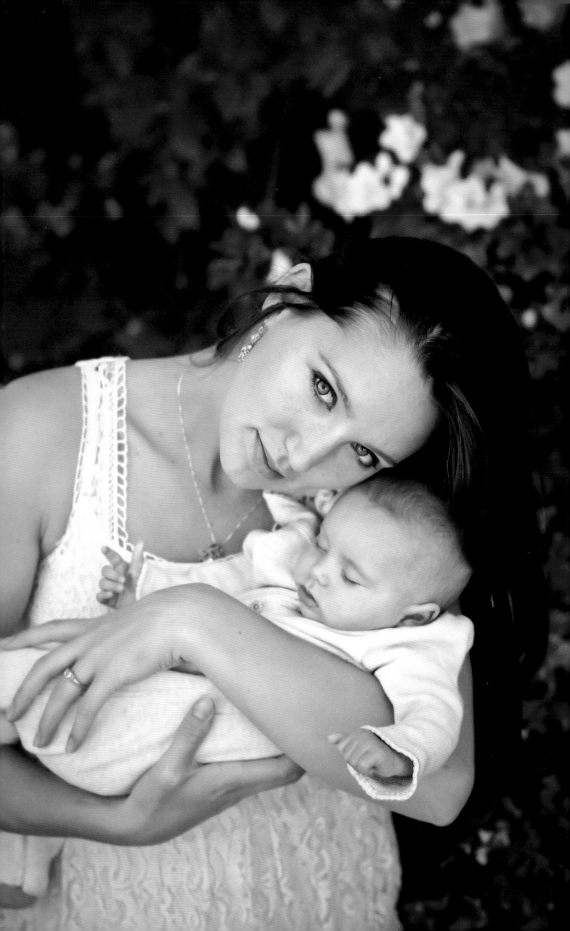

Making babies is so much fun! Step by step you have nourished and taken good care of your baby. Now it is time for you to introduce your baby to the world. Relax and enjoy your birth. The baby that you have carried for nine months will be in your arms soon, holding your finger and staring up at you. You are a mama.

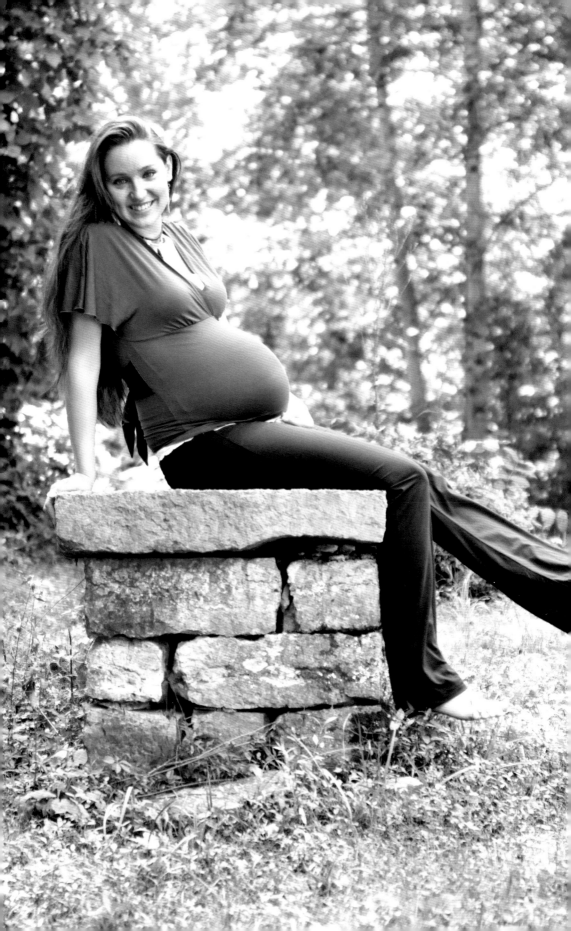

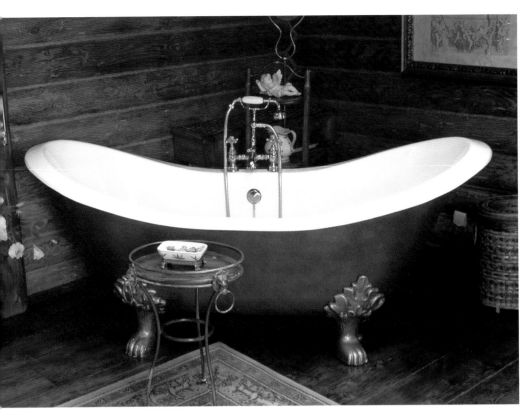

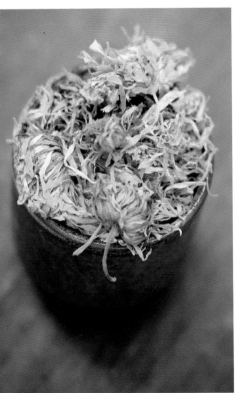

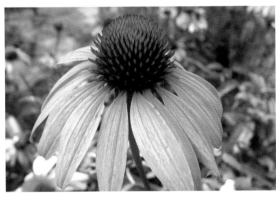

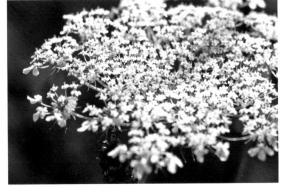

Sitz Bath
Warm, Relaxing, and Healing

To take a sitz bath, sit in water up to your hips, in a squat-like position. Sitz baths clean, increase blood flow, heal, and are used to relieve pain from the area starting at your belly button and continuing around to your lower back bone. They are done in a bathtub or a large basin, using things like herbs, salt, baking soda, or vinegar.

1 cup lavender flowers, whole

1 cup plantain leaf

2 cups comfrey leaf

½ cup rose petals

2 cups rosemary leaf

1 cup calendula flowers, whole

2 cups yarrow flowers

1 cup echinacea herb

4 cups sea salt

Water

Prep: 5 min.   Cook: about 45 min.   Yield: 14½ cups Bath Mix

1. Fill a four-quart pot with water and bring to boil.

2. Remove from heat. Add 4-7 cups of herb mix and cover. Let sit until warm, and strain liquid into bathtub or large bowl.

3. Sit and relax in tub for 20 minutes or more, or squat in bowl for 5-10 minutes.

For more info, see *Making Babies DVD* - Vol. 3

Granola From Heaven

So Good You Might Believe It!

My five-year-old son started calling this Granola From Heaven because it is so good!!

2 cups pecans

1 cup walnuts

1 cup cashews

¼ cup flax seeds

¼ cup sunflower seeds

1 cup almonds

¼ cup pumpkin seeds

¼ cup hazelnuts

¼ cup pine nuts

4 cups unsweetened coconut flakes

1 T. sea salt

¼ tsp. coriander

1 T. cinnamon

2 tsp. vanilla

½ cup maple syrup

¾ cup brown sugar or Sucanat

Prep: 10 min. Cook: 2 hours Yield: 10 cups

1. Place all ingredients in a large mixing bowl and mix until thoroughly combined.

2. Split and spread granola on 2 baking sheets lined with parchment paper.

3. Bake at 275° F for 2 hours, stirring every 30 minutes.

For more info, see Making Babies DVD - Vol. 3

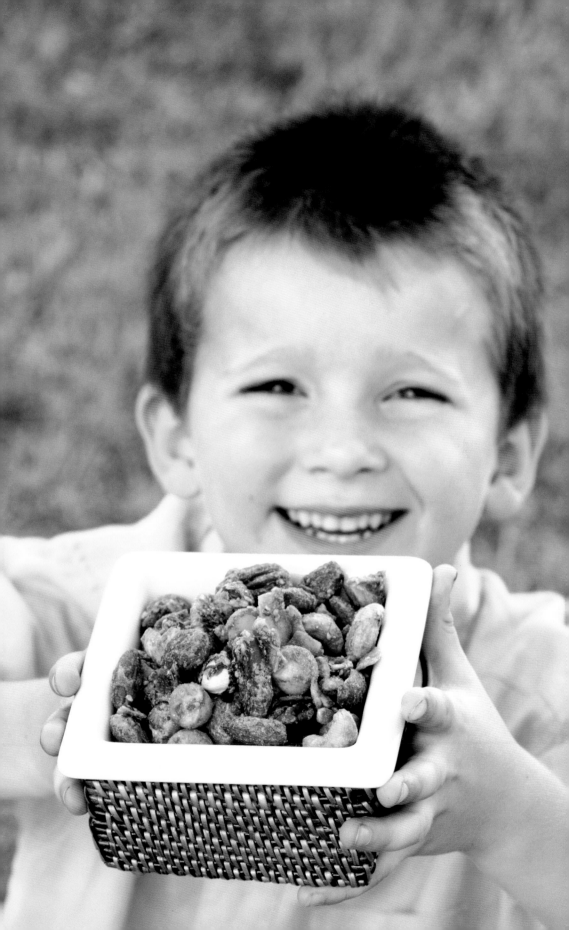

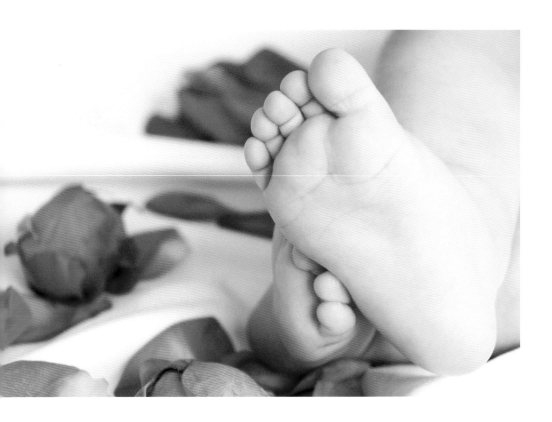

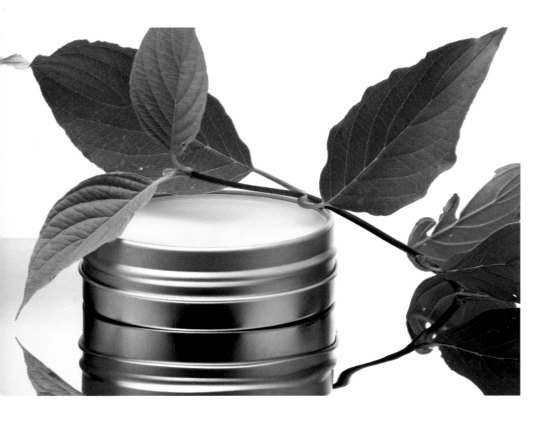

Herban Baby Oil

This Is Great for the Bath or Skin.

1 cup calendula flowers

1 cup rose petals

1 cup lavender flowers

4 cups coconut oil

Herbs can be fresh or dried.

For a bath, add ¼ cup to water in tub.

Prep: 5 min.   Cook: 3 days   Yield: 4 cups

1. Place herbs in a quart jar.

2. In a small saucepan, warm coconut oil until just melted.

3. Pour coconut oil over herbs in jar and cover tightly with lid.

4. Place jar in Crock-Pot with a small towel underneath to keep the jar from breaking.

5. Fill the Crock-Pot with water up to the top of the jar (not touching the lid), and leave it on the lowest setting for 3 days, keeping the oil hot but not boiling and adding water as necessary.

6. Cool and strain out herb solids and place oil into glass jar with lid.

See page 22 for Crock-Pot safety instructions.

Baby Salve

You Can Add Some Essential Oils for Scent.

2 cups **Herban Baby Oil** (above)

½ cup beeswax pastilles, found at Bulk Herb Store

20 drops grapefruit seed extract

Prep: 2 min.   Cook: 8 min.   Yield: 2¼ cups

1. In a small saucepan, heat oil and wax on low heat until wax is melted. (About 8 min.)

2. Take off heat and stir in grapefruit seed extract.

3. Pour liquid in jars or cans for salve, or glass 9x11 baking dish for making cream. (See page 134.)

Baby Cream
Moisturizing and Healing

1 ½ cups **Baby Salve** (page 133)

6-8 oz. organic aloe vera juice or water

1 tsp. vitamin E

10 drops grapefruit seed extract

Prep: 5 min.   Yield: 2 cups

1. Blend all ingredients together in an electric blender. Stir and scrape edges of blender with a spatula and continue blending until smooth, white, and creamy.

2. Store in a glass jar with lid.

Read more about aloe on page 381.

For more info, see *Making Babies DVD - Vol. 3*

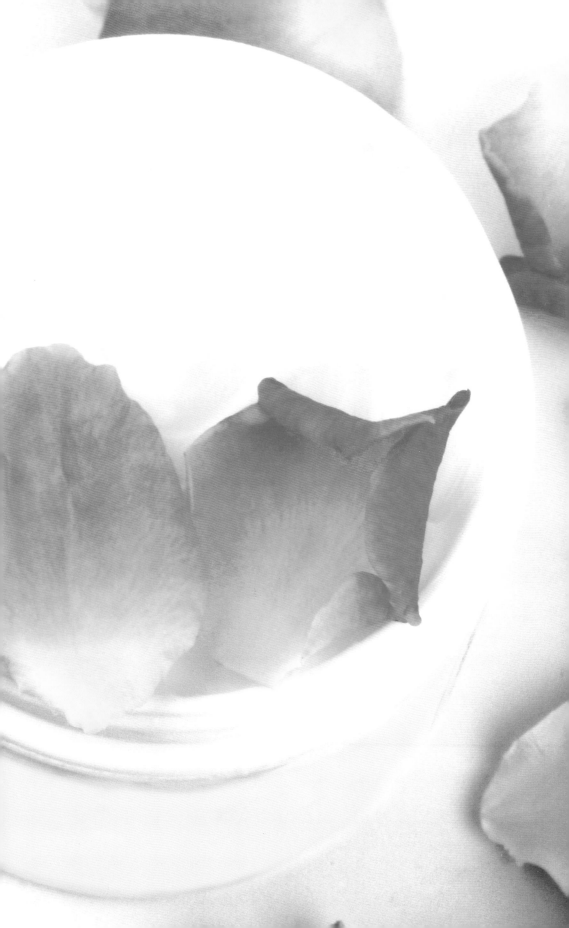

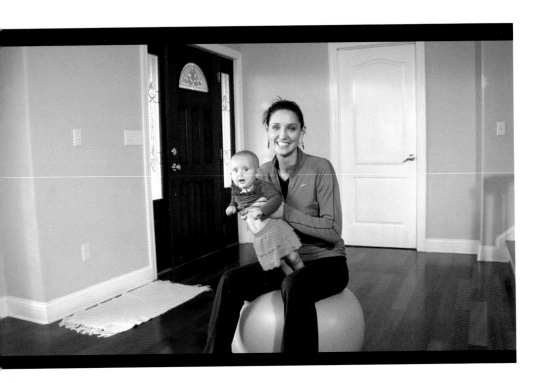

Spend time every day playing with, talking to, working with, and stimulating your baby. This will help her grow and develop into a smart, strong, and healthy child.

Bouncing My Butt Away
Fun and Easy to Do Every Day

After Penelope Jane was born I was so busy. I was nursing, burping, changing diapers, playing with Penelope, and putting her to sleep. When I was not doing that, I had the house, work, my husband, and our son to take care of.

Before I had Penelope Jane, I bought an exercise ball. I had planned to use it, and I did - just not like I thought I would. Exercise is very important to health. It helps to level your hormones and gives you energy. So I knew I wanted to add it to my life. The ball quickly became my seat. I used it when I was nursing, burping, playing, and putting Penelope Jane to sleep. She loved it, and so did I! Everyday, throughout the day, I was bouncing my butt away and toning up. I sat on the ball and tightened up my butt, making us bounce. I tightened, and we bounced again and again! Two weeks later, my butt had shrunk in half. In no time I was back at full throttle, passing up the energizer bunny.

Making exercise a part of your life activities really makes a difference. It keeps you consistent and distracted, and before you know it, you are in shape and feeling great! Find ways to make your daily life a workout that keeps you feeling GREAT!!

For more info, see Making Babies DVD - Vol. 3

GF/CF Pancakes
You Would Never Know These Are GF/CF.

⅛ cup arrowroot powder

⅔ cup oats

⅔ cup brown rice flour

⅔ cup almond meal

⅔ cup pecan meal

1 T. baking powder

½ -1 tsp. lemon zest

½ tsp. cinnamon

1 tsp. sea salt

¾ cup water or coconut milk

6 T. butter, melted

2 eggs

1 tsp. vanilla

2 T. raw honey (*optional*)

1 cup blueberries, fresh (*optional*)

Prep: 7 min.   Cook: 20 min. Yield: 12-18

1. In a medium-size bowl, whisk together all dry ingredients until thoroughly combined.

2. In a separate bowl, crack and beat eggs until fluffy. Add all liquid ingredients and zest. Whisk together.

3. Add liquid ingredients to dry ingredients, and mix until just combined.

4. Heat a slightly oiled griddle or frying pan to medium-high heat. Using a ¼ measuring cup, pour batter onto the griddle.

5. When tiny holes appear all over the top of the uncooked pancake, flip and cook until browned on both sides. Serve pancakes hot! Enjoy!

Banana Syrup
My Family Loves This!

2 bananas, sliced

4 T. butter

¼ cup maple syrup or Sucanat

¼ cup brown sugar or Sucanat

¼ tsp. sea salt

½ tsp. cinnamon

¼ tsp. fresh nutmeg

Prep: 3 min.   Cook: about 10 min.   Yield: 1½ cups

1. Slices bananas diagonally, about a half inch thick.

2. Fry bananas in a frying pan with butter on medium-high until golden. Flip and fry other side.

3. Add rest of ingredients. Reduce heat to medium-low and cook 5 minutes, stirring gently twice. Pour over pancakes.

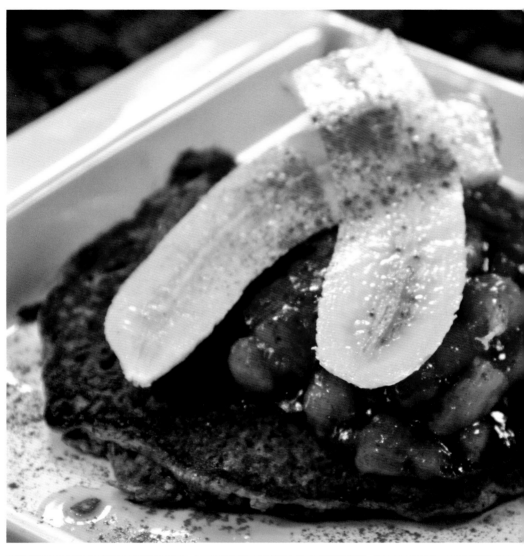

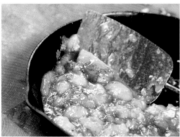 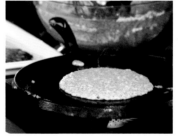 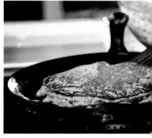

For more info, see *Making Babies DVD* - Vol. 3

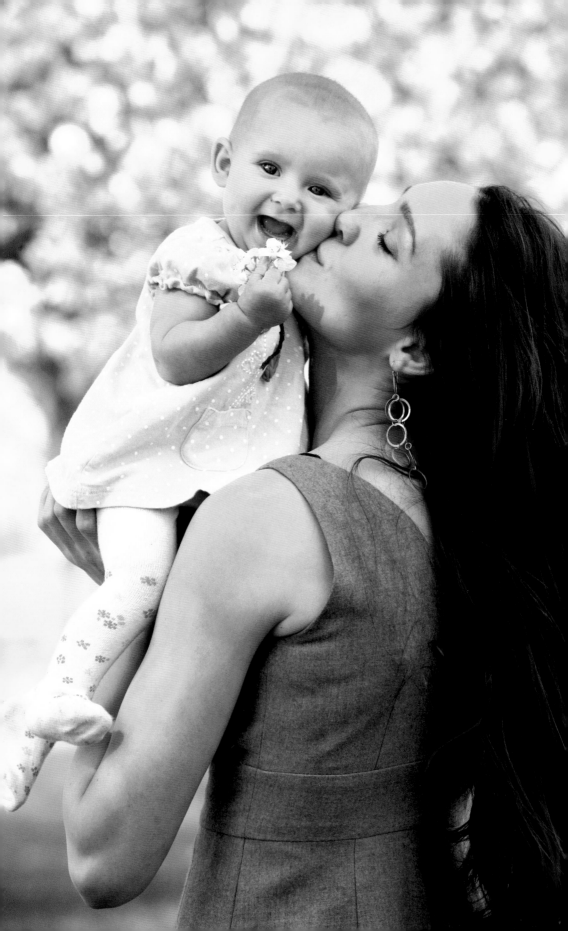

My Vitamin Tincture

Nursing Takes a Lot Out of You. Put Some back!

Hot water

Glycerine

2 cups raspberry leaf

1 cup gingko leaf

1 cup rose hips

¾ cup dandelion root

1 cup ginger root

1 cup chamomile flowers

½ cup fenugreek seeds

2 cups oat straw

2½ cups alfalfa

Herbs can be fresh or dried.

Prep: 8 min.   Cook: 3 days   Yield: about 3 cups

1. Place herb ingredients inside a clean, quart canning jar.

2. Fill herb jar 40% (not including 1-2 inches from top of jar) with hot water.

3. Fill the rest of the jar with glycerin, up to 1-2 inches from top of jar.

4. Close jar tightly. Place in a Crock-Pot with a small towel underneath to keep the jar from breaking.

5. Fill the Crock-Pot with water up to the top of the jar (not touching the lid), and leave it on the lowest setting for 3 days, keeping the glycerin hot, but not boiling, and adding water as necessary.

6. Strain out herb solids and place liquid into tincture bottle.

I like to take 1-2 droppers twice a day. (1 dropper is equivalent to about ¼ teaspoon.)

For more info, see *Making Babies DVD* - Vol. 3

Fried Rice

I Learned How to Make This in Thailand.

1½ cups **Simple and Basic Brown Rice** (page 339)

2 T. olive oil

1 cup raw chicken, chopped

1 cup carrots, chopped small

2 cups asian vegetables, frozen

Sea salt, to taste

3 garlic cloves, chopped

½ cup cilantro

½ tsp. fresh lime juice

⅛ tsp. lime zest

Lime wedge

Cilantro

Prep: 8 min.   Cook: about an hour   Serves: 4-6

1. Cook rice according to directions on page 339.

2. In a frying pan, heat oil on medium-high.

3. Add chicken and carrots. Cook 5 minutes.

4. Add Asian vegetables and salt, and cook another 5-8 minutes or until chicken is done and vegetables are cooked to desired tenderness.

5. Add rice, garlic, lime juice, zest, and cilantro. Mix.

6. Garnish with lime wedge and cilantro and serve. One of my favorites!

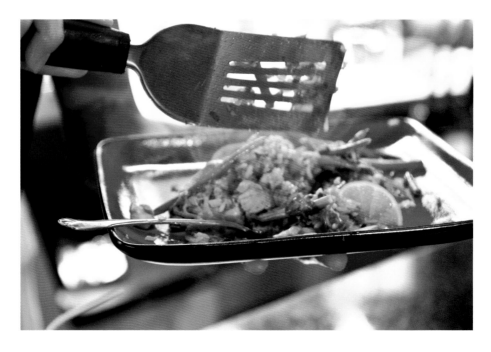

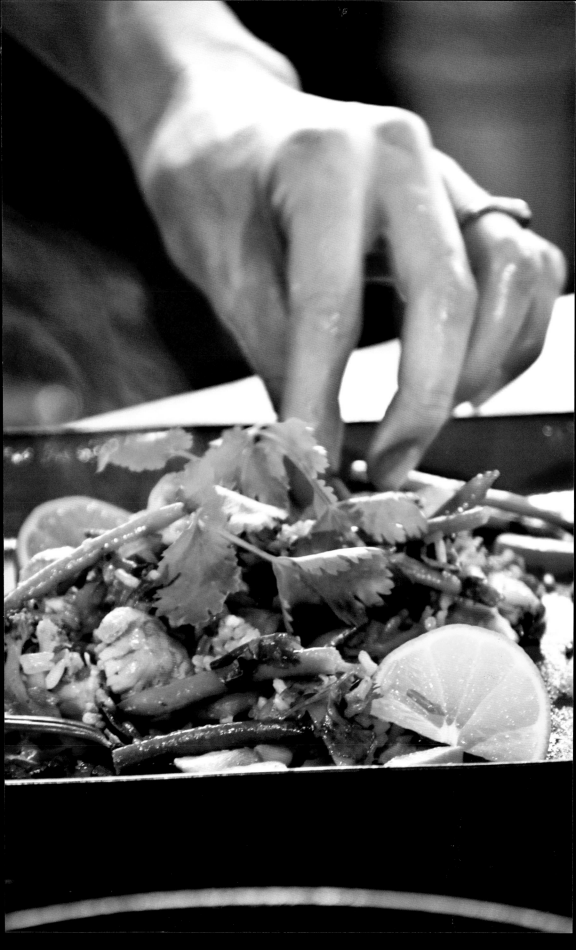

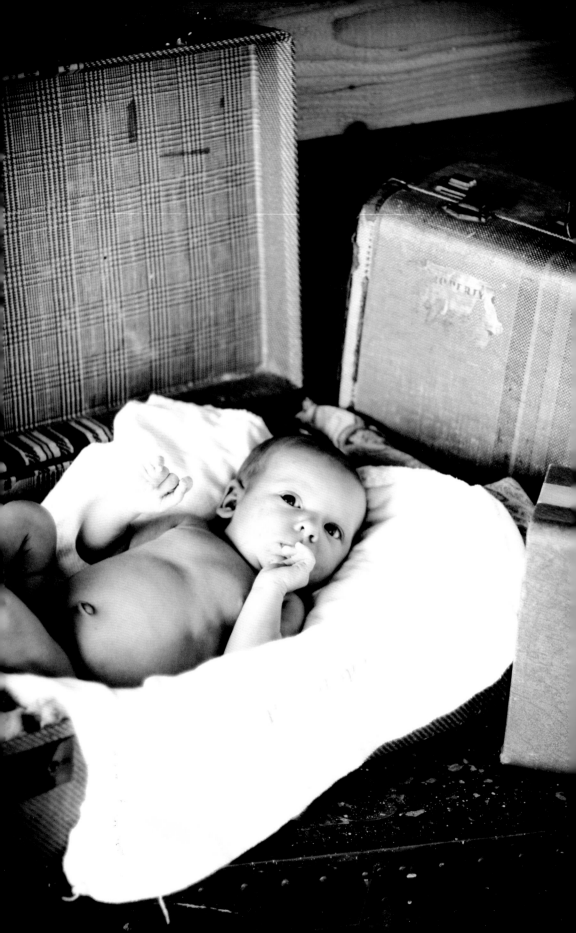

Belly Button Tincture

So Simple and Does a Great Job

½ cup rosemary

⅓ cup calendula

1 cup comfrey

about 2¼ cups rubbing alcohol

Herbs can be fresh or dried.

Prep: 5 min.   Yield: 2 cups

1. Place herbs in a pint canning jar and cover with alcohol, leaving about 1½ inches from top of jar.

2. Screw on lid and let sit for 5 to 7 days.

3. With an old but clean T-shirt, strain off herbs.

4. Pour tincture in a tincture bottle and clearly mark what it is.

5. I put 3 drops on my baby's belly button 3 times a day, until cord fell off.

Caution: Do not rub, move, or pull at cord. Allow it to fall off naturally.

External use only.

For more info, see Making Babies DVD - Vol. 3

Big Portobellos, Stuffed

Melt-in-Your Mouth Goodness, Vitamin C, Iron ...

1 lb. ground turkey

1 onion, chopped

1 pepper, chopped and sautéed

2-4 T. Bragg's Liquid Aminos, to taste

2 garlic cloves, crushed

½ tsp. sea salt

½ tsp. peppercorns, freshly ground

¼ cup parsley, washed and chopped

4 portobello mushrooms, large

⅓ cup olive oil

¼ cup fresh green onion, chopped

8 thin slices red pepper per mushroom

Prep: 10 min.   Cook: about 30 min.   Serves: 4

1. Brown ground turkey in a large frying pan with 2 tablespoons of olive oil on medium-high.

2. Pour cooked turkey in a bowl. Use the same pan to sauté onions in 1 tablespoon of olive oil until golden brown.

3. Pour cooked onions in the bowl with turkey. In same pan, sauté peppers in 1 tablespoon of olive oil until golden brown.

4. Pour peppers in the bowl, and add parsley, Bragg's, garlic, salt, and pepper. Mix.

5. Clean large portobellos. Flip mushrooms upside down and cut out craters of meat and stock from mushrooms.

6. Lay mushrooms upside down on a baking dish, drizzle with olive oil, and fill with meat mixture.

7. Add 1 tablespoon of green onions and 2 thin slices of red pepper on top of each mushroom.

8. Bake at 375° F for 10 to 15 minutes.

9. Garnish with parsley.

10. Serve by itself or on a bed of mashed potatoes (page 149), quinoa, or rice.

For more info, see *Making Babies DVD - Vol. 3*

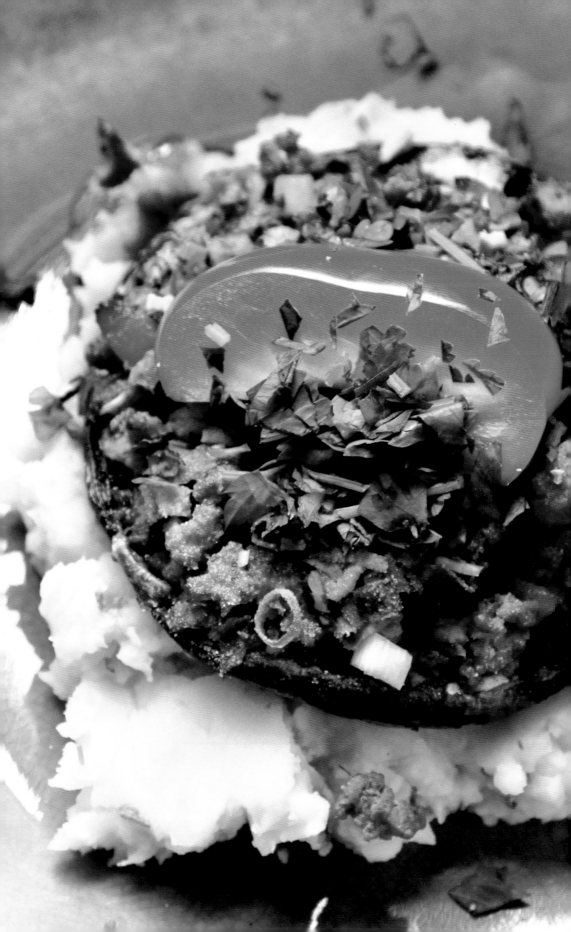

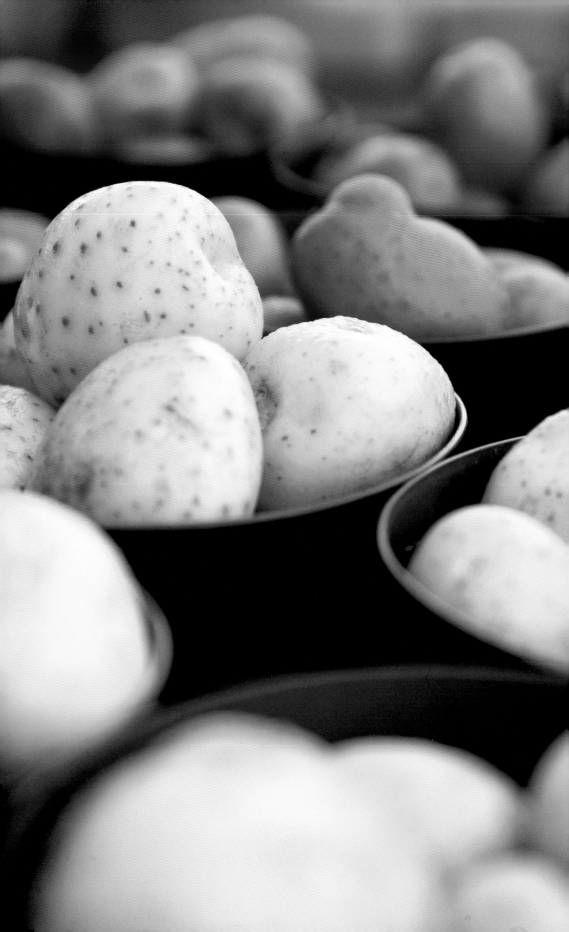

Mashed Potatoes
Creamy With Great Flavor

4 red potatoes, washed and chopped

2 white potatoes, washed and chopped

6-8 cups water, boiling

½ tsp. garlic powder

1 tsp. onion powder

½ tsp. sea salt

½ cup chicken broth

3 T. parsley, chopped

Prep: 10 min.   Cook: 25 min.   Serves: 4-6

1. Place potatoes in a pot with boiling water and cook for 20-25 minutes or until potatoes are soft.

2. Pour water off of potatoes, and put potatoes in a mixer.

3. Add garlic, onion powder, salt, broth and parsley. Mix on low speed for 30 seconds, then on medium speed for one minute. Add more broth if desired to add creaminess.

For more info, see *Making Babies DVD - Vol. 3*

After Birth Cramping Tincture

You Are Going to Be Glad You Made This.

2 T. chamomile flower

1 T. lavender flower

1 T. lemon balm leaf

4 T. cramp bark

3 T. passion flower

Vodka

Herbs can be fresh or dried.

Prep: 5 min. Soak: 6 weeks Yield: about 1½ cups

1. Place all herbs in a pint jar.

2. Cover herbs with alcohol, close it, and store for 2-6 weeks in a dry, cool place, shaking the jar daily.

3. When you are ready to pour your tincture up, strain off herbs with an old but clean T-shirt.

4. Pour tincture in a tincture bottle and clearly label it.

5. To evaporate the alcohol for pregnant or nursing mamas, place your dose in a hot liquid, such as tea or water before taking.

6. I take 2 droppers as needed throughout the day.

You can also make this with glycerin instead of vodka.

For more info, see *Making Babies DVD - Vol. 3*

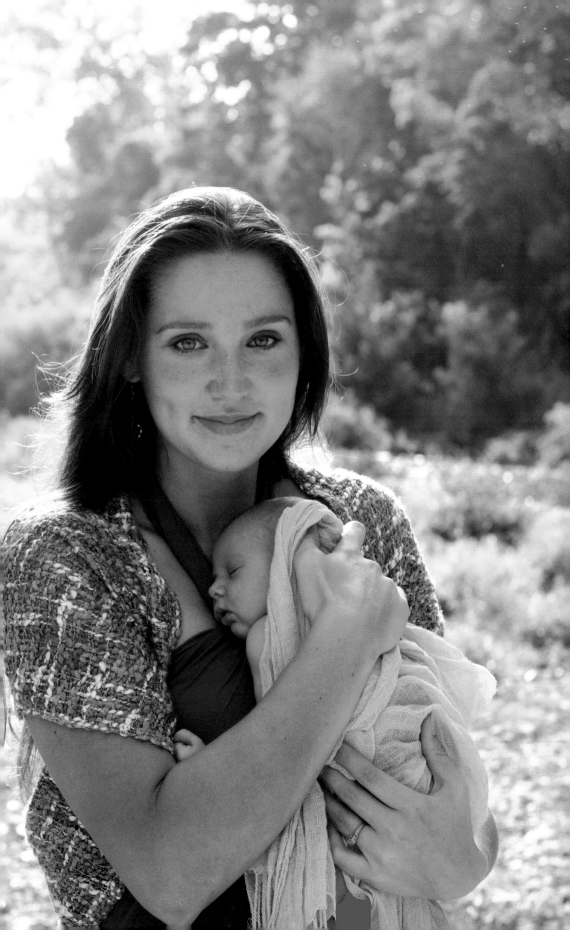

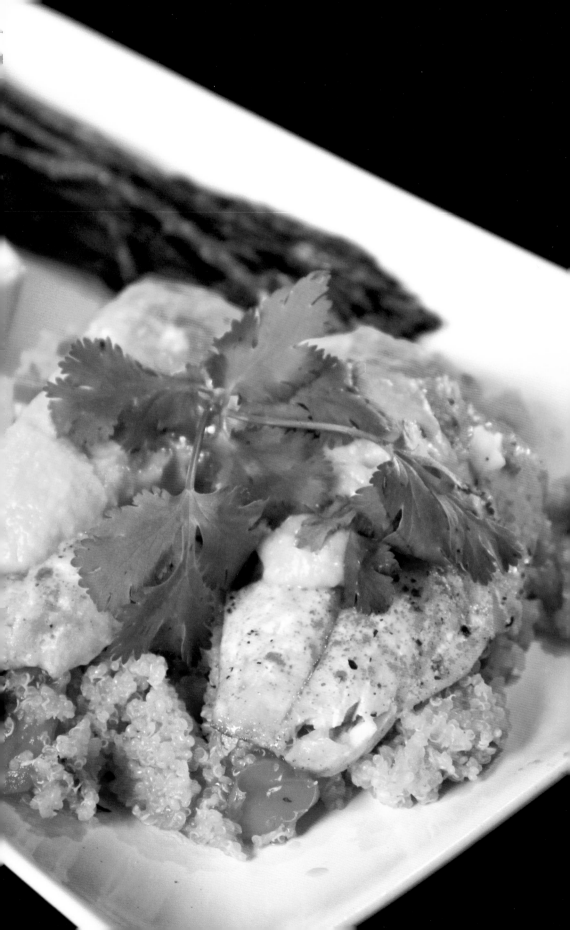

Snapper on a Bed of Quinoa With Hummus on Top

This Is so Good for You and Baby.

Prep: 15 min.   Cook: 25 min.   Serves: 4

Snapper

4 snapper fillets

1 lemon, juiced

½ tsp. peppercorns, freshly ground

½ tsp. sea salt

2 T. butter, softened

1 tsp. onion powder

¼ tsp. paprika

Bed of Quinoa

1 ½ cups quinoa

3 cups water or **Chicken Broth** (page 38)

½ tsp. sea salt

1 T. basil, chopped

1 T. mint, chopped

1 tomato, chopped

½ cup cilantro, chopped

1 tsp. onion powder

Bean Hummus

Can of garbanzo beans, rinsed

½ to ¾ cup **Chicken Broth** (page 38)

2-4 cloves garlic

½ small onion

Sea salt, to taste

Snapper

1. Preheat oven to 450° F.

2. Rub snapper with butter and place in a medium-size, rectangular, oven-proof dish. Drizzle fish with lemon juice.

3. Sprinkle with sea salt, onion powder, pepper, and paprika.

4. Bake for 15 minutes or until fish is flaky.

Quinoa

1. To a saucepan, add broth or water, quinoa, and salt.

2. Cook on medium-low for 20 to 25 minutes.

3. When quinoa is done, let rest for 10 minutes.

4. Mix in the rest of ingredients and you have your bed!

Bean Hummus

1. Add ingredients to blender.

2. Blend, stir, blend, and stir until smooth.

For more info, see *Making Babies DVD* - Vol. 3

Asparagus Made With Broth
I Love to Cook Veggies This Way!

1 bunch asparagus

1 cup **Chicken Broth** (page 38)

Prep: 3 min.   Cook: 5-8 min.   Serves: 4-6

1. Wash asparagus and cut one inch off of cut end.

2. Place ingredients in a large skillet.

3. Cook on medium-high for 5-8 minutes.

Stuffed Tomatoes
Fresh and Full of Flavor and Texture

1 avocado, spooned out

¼ cup green onions

¼ cup cilantro

1 tsp. lemon juice

½ tsp. onion powder

Sea salt, to taste

1 cup bean sprouts

4 to 6 Roma tomatoes (canning tomatoes)

Prep: 10 min.   Serves: 4-6

1. Wash tomatoes and cut them in half. Gut the insides. Pat dry.

2. Wash and chop onions and cilantro. Mix first 6 ingredients together.

3. Add bean sprouts and lightly stir.

4. Stuff tomato halves with avocado mixture.

5. Garnish each tomato half with cilantro and a bean sprout.

For more info, see *Making Babies DVD - Vol. 3*

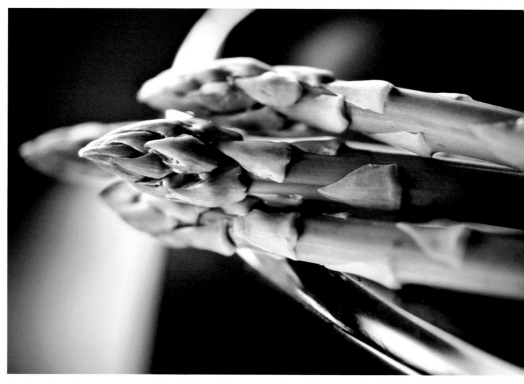

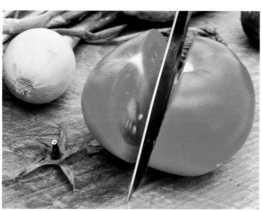

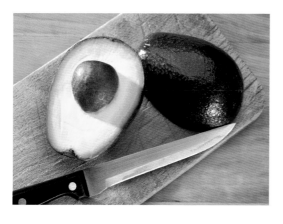

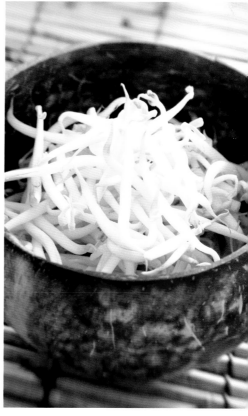

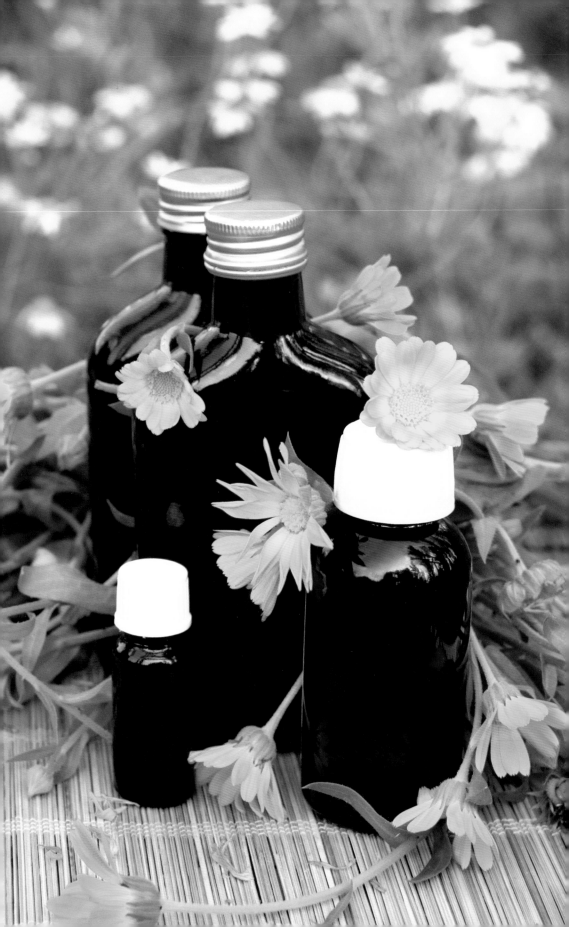

Healing Oil for Circumcision

Great Soothing Herbal Oil

Prep: 5 min.   Cook: 3 days   Yield: 2 cups

2 T. lavender

2 T. calendula

4 T. rosemary

½ cup comfrey

2 cups coconut oil

Herbs can be fresh or dried.

1. Place all herbs in a pint jar.

2. In a small saucepan, heat coconut oil over low heat until just melted.

3. Pour coconut oil over herbs in jar. Cover jar tightly with a lid.

4. Place in a Crock-Pot with a small towel underneath to keep the jar from breaking.

5. Fill the Crock-Pot with water up to the top of the jar (not touching the lid).

6. Set Crock-Pot to lowest setting for 3 days. Add water as necessary.

7. After the 3 days, allow the oil to cool, then use a cheesecloth or T-shirt to strain out herb solids. Store in glass jar.

This can also be made into a great salve. See page 133 for instructions on how to make oil into a salve.

For more info, see *Making Babies DVD - Vol. 3*

Frozen Chocolate Banana

No Need to Go Out; It's Better In!

1 banana

⅛ to ¼ cup **Chocolate Syrup** (page 161)

⅛ cup shredded coconut, unsweetened

⅛ cup pecans

Prep: 2 min.   Cook: 10 min.   Serves: 1

1. Cut a fresh banana in half lengthwise.

2. Freeze bananas in the freezer 2 hours or overnight.

3. Take bananas out and place them in a pretty bowl.

4. Drizzle frozen banana with chocolate syrup.

5. Sprinkle with shredded coconut, and chopped pecans.

6. Enjoy!

Banana Split

Yum, Yum! Should I Say More?

1 banana

¼ cup Purely Decadent chocolate ice cream

3 T. fresh raspberries, crushed

3 T. blackberries, crushed

⅛ cup **Chocolate Syrup** (page 161)

1-2 T. **Granola From Heaven** (page 130)

Prep: 5 min.   Cook: 10 min.   Serves: 1

1. Wash and crush berries.

2. Follow steps 1-3 above.

3. Place spoonfuls of ice cream around banana.

4. On one side of banana, drop spoonfuls of raspberries; on other side, do the same with blackberries.

5. Follow steps 4 and 5 above.

6. Top with granola and enjoy every delicious bite.

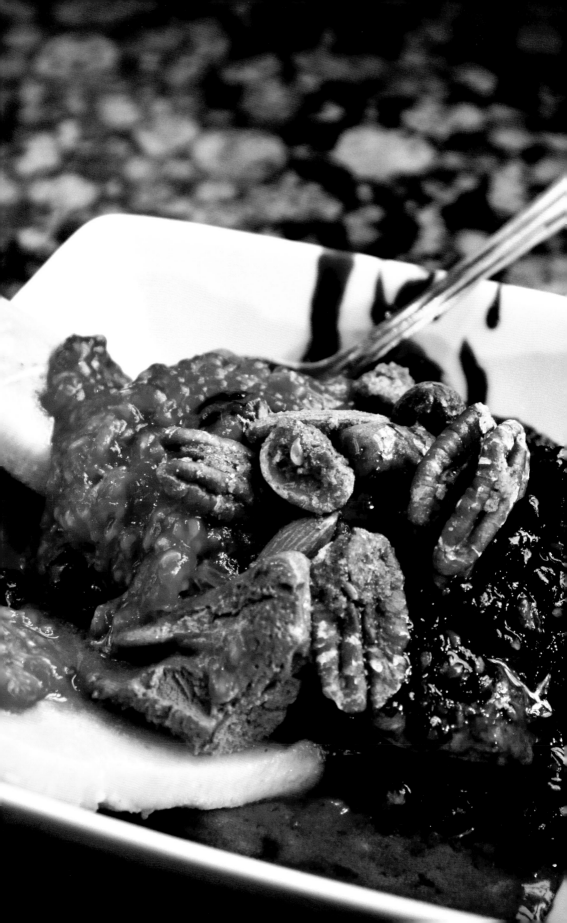

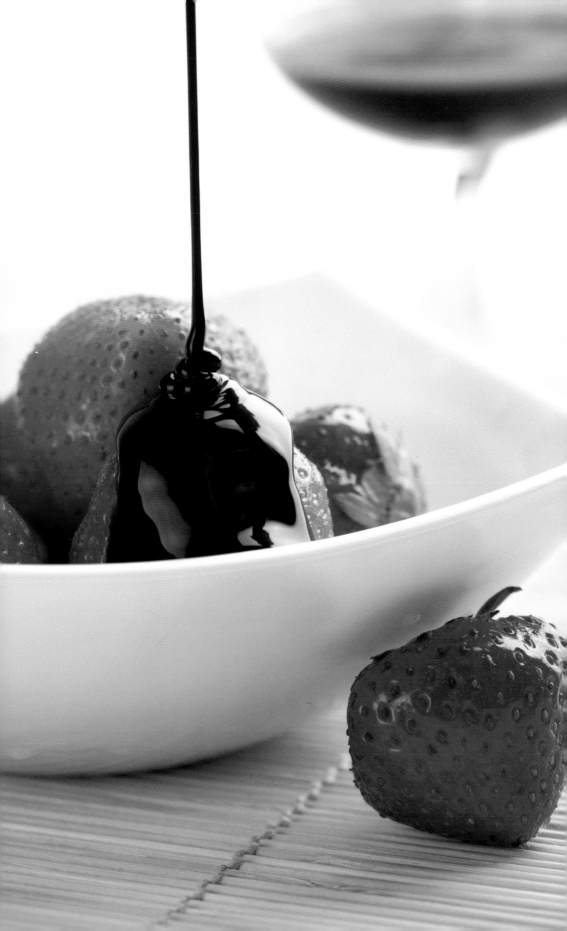

Chocolate Syrup
Gooey, Chewy, Oh-So-Good!

2 T. butter or coconut oil

1 cup raw sugar

⅔ heaping cup cocoa powder

1 T. water

½ tsp. vanilla (*optional*)

Prep: 1 min.   Cook: 10 min.   Serves: 4

1. Melt butter or oil in a small saucepan over medium-low heat.

2. Mix in remaining ingredients, and heat until simmering.

3. Cook 7-10 minutes, stirring off and on.

4. Drizzle over banana splits and ice cream. Enjoy!

For more info, see *Making Babies DVD - Vol. 3*

Baby Calm Tincture

Sleeping Baby, Lullabye, Hush Now, Don't Cry

1¾ cups chamomile
flowers, whole

¾ cup lemon balm, leaf

¾ cup passion flower

½ cup hops (*optional*)

3½ cups glycerin

1 cup water

Herbs can be fresh or dried.

Prep: 5 min.   Cook: 1 day   Yield: 4 cups

1. Put herbs into quart-size glass canning jar. Add water and glycerin. Make sure your tincture mix is at least one inch from top of jar. Screw a lid tightly on and place jar in a Crock-Pot with a small towel underneath to keep the jar from breaking.

2. Fill the Crock-Pot with water up to level of tincture in jar but not over lid. Turn Crock-Pot on lowest setting. Leave it on for 1 day, keeping the glycerin hot, but not boiling. Add more water to Crock-Pot as necessary.

3. After about 24 hours, turn it off and let it cool. Strain the herbal mixture through a cheesecloth into a glass container, squeezing the herbs to release the finished tincture. Throw the used herbs away. Pour tincture in glass tincture bottles, screw lid on, and label the glycerin tincture with date and name. Keep in the cabinet. Tinctures keep for several years.

I use one dropperful for colic or a fussy baby as needed.

For more info, see *Making Babies DVD - Vol. 3*

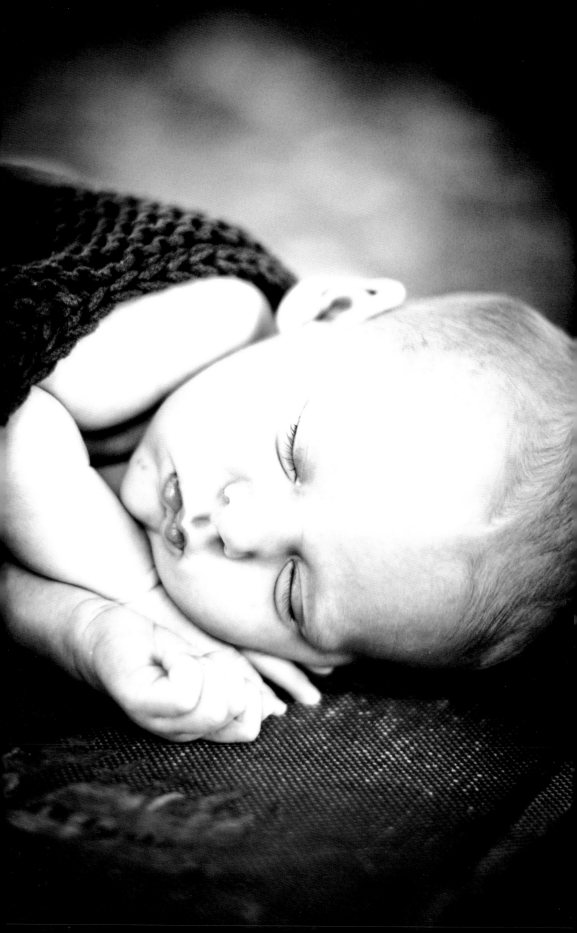

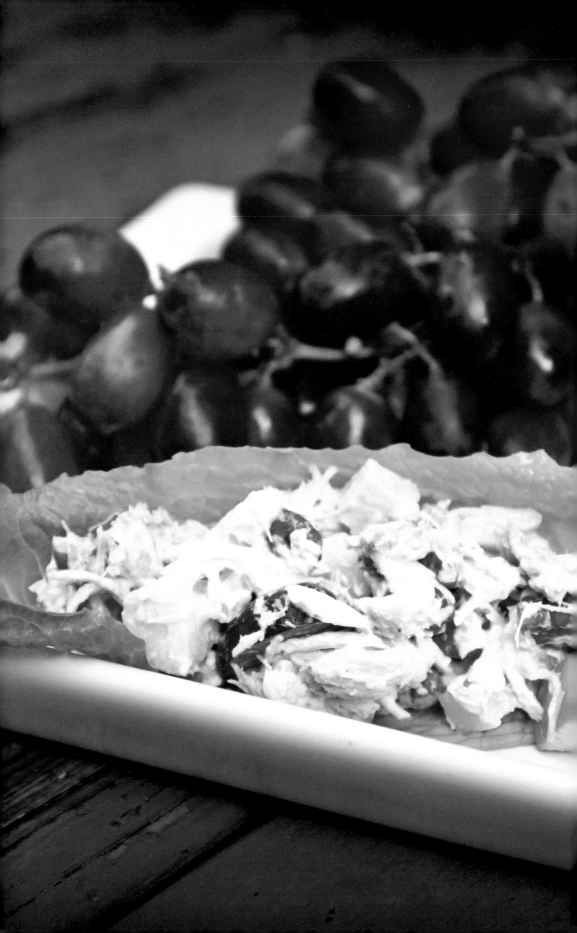

Chicken and Salad Wraps

Lettuce Gives a Nice, Crisp Taste.

2 cups chicken, chopped

3-4 T. Veganaise

¼ cup green apples, chopped

¼ cup toasted pecans, chopped

¼ cup red grapes, halved

⅛ cup Craisins

⅛ cup celery, finely chopped

½ tsp. sea salt

8-12 lettuce leaves, such as romaine, washed

Prep: 10 min.   Yield: 3 cups

1. Wash fresh ingredients, and chop apples, pecans, grapes, and celery.

2. In a bowl, combine all ingredients except for lettuce.

3. Place chicken salad mixture in lettuce leaves, using leaves as wraps.

4. Enjoy the delicious tastes!

For more info, see *Making Babies DVD - Vol. 3*

Potty Training

At age five, ninety percent of the brain is built.

You can start potty training as early as birth. Everything you do with your baby teaches her. When you bring her to the potty and reward her with sweet words of praise, she will quickly learn to potty when you take her. How do you know when your baby needs to go? When she wakes up from her nap or after nursing, just learn to pay attention to her body language. If you see she is needing or starting to go, then take her diaper off and say a special word or sound you reserve for potty time. If she does a job, then praise her! As she learns where to potty, she will start wanting you to take her. She will fuss and cry until you do. She is potty trained!

Ways to take her to the potty:

1. Set her on a little potty chair.

2. Hold her over a bowl or toilet, your hands holding her thighs, giving her a squat/sitting position.

For more info, see Making Babies DVD - Vol. 3

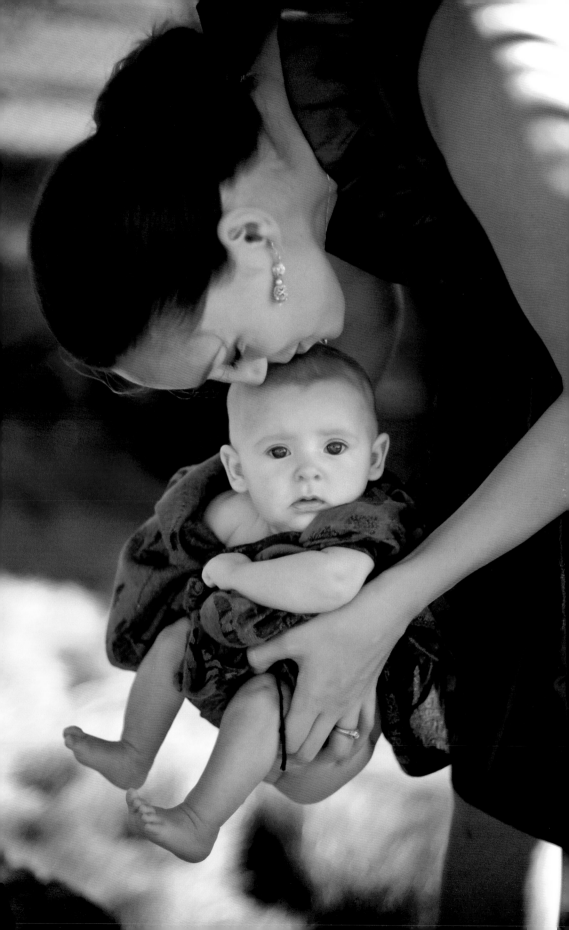

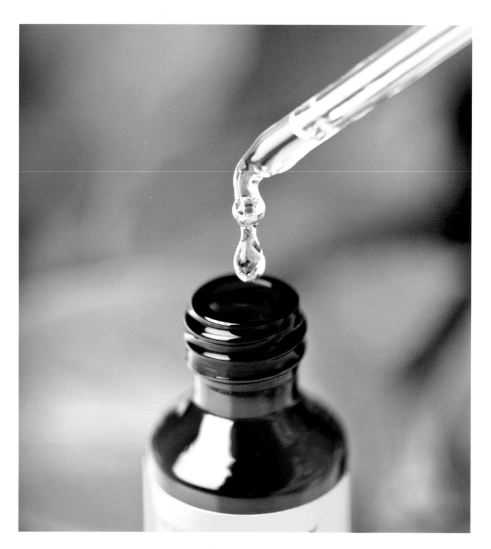

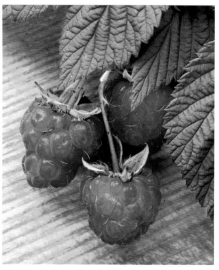

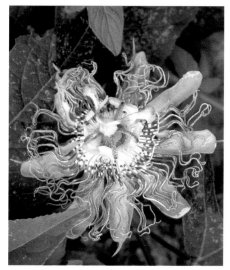

Healing Tincture
Nutritious and Healing

4 T. chasteberry

2 T. oatstraw

2 T. dandelion root

4 T. raspberry leaf

1 T. alfalfa

2 T. passion flower

2 T. nettle leaf

Glycerine

Water

Herbs can be fresh or dried.

Prep: 5 min.   Cook: 3 days   Yield: about 1½ cups

1. Place herbs in a pint canning jar.

2. Fill jar with 40% hot water and 60% glycerin, not including the top 1-2 inches of jar.

3. Close jar lid tightly and place it in a Crock-Pot with a small towel underneath to keep the jar from breaking.

4. Fill the Crock-Pot with water up to the top of the jar (not touching the lid), and turn it on the warm setting for 3 days, keeping the glycerin hot, but not boiling, and adding water as necessary.

5. Strain out herb solids and place the liquid in a tincture bottle.

6. I like to take one dropper twice a day for 3 weeks after birth

Warning: If your Crock-Pot gets too hot and water has boiled down, turn it off and do not touch until cool. Never pour water over a hot glass jar. It can explode.

For more info, see Making Babies DVD - Vol. 3

How to Make Baby Food
Don't Buy It! You Can Make It Better!

1 sweet potato, cooked

½ cup blueberries, heated

2 T. beet powder

¼ to ½ cup **Chicken Broth** (page 38) or **Vegetable Broth** (page 320)

pinch sea salt

Other Ideas

Pumpkin

Squash

Onions

Cabbage

Green beans

Broccoli

Mango

Coconut water

Coconut oil

Apples

Flax

Arrowroot

Prep: 5 min.   Cook: about 20 min.   Yield: 2-3 cups

1. In a small saucepan, boil canning jar lids in water. Meanwhile, thoroughly clean glass canning jars with hot soapy water and rinse well.

2. Fill jars with baby food (veggies or fruit), leaving food one inch from top of jar.

3. With a clean, hot, damp rag, wipe down jar top. Pat dry canning lids and place on jar. Screw rings on tightly.

4. Place a small towel in bottom of pan and place jars on it.

5. Fill water up to one inch from top of jar. Cook until it starts to simmer, then cook 10 minutes more.

6. Take out hot jars with jar tongs carefully and place on a towel on counter. Don't touch or move until completely cooled, about 12-24 hours.

7. To see if jars sealed successfully, press the middle of the lid with a finger or thumb. If the lid does not spring up when you release your finger, the lid is sealed.

Tip From Shoshanna:

Keep in fridge for 1-2 weeks.

Try to nurse for at least 12-15 months. You can start adding foods to your baby's diet at 6 months.

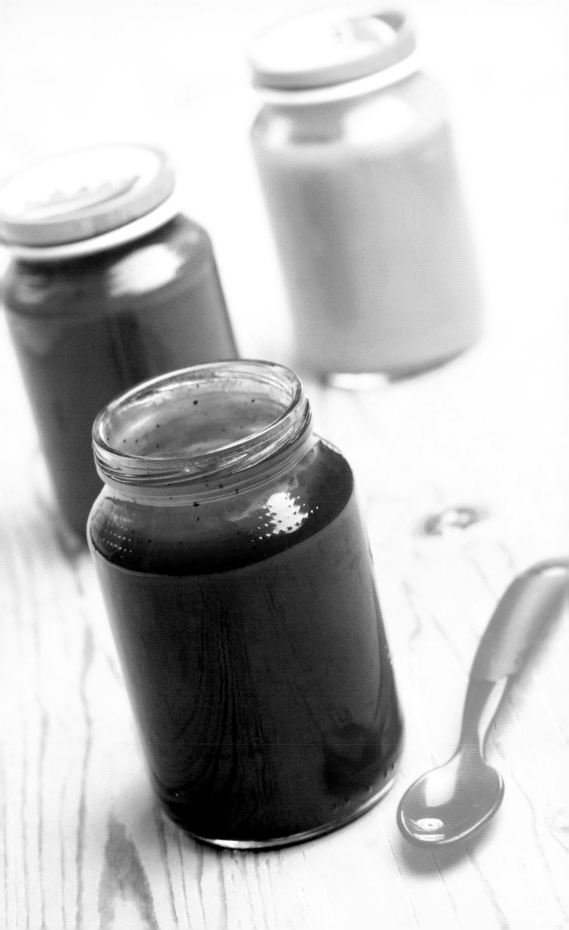

Meat Loaf Patties

Lean and Mean

⅛ tsp. sage

½ tsp. garlic, crushed

⅛ tsp. thyme

1 tsp. salt

1 egg

1 lb. ground turkey

2 T. olive oil or butter

4 T. gluten-free bread crumbs (*optional*)

Prep: 5 min.   Cook: 10 min.   Yield: 4-6

1. Mix first six ingredients and make into palm-size patties.

2. Cook on medium-low in olive oil for 3-5 minutes on each side or until done.

3. Great on a plate or on a bun!

Green Beans

Simple and Green. Yum!

About 4 cups green beans, fresh or frozen

¼ cup water

½ tsp. sea salt

2 T. butter

Prep: 2 min.   Cook: 8 min.   Serves: 4-6

1. In a pan combine all ingredients.

2. Cook on medium-high for 5-8 minutes, or until desired tenderness.

Sweet Potatoes

Simple, Sweet, and Awesome!

4 cups sweet potatoes, chopped into one-inch squares

2 cups water

¾ tsp. sea salt

4 T. butter

Prep: 7 min.   Cook: 15 min.   Serves: 4-6

1. Place potatoes and water in a saucepan.

2. Cook on stove top for 10 to 15 minutes or until tender.

3. Sprinkle with sea salt and add butter.

4. Enjoy!!

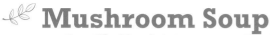

Mushroom Soup
So Full of Vitamin C. Delicious!

1 large onion, peeled and chopped

1 lb. portobello mushrooms

¼ cup olive oil

3 cups **Chicken Broth** (page 38)

Sea salt

Shiitaki mushrooms, cleaned and trimmed

Prep: 7 min.   Cook: 30 min.   Serves: 6-8

1. Clean all mushrooms, trim ends, and chop.

2. In a large frying pan with ⅛ cup oil, sauté onion on medium-high about 10 minutes until golden brown.

3. Pour onions in a blender. Sauté portobello mushrooms with ⅛ cup oil for about 5-8 minutes.

4. Puree onions and portobello mushrooms.

5. Pour mixture in a pot and add broth, salt, and cleaned, trimmed shiitaki mushrooms.

6. Cook 10 minutes and serve. Yumm!!

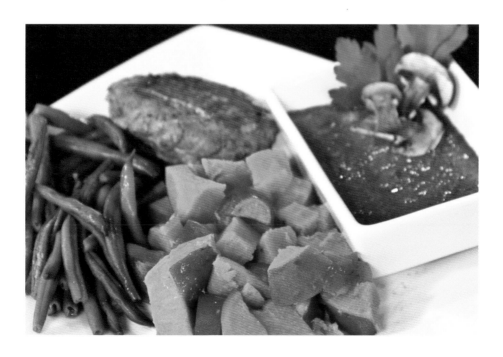

Pregnancy
TIPS

Baby Wrap

Snug as a bug in a rug!

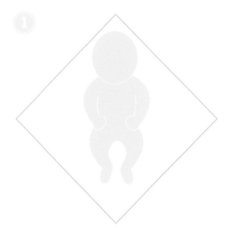

Lay baby on back in upper center.

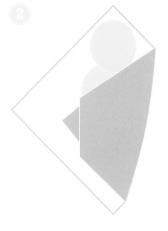

Wrap one edge of blanket around baby and tuck underneath.

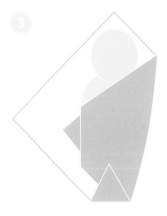

Fold bottom of blanket over baby's feet.

Wrap other edge around baby and tuck.

Rash-Free

½ cup aloe vera juice, organic

1 cup witch hazel, organic

½ cup spring water,

1 T. vitamin E oil

Herbs can be fresh or dried.

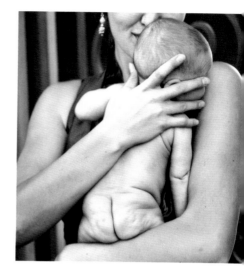

1. Mix all ingredients together and pour into a spray bottle. If needed, spray on baby's bottom and wipe with an organic cotton cloth.

Read more about aloe on page 381.

Cracks

With a new baby, a lot of times we forget to wash and dry between all the cracks. Don't overdo it with lots of soap and scrubbing. Just give a simple wash and pat dry. A little *Baby Powder* (page 120) in the clean, dry cracks can keep your baby from developing any rashes.

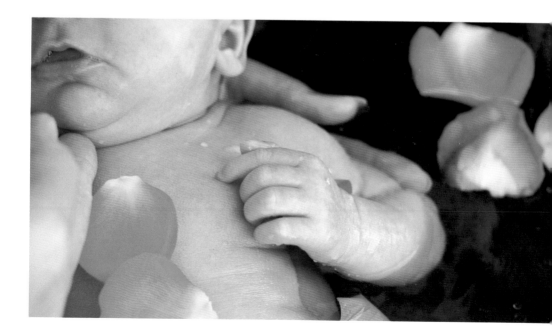

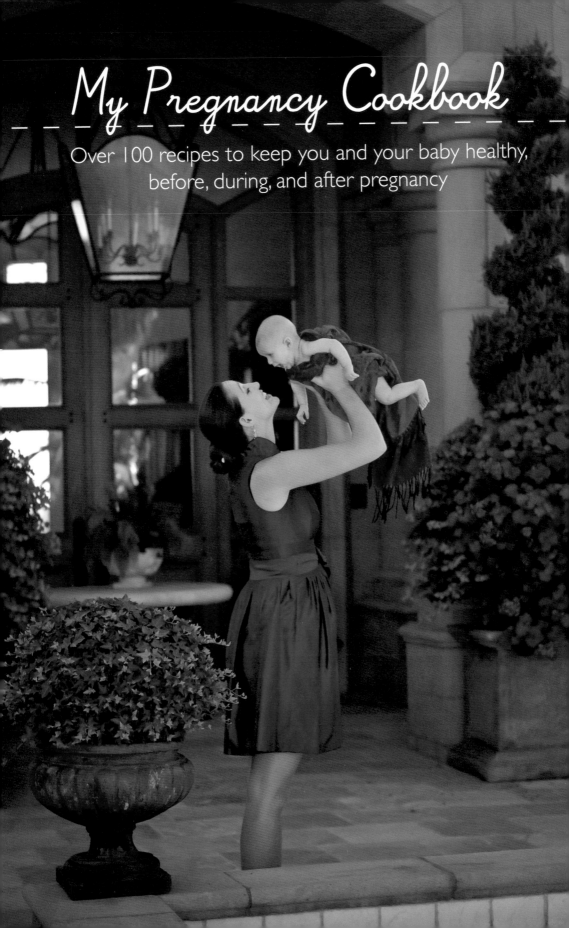

My Pregnancy Cookbook

Over 100 recipes to keep you and your baby healthy,
before, during, and after pregnancy

Beverages

Making Babies is in everything you drink. Stay hydrated with drinks that quench your thirst and build your baby. Here are some awesomely refreshing, ice-cold drinks that not only taste amazing but make you feel amazing too!

🌿 = Gluten-Free/Low-Casein or Casein-Free Recipe*

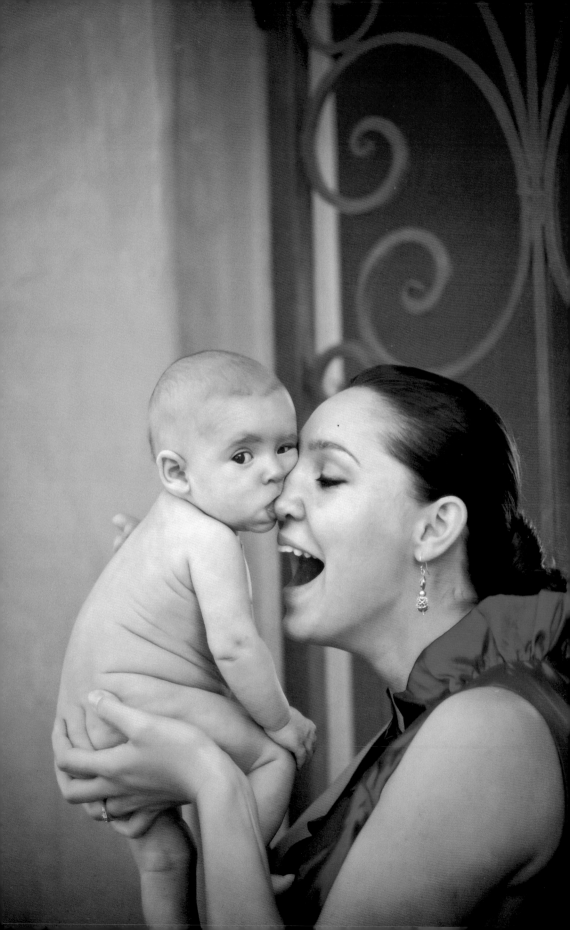

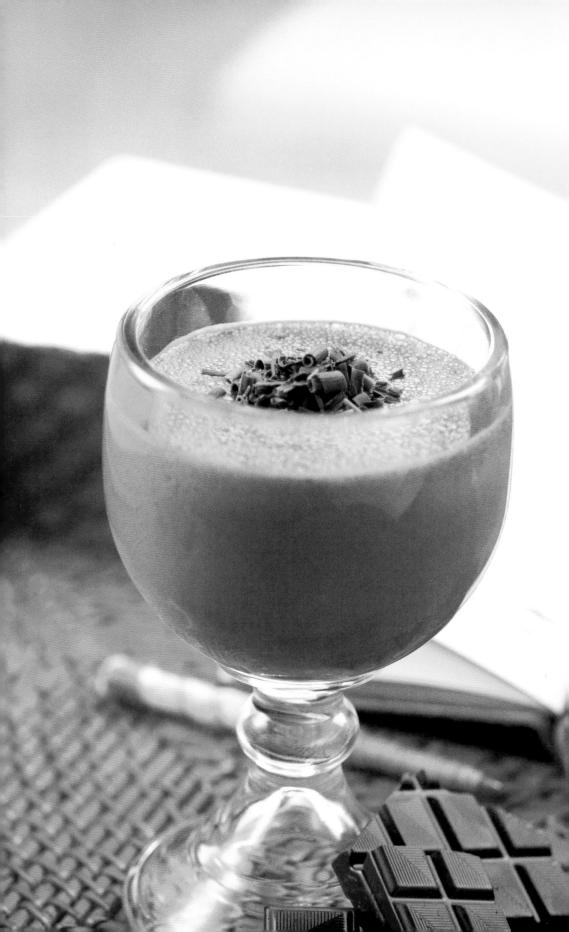

Chocolate Milk

Yum-yum, you gotta have some!

2 cups Purely Decadent Coconut Milk or almond milk

3 T. cocoa powder

4 T. maple syrup

pinch sea salt

dash vanilla

¾ cup Purely Decadent Coconut Vanilla Bean Ice Cream

1 banana, *optional*

2 tsp. New Zealand Colostrum

Prep: 5 min.   Serves: 2

1. Blend all ingredients in a blender until smooth. Yum!

Tip From Shoshanna:

New Zealand Colostrum is bovine colostrum from New Zealand. It is the best colostrum on the market. It gives great support to your immune system and gut.

Beverages

Herban Virgin Mojito

This Is Truly a Spectacular Drink.

2 limes

¼ cup basil

½ cup mint

2 cups sparkling water

¼ to ½ cup honey or maple syrup

Ice

Garnish

Prep: 5 min. Serves: 2

1. Wash limes. Cut one into quarters and one in half. Juice the halved lime.

2. Blend the lime juice, remaining lime, and remaining ingredients on high speed for one minute.

3. Strain drink from pulp, add ice, and garnish. Enjoy!

Tip From Shoshanna:

Basil, an aromatic herb belonging to the mint family, contains many antiviral substances. In traditional Indian medicine, it is used as a remedy for relieving cramps, headaches, fevers, colds, anxiety, indigestion, nausea, and more. Basil, mint, parsley, cilantro, rosemary, and all the kitchen herbs we use are so full of vitamins and nutrients and high in antioxidants and blood purifying properties. I love using lots of fresh herbs in my food!

Beverages

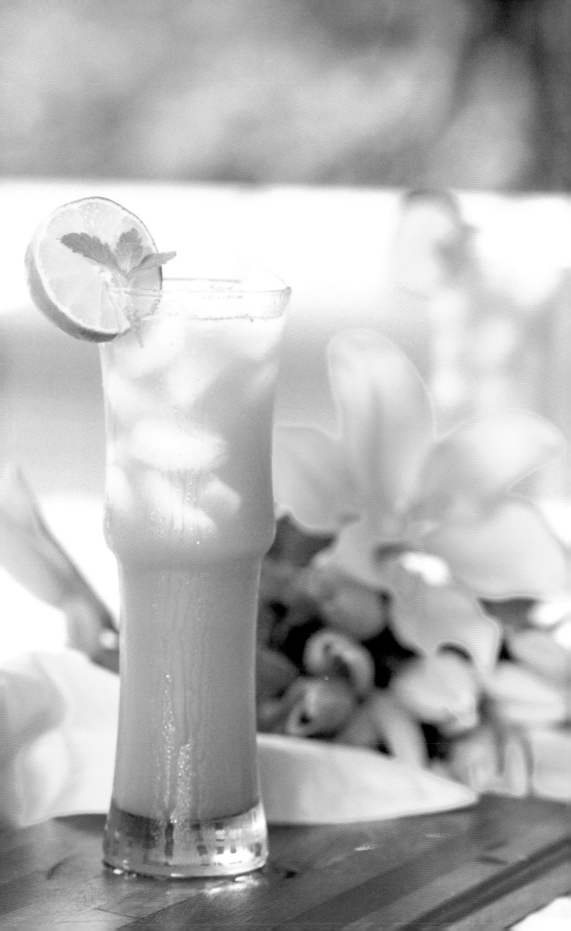

Healthy Soda
Toast to Healthy Delights

Lime Soda

2 cups sparkling water

1 lime, juiced

1 T. honey

2 cups ice

Prep: 3 min.   Serves: 2

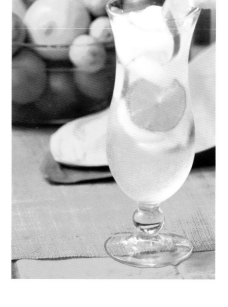

1. Blend lime juice and honey.

2. Add sparkling water and ice.

3. Garnish with lime wedge. Enjoy!

   To make a frozen beverage, blend all ingredients.

Cherry Soda

¼ cup cherry concentrate

1½ cups sparkling water

1 cup ice

Prep: 3 min.   Serves: 2

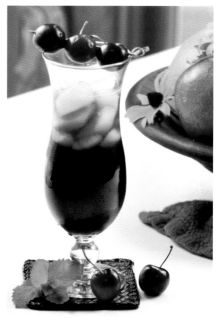

1. Mix cherry concentrate and sparkling water.

2. Pour over ice.

3. Garnish with cherry and enjoy.

   To make a frozen beverage, blend all ingredients.

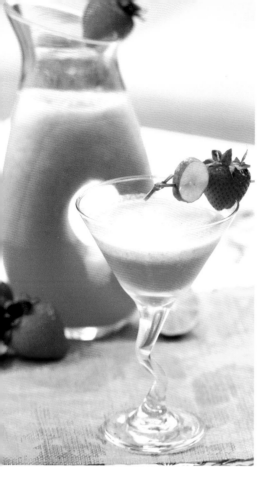

Strawberry-Lime Soda

5 large strawberries, fresh
or frozen

1 lime, juiced

1 cup sparkling water

2 T. honey

Pinch of salt

¼ tsp. vanilla

1 cup ice

Prep: 3 min.   Serves: 2

1. Blend ingredients.

2. Garnish with a strawberry and
lime curl and enjoy.

Blue-Cherry Soda

⅛ cup blueberry
concentrate

1½ cups sparkling water

⅛ cup cherry
concentrate

1 cup ice

Prep: 3 min.   Serves: 2

1. Mix liquids and pour over ice.

2. Garnish with fruit stick and
enjoy.

*To make a frozen beverage, blend
all ingredients.*

Smoothie Boost
Drink to Immune-Boosting Energy!

½ banana, frozen

5 large strawberries, frozen

8 oz. orange juice

2 tsp. New Zealand Colostrum (See tip on page 181.)

Pinch sea salt (*optional*)

⅛ tsp. vanilla (*optional*)

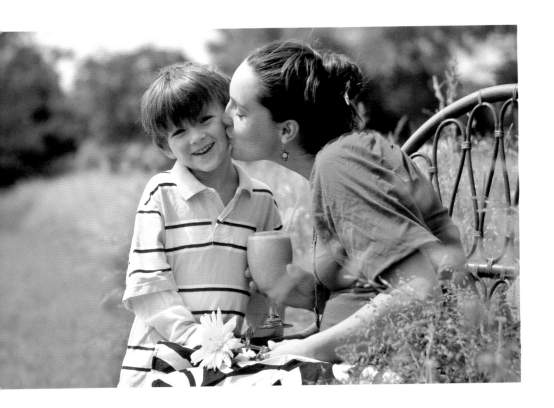

Simply blend all ingredients in a blender until smooth and enjoy every sip!

Beverages

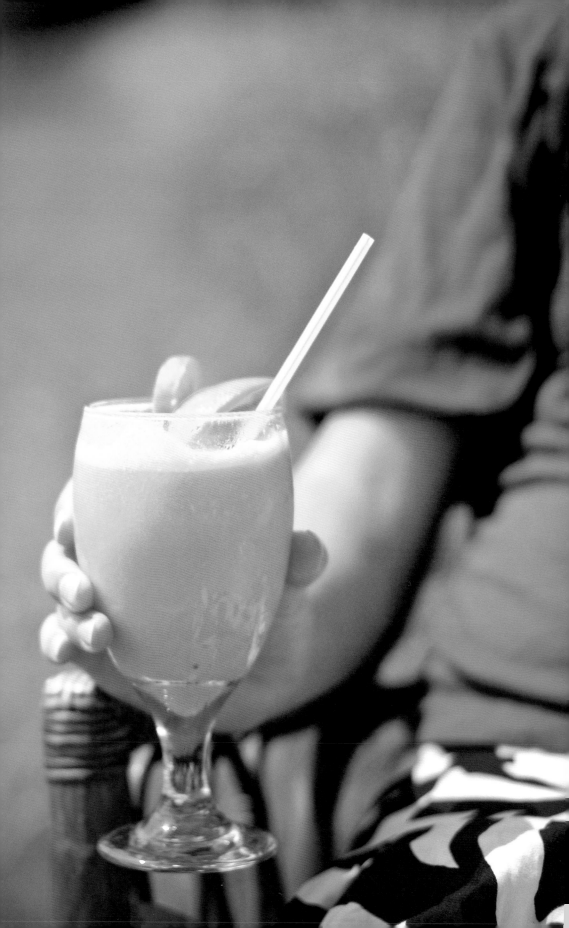

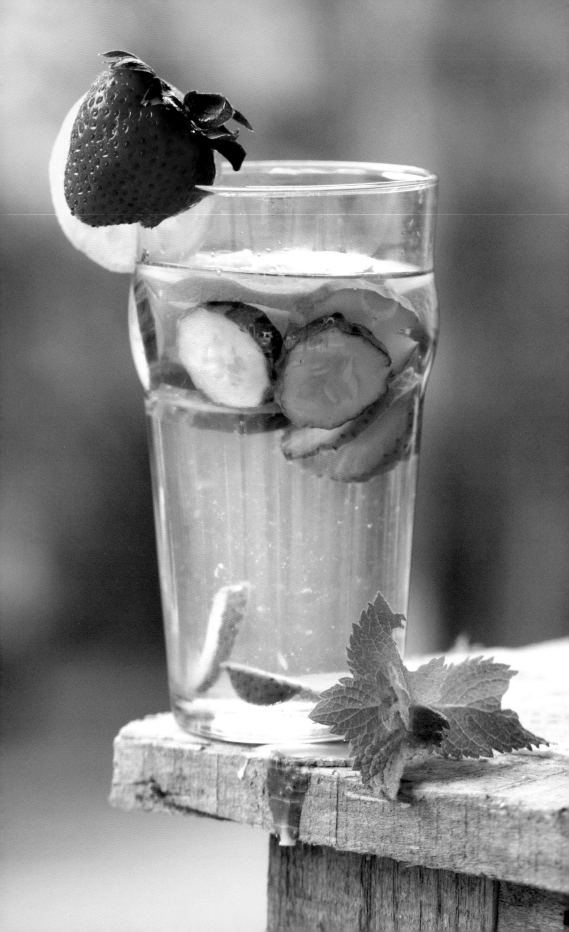

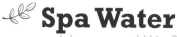

Spa Water
Hydrate With Beauty and Taste

1 cucumber, sliced

5 strawberries, sliced

2 lemons, sliced

2 quarts water

Prep: 5 min.   Serves: 4

1. Fill a glass pitcher with ice-cold water.

2. Layer sliced cucumbers, strawberries, and lemon in water.

3. Chill in fridge for about 1 hour and serve. *Keep refilling water all day.*

Variations

* **Fresh Cucumber Spa Water:** Omit strawberries and lemons.
* **Tropical Spa Water:** Omit strawberries. Add oranges and limes.

Beverages

Breads

Making Babies with baked goods never tasted so fine. Made with nutritious ingredients, these recipes are "corner shop bakery" quality and full of protein and fiber to build a healthy mama and baby.

🌿 = Gluten-Free/Low-Casein or Casein-Free Recipe*

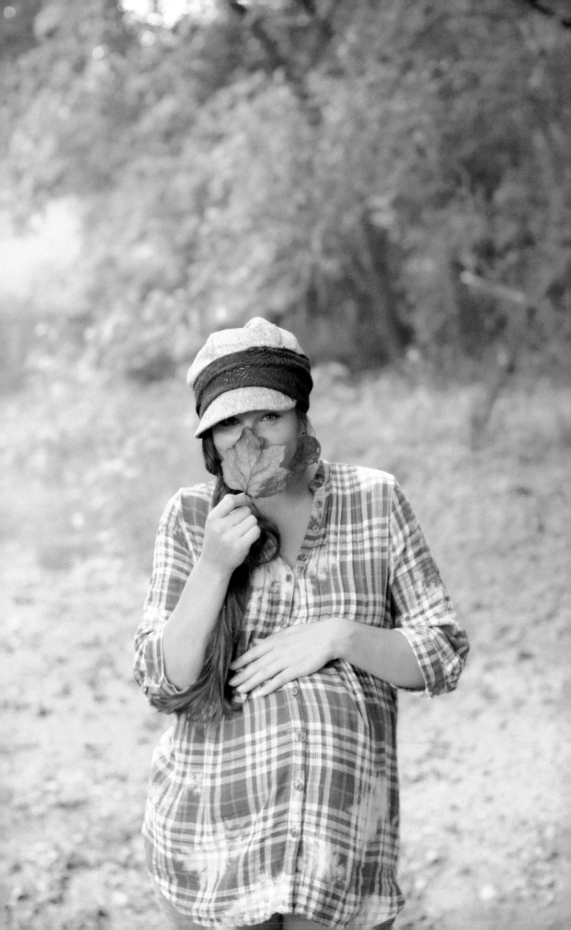

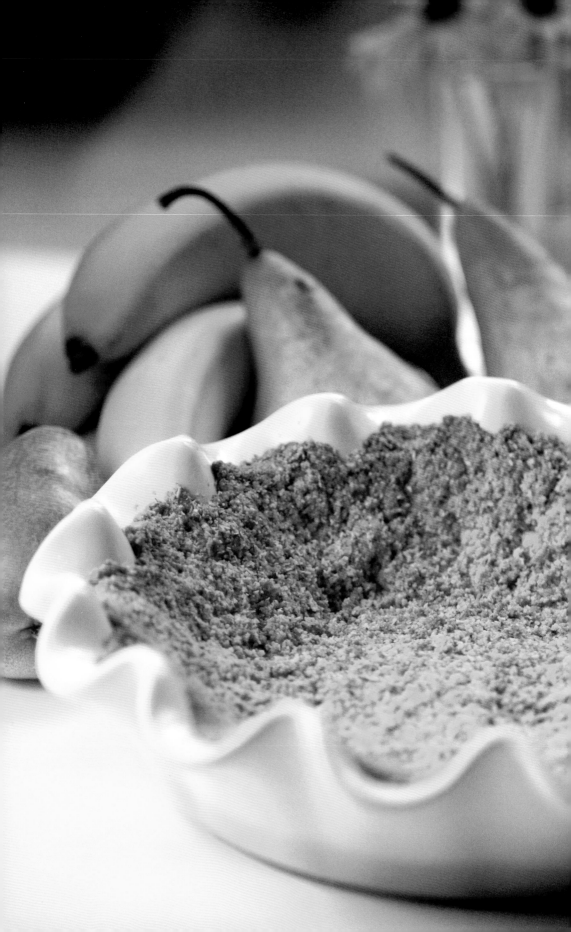

Almond Pie Crust
Almost Too Good to Be True

1½ cups blanched almond flour

¼ cup arrowroot powder

¼ tsp. sea salt

¼ tsp. baking soda

¼ cup grapeseed oil

2 T. honey or maple syrup

1 tsp. vanilla extract

Prep: 8 min. Cook: 15 min. Yield: 1-9½ inch crust

1. Preheat the oven to 350° F.

2. In a large mixing bowl, combine the almond flour, arrowroot, salt, and baking soda. In a medium bowl, whisk together the grapeseed oil, maple syrup, and vanilla extract.

3. Stir the wet ingredients into the almond flour mixture until combined.

4. Press the dough into a 9½-inch pan or deep-dish pie pan.

5. Bake for 10 to 15 minutes, until golden brown. Remove from oven and let cool completely before filling.

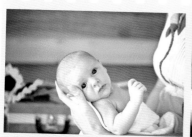
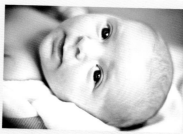
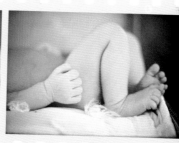

Breads

Banana Nut Muffins
Mouth-Watering, Melt-in-Your-Mouth Muffins

¾ cup coconut oil

1⅓ cups Sucanat

4 eggs

1 tsp. sea salt

1⅔ cups almond meal

⅔ cup brown rice flour

1 tsp. xanthan gum

1 T. cinnamon

1 tsp. baking soda

1 T. baking powder

2 T. arrowroot powder

1½ cups bananas (3 bananas), ripe and chopped. *(Substitute with zucchini, chocolate, apples, strawberries, blueberries, or carrots.)*

⅔ cup pecans

1 tsp. vanilla

⅔ cup chocolate morsels, *(optional)*

additional ⅔ cup pecans, *(optional)*

Prep: 10 min.   Cook: 25 min.   Serves: 20

1. Preheat oven to 350° F. Line muffin tin with paper cups.

2. Blend oil and Sucanat together. Beat in eggs one at a time on medium to high speed for one minute.

3. In another bowl mix salt, flours, xanthan gum, cinnamon, baking powder, baking soda, and arrowroot. Slowly add to sugar mixture.

4. Add vanilla, pecans, and banana and mix for one minute.

5. Pour into lined muffin tin. If desired, sprinkle chocolate morsels and additional pecans on top. Bake at 350° F for 25 minutes or until a toothpick comes out clean.

Breads

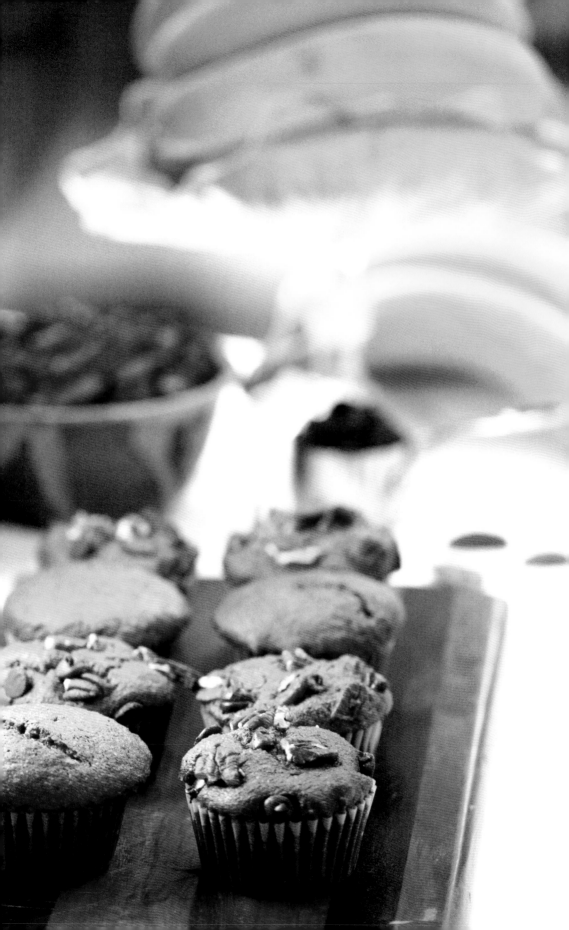

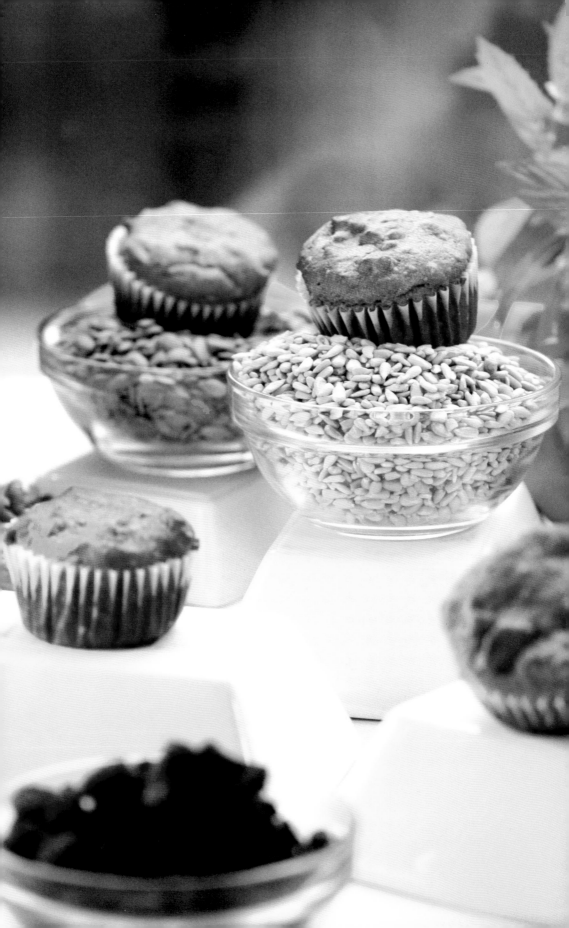

Breakfast Bran Muffins
Delicious, but I Gotta Go ...

A muffin could never be more nutritious for your body. It is packed with health in the form of nuts, seeds, and dried fruits. Skip the no-nutrition, preservative-packaged, breakfast and granola bars, and replace them with these muffins. It's cost-effective, yet delicious.

½ cup blanched almond flour

½ cup flax meal

1 tsp. sea salt

1 T. cinnamon

2 tsp. baking soda

15 Medjool dates, pitted and chopped

8 large eggs

¼ cup olive oil, grapeseed oil, or coconut oil

1 cup almond butter

1½ cups coconut milk

1½ tsp. vanilla

¼ cup water

½ cup pumpkin seeds

½ cup sesame seeds

½ cup sunflower seeds

1 cup pecans or walnuts, chopped

1 cup currants or raisins

Prep: 15 min. Cook: 20 min. Yield: 24 muffins

1. Preheat the oven to 350° F. Line 12 muffin cups with paper liners.

2. In a large bowl, combine the almond flour, flax meal, salt, cinnamon, and baking soda.

3. In a high-powered blender, puree the dates, eggs, olive oil, almond butter, coconut milk, vanilla, and water on high speed until completely smooth.

4. Stir the wet ingredients into the almond flour mixture until blended, then stir in the seeds, walnuts, and currants.

5. Scoop ¼ cup of batter into each prepared muffin cup. Bake for 15 to 20 minutes, until a toothpick inserted into the center of a muffin comes out with just a few moist crumbs attached.

6. Let the muffins cool slightly in the pan for 20 minutes, then serve warm.

Breads

Dinner Pie Crust
Flaky Bites of Yumminess!

Would you ever guess that a chicken pot pie or quiche could be made gluten- and dairy-free? This recipe with almond flour makes it possible.

1½ cups blanched almond flour

½ tsp. sea salt

½ tsp. baking soda

1 T. green onion, minced

½ cup grapeseed oil

1 T. water

Prep: 8 min. Cook: 15 min. Yield: 1-9½ inch crust

1. Preheat the oven to 350° F.

2. In a large mixing bowl, combine almond flour, sea salt, baking soda, and scallions.

3. In a medium mixing bowl whisk the grapeseed oil and water together.

4. Now mix the liquid ingredients into the almond flour mix until completely combined.

5. Press dough into 9½-inch pan or deep-dish pie pan.

6. Bake for 12 to 15 minutes or until golden brown. Remove from oven and allow to cool completely.

Breads

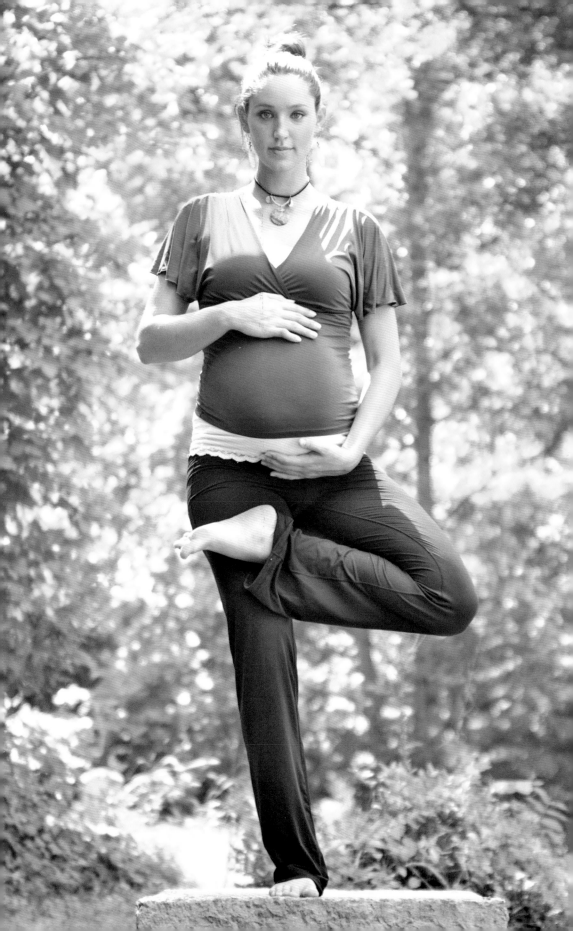

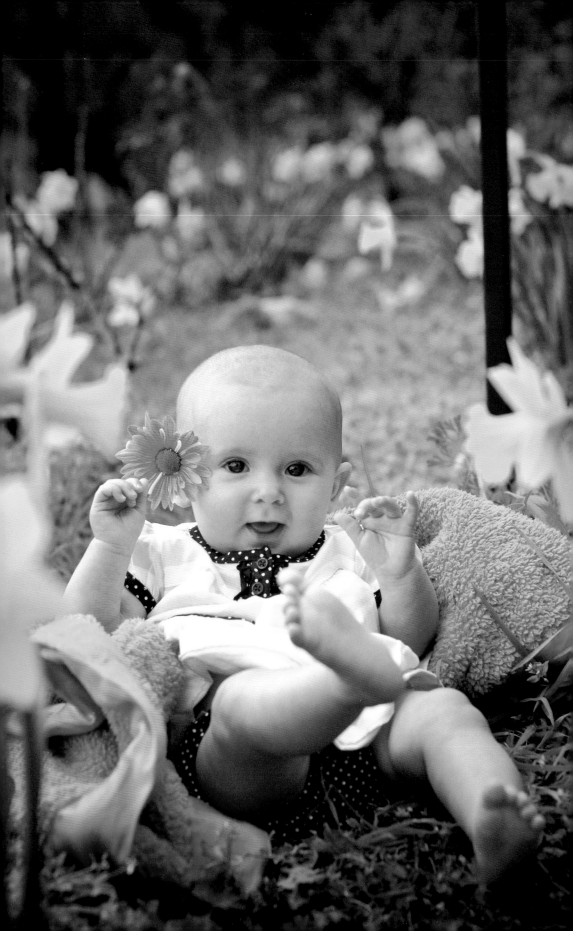

Gluten-Free Flour Mix

Great for the Whole Family!

5 cups brown rice flour

3 cups sorghum flour

2 ⅔ cups arrowroot powder

1 cup potato starch

⅓ cup potato flour or tapioca flour

2 T. xanthan gum

Prep: 5 min.   Yield: 12 cups

1. Mix all ingredients.

2. Store flour mix in the refrigerator in an airtight container.

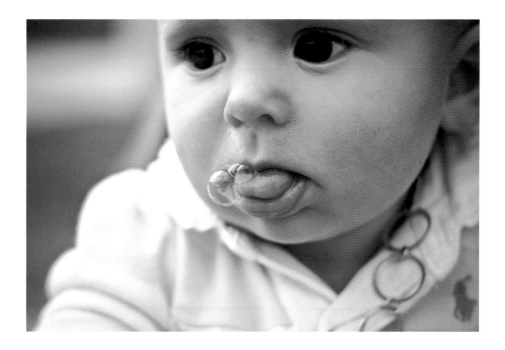

Breads

Scrumptious Sandwich Bread

Protein Packed, Keeping You Going All Day Long

You don't have to say goodbye to sandwich bread when going gluten-free, and definitely not with this sandwich bread recipe. This uncomplicated recipe requires no rising time, no yeasts, and no kneading. This bread will work great for making sandwiches, french toast, and more. It keeps for up to 6 days.

1 cup creamy, roasted almond butter, at room temperature

5 large eggs

½ cup blanched almond flour

½ cup arrowroot powder

¾ tsp. sea salt

1 tsp. baking soda

1 T. flax meal

¼ cup water

Prep: 10 min.   Cook: 45 min.   Yield: 1 Loaf (About 12 slices)

1. Preheat your oven to 350° F. Grease a 9x4-inch loaf pan with grapeseed oil and dust with almond flour.

2. In a large mixing bowl, mix the almond butter with a handheld mixer until smooth; then blend in the eggs.

3. In a medium mixing bowl, mix all the dry ingredients together.

4. Alternately mix dry ingredients and water into egg mixture and blend until thoroughly combined.

5. Pour the batter into the loaf pan.

6. Bake for 40 to 45 minutes on the bottom rack of the oven, or until a knife inserted into the center of the loaf comes out clean.

7. Let the bread cool in the pan for 1 hour, then serve.

Breads

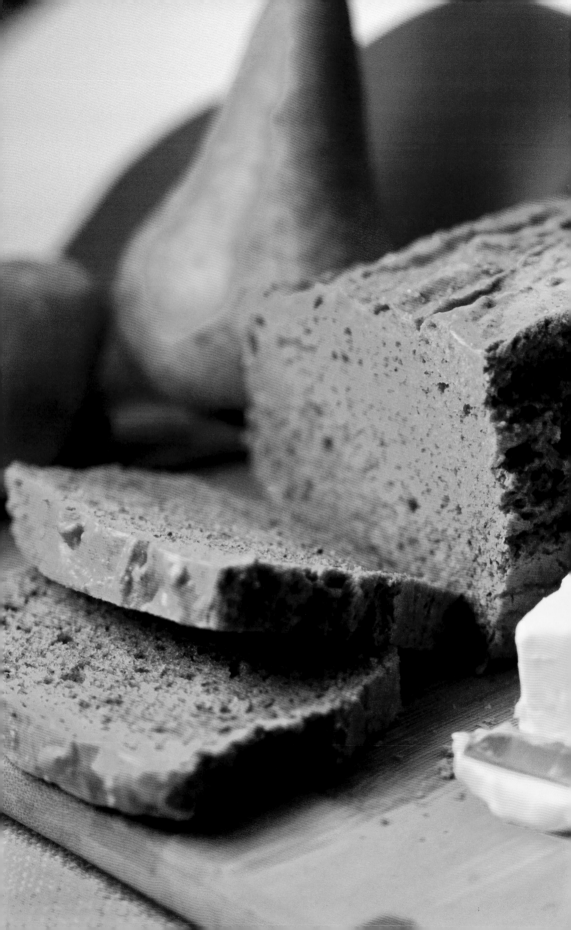

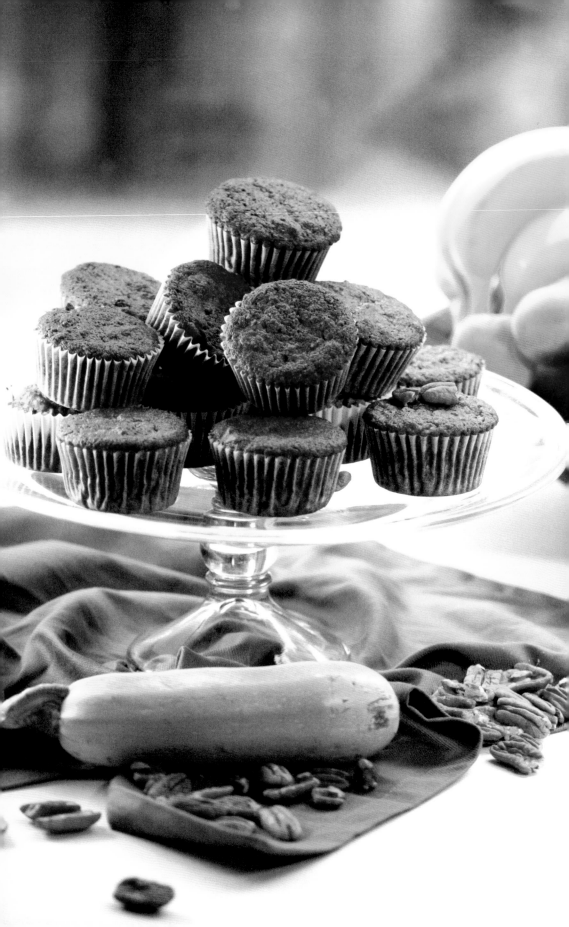

Zucchini Muffins
Soft and Moist Bites of Goodness

1 cup almond flour

1 tsp. ground cinnamon

1 cup Sucanat

½ tsp. allspice

1½ cups **Gluten Free Flour Mix** (page 201)

1 T. baking powder

1 tsp. baking soda

¼ tsp. xanthan gum

1 tsp. salt

5 large eggs

½ cup raw honey or maple syrup

2 cups zucchini, grated

½ cup walnuts or pecans, chopped

¾ cup butter, set out for one hour

Prep: 8 min.   Cook: 25 min.   Yield: 24 muffins

1. Preheat the oven to 350° F. Line 24 muffin cups with paper liners.

2. In a large mixing bowl, combine first 9 ingredients.

3. In a large mixing bowl, combine butter, Sucanat, and honey or maple syrup. Mix on medium-high until light and fluffy or about 3 minutes.

4. Add eggs, one at a time, mixing for 30 seconds before adding another.

5. Add dry ingredients and mix for one minute.

6. Stir in zucchini and nuts. Using a ⅓ measuring cup, scoop batter into lined muffin cups. Bake 20-25 minutes or until a toothpick inserted into the center of the muffin comes out with just a few moist crumbs attached.

Breads

Desserts

Making Babies can be deliciously tasty. I love good food and want to eat food that is good for Baby and me. It is hard to find delicious recipes that have both of these qualities. Cooking is one of my things, so I came up with my own.

🌿 = Gluten-Free/Low-Casein or Casein-Free Recipe*

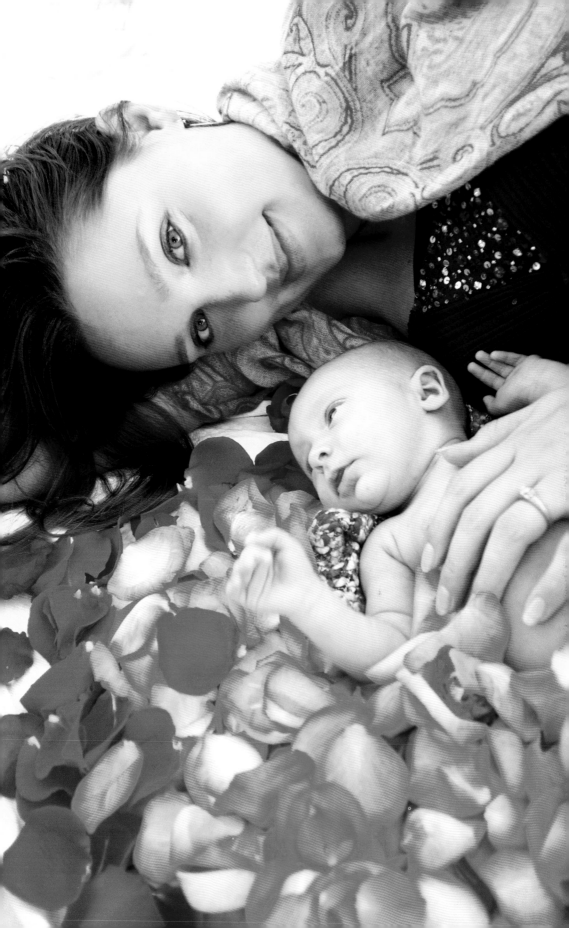

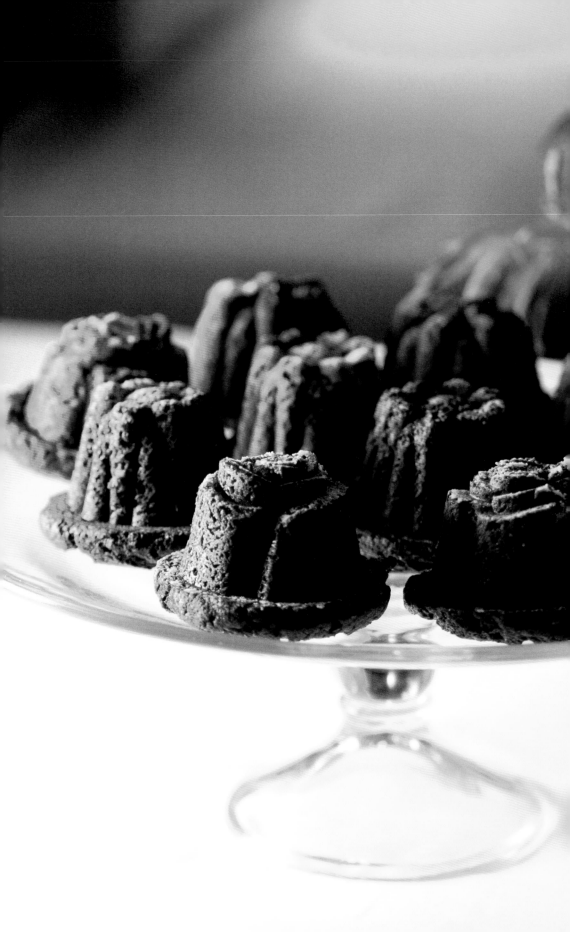

Cocoa Lovers' Cupcakes

Bites of Awesomeness You Will Not Want to Share

5 egg whites

1 cup cocoa powder

1 cup rice flour

½ cup oat flour

1½ tsp. sea salt

2 tsp. baking soda

1 tsp. xanthan gum

¼ cup arrowroot powder

1 T. baking powder

1 cup butter, softened

1 cup Sucanat

1 cup brown sugar

2 tsp. vanilla

2 egg yolks

1¼ cups water

1 recipe **Maple Cream Icing** (page 217), (*optional*)

Prep: 10 min.   Cook: 30 min.   Yield: 24

1. Preheat oven to 350° F. Grease and flour cupcake pan or cupcake flower molds.

2. Beat egg whites until a stiff peak forms. Set aside.

3. Sift dry ingredients together and set aside.

4. In a separate bowl, mix butter, sugars, and vanilla for 2 minutes. Add yolks one at a time and beat until well mixed.

5. Alternately mix dry ingredients and water into butter/sugar combination. Blend until smooth (about 2 minutes).

6. Fold egg whites into batter.

7. Pour batter into pan or molds.

8. Bake in preheated oven for 30 minutes, or until toothpick inserted in center comes out clean.

9. Cool and frost with Maple Cream Icing, if desired.

Desserts

Cracker Jack Unboxed
You Will Be Back on Grandma's Porch.

1 cup popcorn kernels

¼ cup coconut oil or butter

⅔ cup Sucanat

⅔ cup brown sugar

⅓ cup blackstrap molasses

1 T. water

½ tsp. sea salt

½ tsp. baking soda

Prep: 5 min.   Cook 10 min.   Serves: 6-10

1. Pop popcorn in coconut oil or butter in a 4-quart pot, shaking constantly until popping stops.

2. Combine remaining ingredients in a small to medium saucepan. Cook over low to medium heat.

3. Stir frequently, until sugar dissolves, approximately 10 minutes.

4. Add baking soda, stirring well to combine.

5. Pour over popcorn and you have delicious, homemade Cracker Jack that is not a preservative-filled box from the store!

Desserts

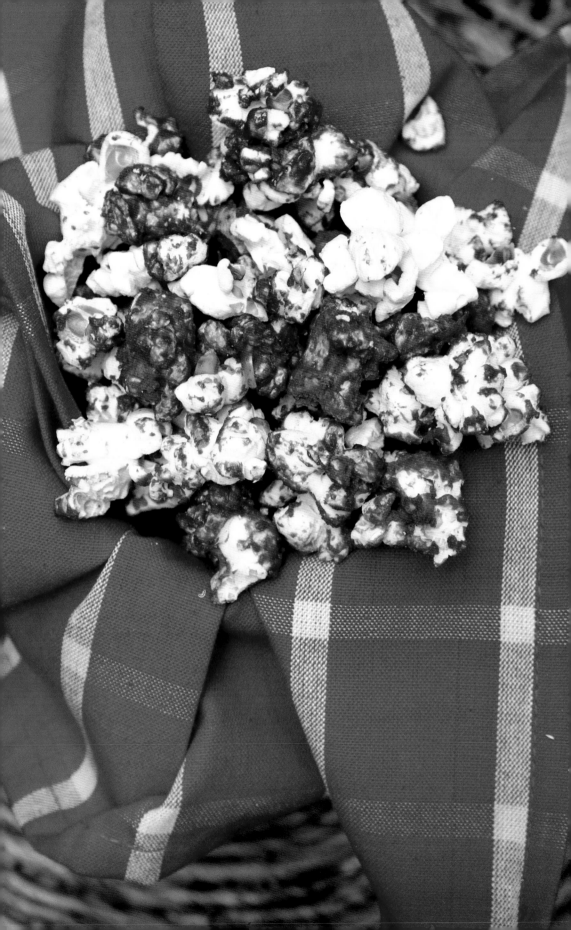

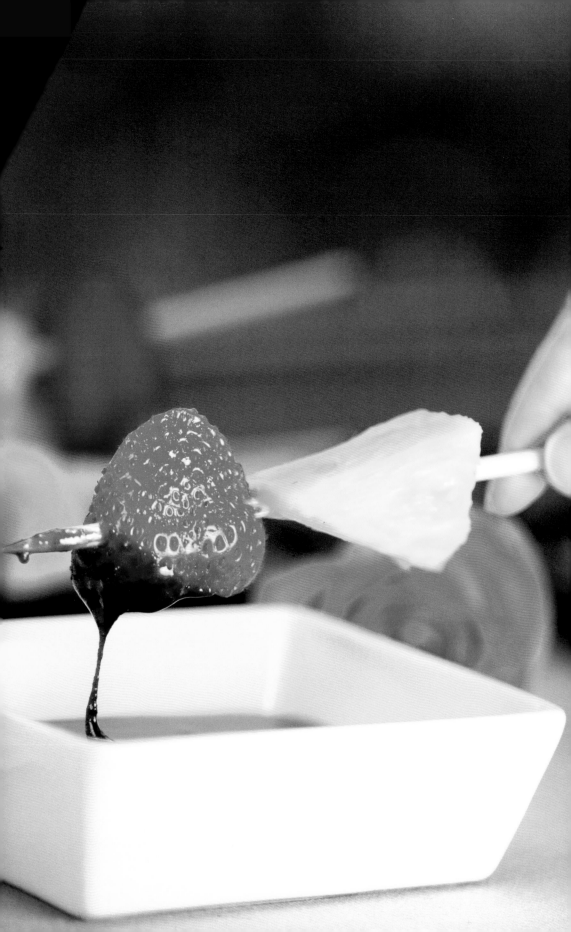

Fruit Skewers

Chunks of fruit, such as apricots, peaches, figs, strawberries, mangoes, pineapple, bananas, dates, and papaya

Maple syrup

1 recipe **Raw Chocolate Sauce** (below) or **Chocolate Syrup** (page 161)

Prep: 25 min. Cook 3 min.   Serves: 4

1. Soak 4 skewers in water for 25 minutes.

2. Preheat the broiler to high and line the broiler pan with foil.

3. Thread alternate pieces of fruit onto each skewer. Brush each fruit with a little maple syrup.

4. Cook the fruit-threaded skewers under the preheated broiler for 3 minutes, or until caramelized.

5. Drizzle fruit with *Raw Chocolate Sauce* as a finishing touch.

Raw Chocolate Sauce

Raw Energy That Tastes Sweet.

¼ cup raw honey

¼ cup cocoa powder

Pinch sea salt

Dash vanilla

2 T. butter

¼ cup maple syrup

Prep: 5 min.   Serves: 4

1. Place all ingredients in a small to medium saucepan. Stir well.

2. Heat over low heat until warm and thoroughly combined.

For another delicious snack, pour this sauce over frozen bananas and top with toasted pecans and coconut.

Desserts

Fruit Kabobs With Yogurt

Fresh and Scrumptious, Enzyme Packed

4 cups assorted fresh fruit such as pineapple, cantaloupe, strawberries, oranges, or kiwifruit, cut into bite-size pieces

3 cups strawberry yogurt

Prep: 20 min. Serves: 8

1. Thread 5 pieces of fruit on each of 8 bamboo skewers.

2. Serve and dip fruit kabobs in yogurt or spoon yogurt over fruit.

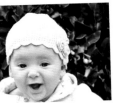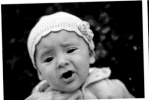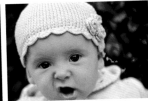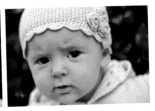

At five months, Penelope Jane was so talkative. She would look at you and carry on a conversation like a fifty-year-old woman talking about her neighborhood. She is always keeping us in stitches!

Desserts

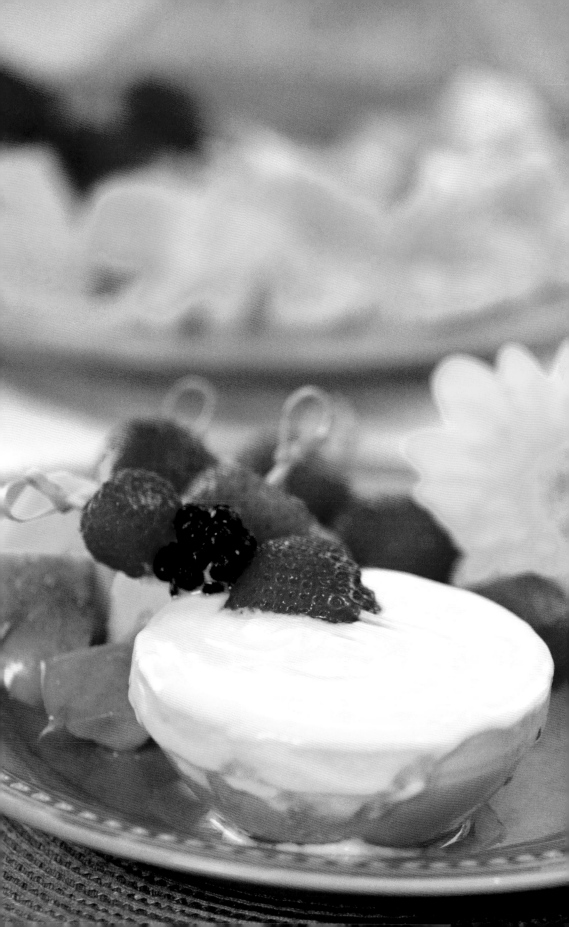

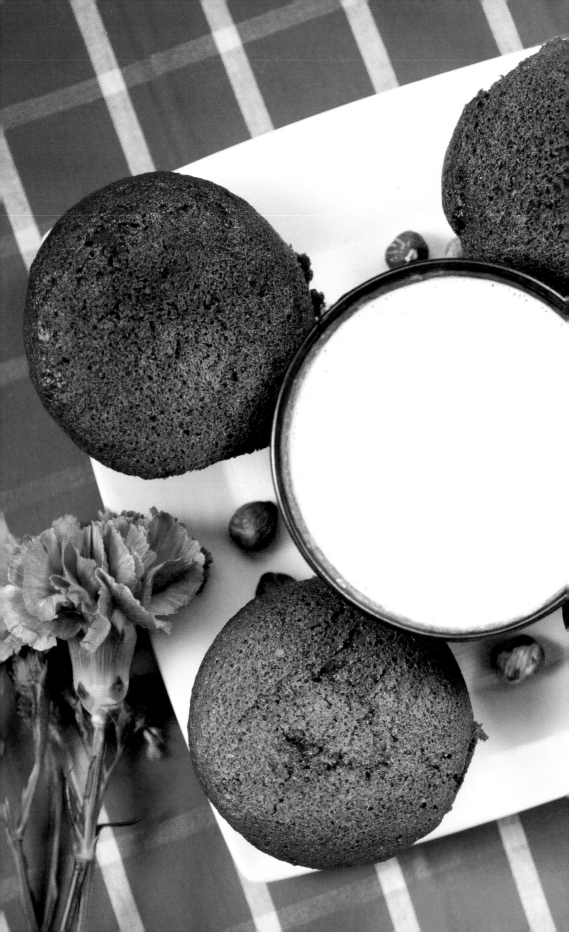

Maple Cream Icing
You Can't Believe There Is No Cream in It.

2 cups cashews, raw

3 cups water

½ cup maple syrup

½ tsp. sea salt

Prep: 3 min. Soak: 2 hours   Serves: 6

1. Soak cashews in water for two hours.

2. Strain water from cashews.

3. Add maple syrup and salt.

4. Blend well until smooth and creamy.

If you want a more liquid cream, add two cups of Purely Decadent Coconut Milk and blend.

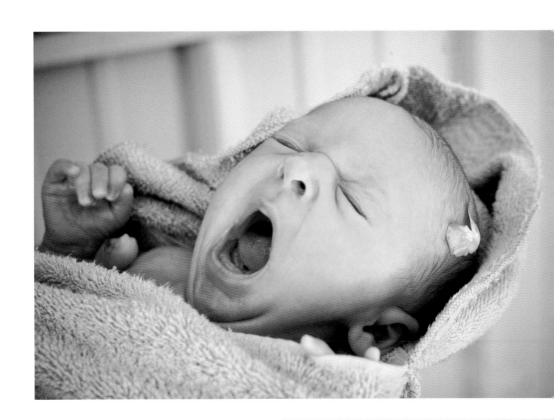

Desserts

Old-Fashioned Carrot Cake

Who Knew Making Babies Could Taste So Good?

Cake

1 cup walnuts

½ cup raisins

3 cups carrots, shredded

1 cup buckweat flour

1 cup wheat flour or **Gluten-Free Flour Mix** (page 201)

2 cups Sucanat

2 tsp. baking powder

1 tsp. baking soda

2 tsp. ground cinnamon

1½ tsp. sea salt

4 large eggs, lightly beaten

¾ cup grapeseed oil

1 tsp. vanilla extract

Cream Cheese Frosting

1- 8oz. package cream cheese, softened

½ cup butter, softened

1-16oz. package powdered sugar, sifted

1 tsp. vanilla extract

Cake

1. Preheat oven to 350° F. Butter three, 9-inch, round cake pans and line with parchment paper; then butter and flour parchment paper.

2. Combine first 10 ingredients in a large bowl. Add eggs, oil, and vanilla, stirring until blended. Pour into prepared pans.

3. Bake for 25 minutes or until a toothpick inserted in center comes out clean.

4. Cool in pans on racks for 10 minutes. Remove from pans and cool completely on wire racks.

5. Spread *Cream Cheese Frosting* between layers, on top and sides of cake. Chill.

Cream Cheese Frosting

1. Mix thoroughly or blend on low all ingredients.

2. Spread evenly on cake, as desired.

3. *This cake also tastes great with Maple Cream Icing (page 217) instead of the Cream Cheese Frosting.*

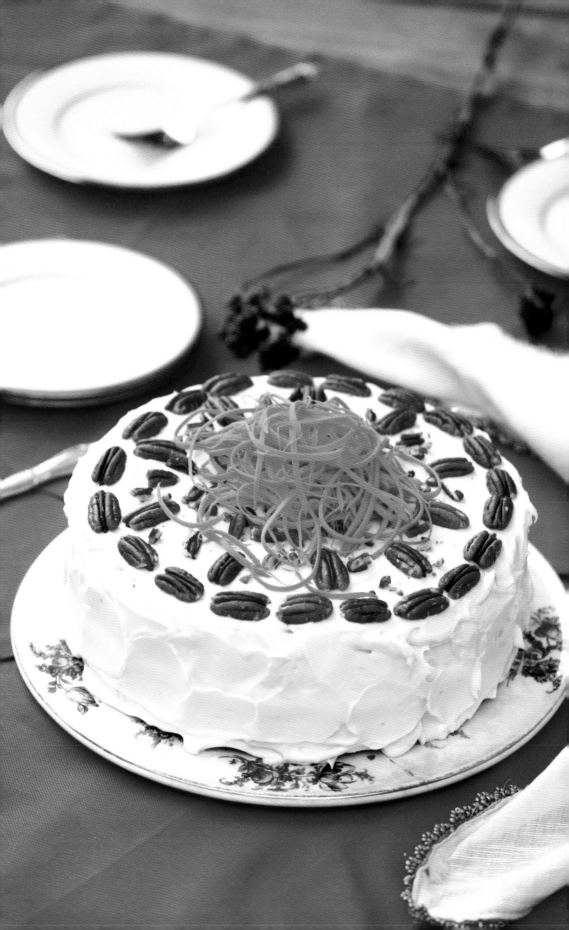

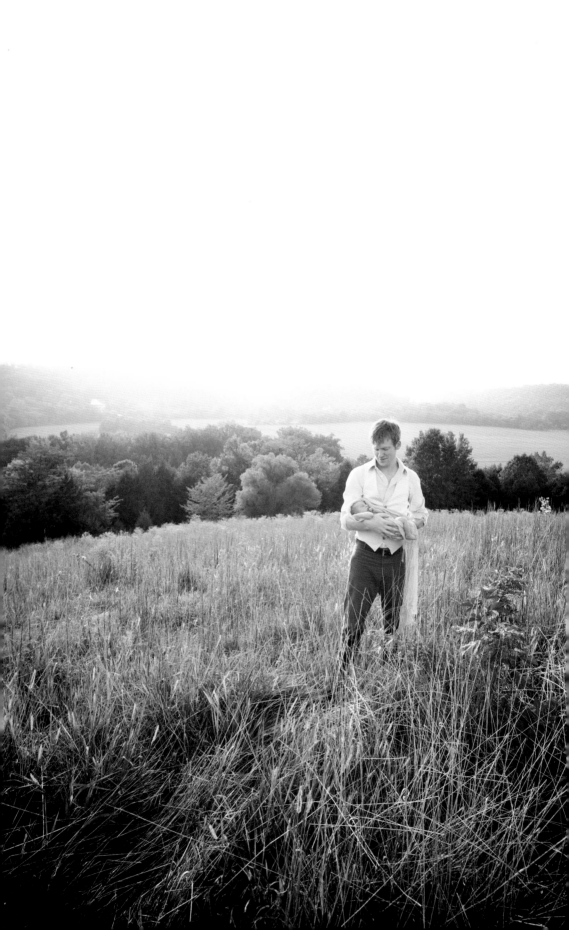

Rhubarb Sauce

Makes Your Mouth Pucker and Your Face Smile

This is a versatile sauce that can be served on desserts, over ice cream or cake, or even on pork. It's great with *Yogurt Parfait* (page 29.)

½ - ¾ cup raw sugar

½ cup water

4 cups rhubarb, cut into 1-inch pieces

Ground cinnamon, (*optional*)

Prep: 10 min.   Cook: 12 min.   Yield: 2½ cups

1. Heat raw sugar and water to boiling in a small saucepan, stirring occasionally.

2. Stir in rhubarb; reduce heat. Simmer uncovered for 12 minutes, stirring occasionally, or until rhubarb is tender and slightly transparent.

3. Stir in cinnamon to taste. Serve sauce warm or chilled.

Variations

* Strawberry Rhubarb Sauce: Reduce rhubarb to 3 cups. After step 1, stir in 1 cup of halved strawberries and heat just until it begins to boil. Remove from heat and continue to step 2.

Desserts

Sticky Fruit Oat Squares
Lip-Smacking Good and Sticky Fingers

¾ cup butter, unsalted, plus extra for greasing

¼ cup honey

Generous ¾ cup packed raw brown sugar

¼ cup creamy peanut butter

2¾ cups oats, rolled

Generous ¼ cup dried apricots or apples, chopped

¼ cup sunflower seeds

¾ cup sesame seeds

1 tsp. salt

1. Preheat the oven to 350° F. Grease and line an 8½-inch baking pan (glass is best).

2. Melt the butter, honey, and sugar in a pan over low heat, about 5 minutes.

3. When the sugar has melted, add the peanut butter and mix until all the ingredients are well combined.

4. Add all the remaining ingredients except for ¼ cup of the sesame seeds. Mix well.

5. Press the mixture into the prepared pan and bake in the preheated oven for 20 minutes.

6. Remove from the oven and sprinkle the rest of the sesame seeds on top.

7. Let cool in the pan, then cut into 16 squares.

Desserts

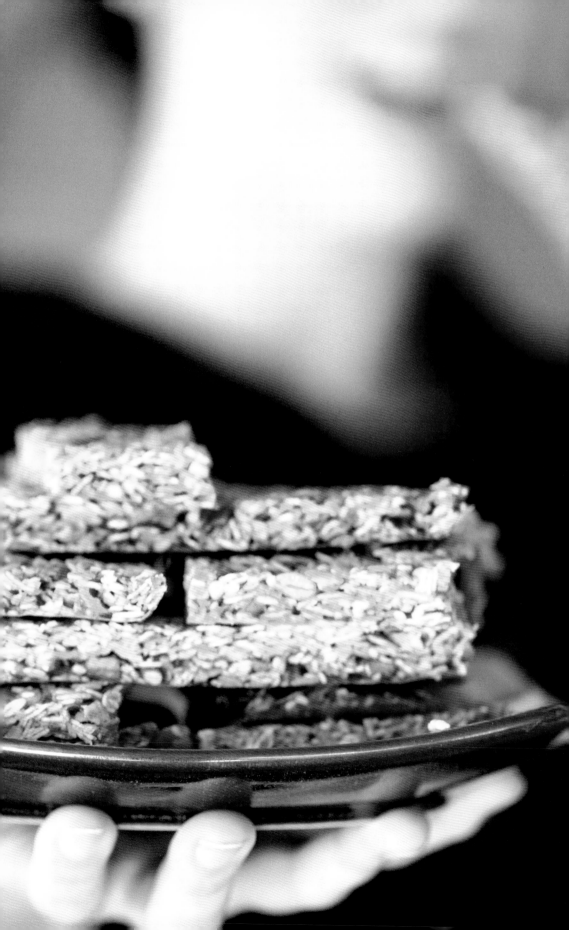

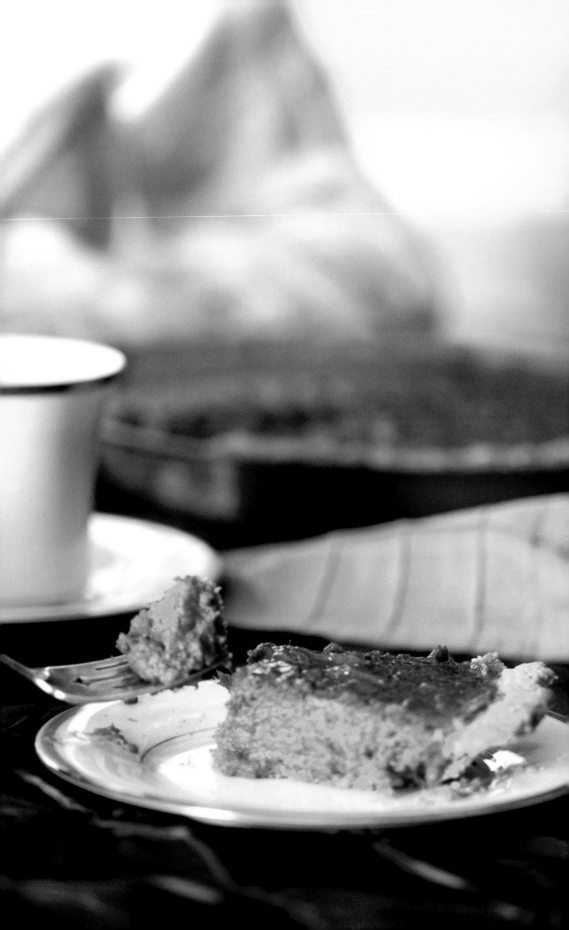

Sweet Potato Pie

Sweet Home Alabama With a Baby on My Knee

2 large sweet potatoes

1 recipe **Almond Pie Crust** (page 193)

½ cup Sucanat

2 T. **Gluten-Free Flour Mix** (page 201)

2 large eggs

½ cup coconut milk

1 tsp. nutmeg, freshly ground

½ tsp. ground allspice

½ tsp. sea salt

½ tsp. ground cinnamon

1 tsp. vanilla extract

⅛ tsp. ginger, freshly ground

Prep: 45 min.   Cook: 57 min.   Yield: 1 9-inch pie

1. Cook sweet potatoes in boiling water, covered, for 45 minutes or until tender. Drain and allow to cool.

2. Meanwhile, place pie crust in a 9-inch pie plate. Fold edges under and crimp. Line pastry with parchment paper, and fill with pie weights or dried beans.

3. Bake at 450° F for 8 minutes. Remove weights. Bake 4 more minutes.

4. Meanwhile, once cooled, peel sweet potatoes and place in a mixing bowl; beat at medium speed with an electric mixer until smooth. Add Sucanat and remaining ingredients, mixing until well blended. Pour into pie crust.

5. Bake at 375° F for 45 minutes or until a knife inserted in center comes out clean. Shield edges with strips of aluminum foil the last 15 minutes to prevent excessive browning. Serve at temperature of choice.

Desserts

Breakfast

Making Babies is a full-time job. Eat less, more often. Your body can digest small amounts of food better than a normal-size meal. Eating six small meals a day is healthier than eating three larger ones.

🌾 = Gluten-Free/Low-Casein or Casein-Free Recipe*

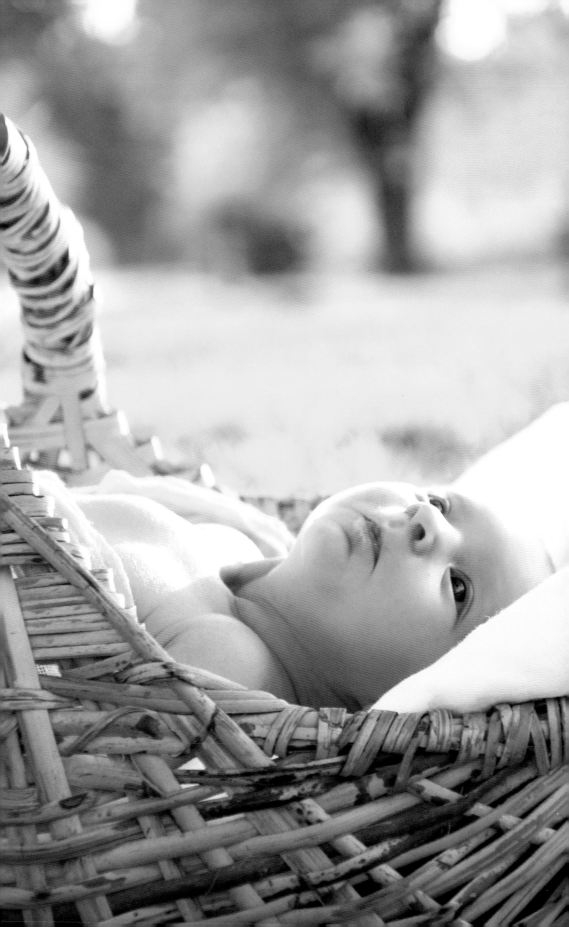

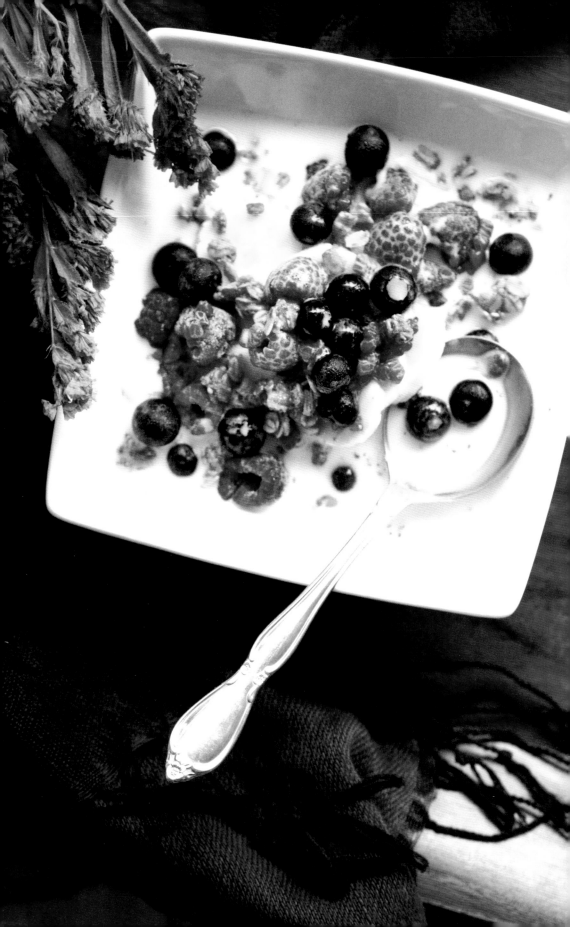

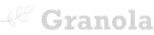

Berry Cereal With Almonds
Fiber and Antioxidants With a Smile

¼ cup **Granola** (below)

2 T. flax meal

¼ cup blueberries

¼ cup almonds, sliced

¼ cup bananas, sliced

½ tsp. cinnamon

Coconut milk or almond milk

Prep: 5 min.   Serves: 1

1. Mix together first six ingredients in a bowl.

2. Serve with almond or coconut milk.

Granola
Simple and Delicious!

1 cup rolled oats, gluten-free

2 T. almond butter

2 T. raw honey

¼ tsp. salt

½ tsp. cinnamon

Prep: 5 min.   Cook: 25 min.   Yield: 1 cup

1. Mix all ingredients together. Pour into a 9x13 baking pan and spread evenly.

2. Bake at 350° F for 25 minutes. Stir 2 or 3 times throughout cooking time.

3. Store in jar with lid.

Makes enough for 8 bowls of cereal.

Breakfast

Florentine Omelet
This Is So-o-o Good and So Good for You!

5 eggs

⅛ cup water

1 T. coconut oil or butter

2 handfuls baby spinach

½ small onion, finely diced

½ cup sun-dried tomatoes

2 garlic cloves, finely chopped

½ tsp. lemon zest, freshly grated

½ tsp. black pepper, freshly ground

1 tsp. sea salt

8 baby portobello mushrooms, halved

3 T. feta cheese, crumbled, (*optional*)

Prep: 7 min.   Cook: 10-12 min.   Serves: 4 to 5

1. Heat oven to 350° F.

2. In a bowl, beat the eggs and water.

3. Sauté onion and spinach in a saucepan with oil on medium-high for 5 minutes.

4. Pour onion-spinach mixture into a bowl; add tomatoes, garlic, lemon zest, pepper, and salt. Stir in eggs.

5. Butter a hot, glass tart pan. Lay mushrooms on bottom of pan and pour egg mixture on top. Sprinkle with cheese.

6. Bake for 10 to 12 minutes or until eggs are set.

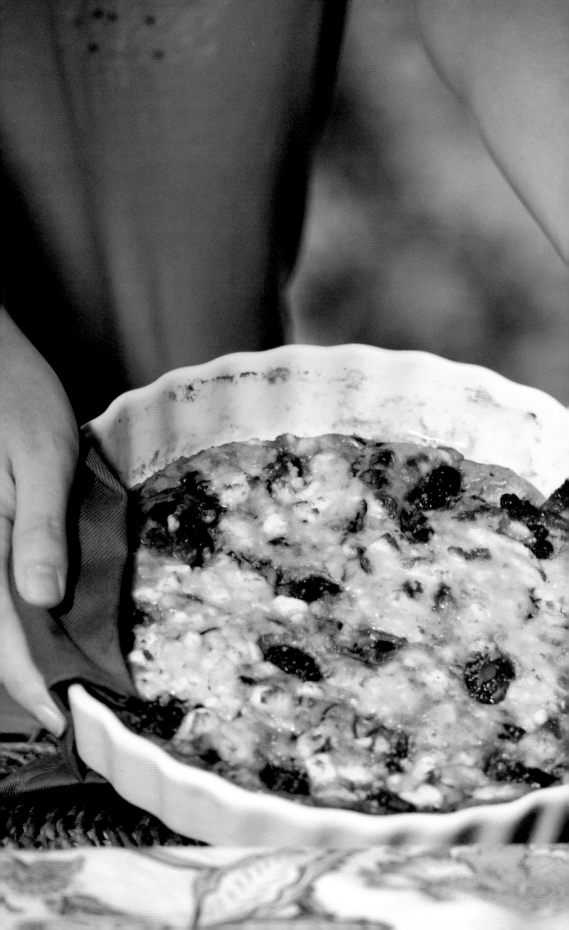

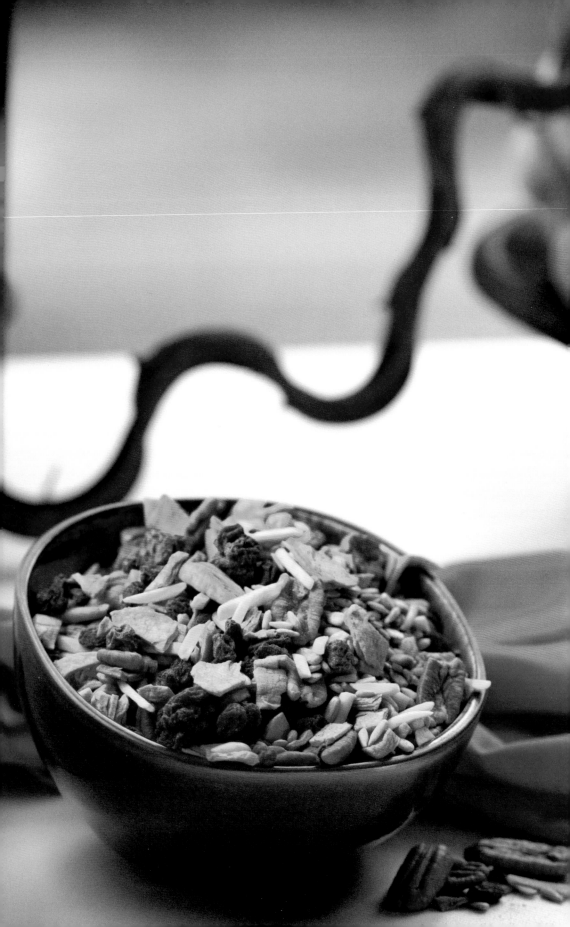

Grainless Granola
We Have All Gone Nutty.

1 cup pecans or walnuts, chopped

1 cup dried apples, chopped

1 cup raisins or dried cherries

1 cup sunflower seeds, raw

½ cup almonds, chopped

Pinch of each: ground cloves, cinnamon, and nutmeg

½ cup rolled oats (*optional*)

Prep: 5 min.   Serves: 6-10

1. Place all ingredients together in a large bowl and mix well.

2. Serve with coconut milk or almond milk and fresh fruit, such as raspberries or blueberries.

Grandma's Breakfast Sausage
Tasty, Juicy Bites of Goodness

2 lb. turkey meat, ground

2 or 2½ tsp. sea salt

1 tsp. pepper, finely ground

½ tsp. marjoram, dried and finely ground

½ tsp. thyme, dried and finely ground

½ tsp. sage, dried and finely ground

2 T. white wine (*optional*)

Prep: 5 min.   Cook: 8 min.   Yield: 2 lb. Sausage

1. In a large bowl combine all ingredients. Mix well using hands.

2. Pat into patties.

3. In a fry pan cook on medium for 4 minutes each side or until done.

You can freeze uncooked leftover meat for 2 months or refrigerate for 3 days.

Afternoon fun, playing together!

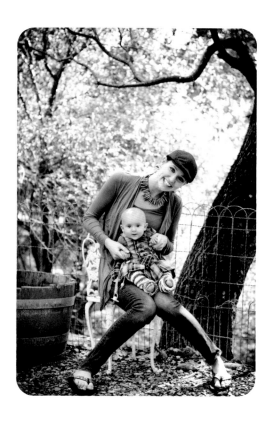

Breakfast

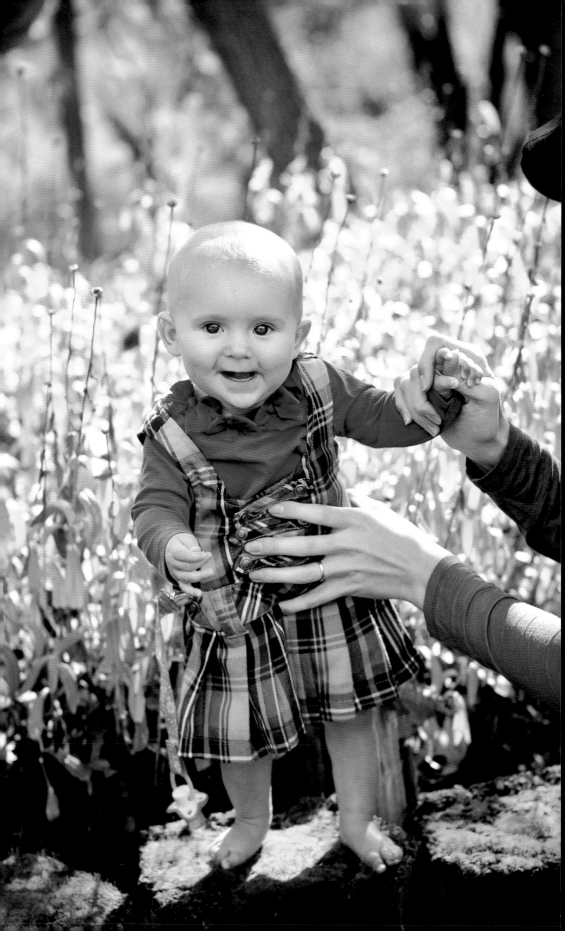

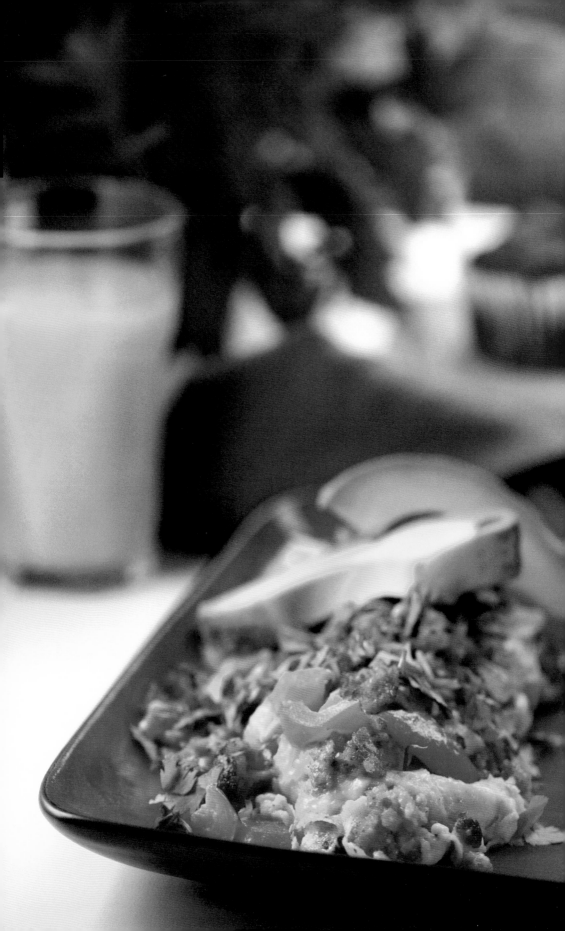

Mexican-Style Scrambled Eggs
Great for Breakfast, Lunch, or Dinner

½ lb. **Grandma's Breakfast Sausage** (page 234)

1 small green bell pepper

1 medium onion

6 large eggs

⅓ cup milk, cream, or water

¼ tsp. sea salt

⅛ tsp. pepper, freshly ground

1 T. butter

Optional Ingredients:

6 tortillas

1 cup fresh salsa

¾ cup cheese

¼ cup sour cream

1 avocado, sliced

Prep: 5 min.   Cook: 10 min.   Serves: 4-6

1. Cook sausage, green pepper, and onion in a 10-inch skillet over medium-high heat for 5 minutes, stirring often or until sausage is no longer pink. Remove mixture from skillet and drain.

2. Beat eggs, milk, salt, and pepper thoroughly with a whisk in a medium-size bowl until well combined.

3. In a 10-inch skillet, bring butter to a sizzle. Pour in egg mixture.

4. As you notice the eggs setting on the side and bottom, carefully lift cooked portions with a spatula, so that the uncooked egg portion can flow to bottom. Do not mix.

5. Add sausage mixture to eggs and cook 3 to 4 minutes or until eggs are thickened.

6. To make breakfast burritos, place Mexican-Style Scrambled Eggs in tortillas. Top with fresh salsa, shredded cheese, sliced avocado, and sour cream.

Breakfast

Pancakes
Great for the Whole Family!

3 eggs

1 cup Purely Decadent Coconut Milk

2 T. honey

2½ tsp. vanilla

¼ cup coconut oil

1 tsp. salt

1 cup almond flour

1 cup *Gluten-Free Flour Mix* (page 201)

1 T. baking powder

½ tsp. baking soda

Nuts (*optional*)

Blueberries (*optional*)

Prep: 5 min. Cook: 15 min.   Serves: 12 3-inch pancakes

1. Melt coconut oil in warm pan.

2. Whisk first four ingredients together in a bowl. Slowly pour in coconut oil, whisking into wet ingredients.

3. Mix dry ingredients, except nuts and blueberries, together in a separate bowl.

4. Whisk mixed dry ingredients into wet ingredients until combined. Do not overmix.

5. Heat a griddle or skillet to medium-high. Grease with butter. Pour the batter into rounds on the hot griddle or skillet using a 2-ounce ladle. Sprinkle on nuts and blueberries as desired. Cook 2 minutes, or until bubbles have formed on the surface of each pancake. Flip and cook until the other sides are golden brown.

Variations

* **Pancake Sandwich Bread:** Omit blueberries and sugar.

Breakfast

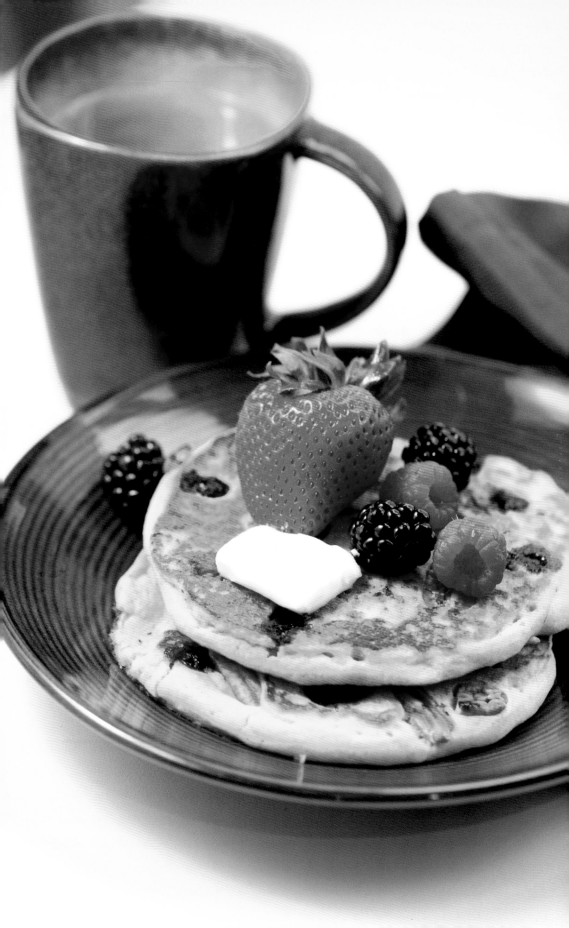

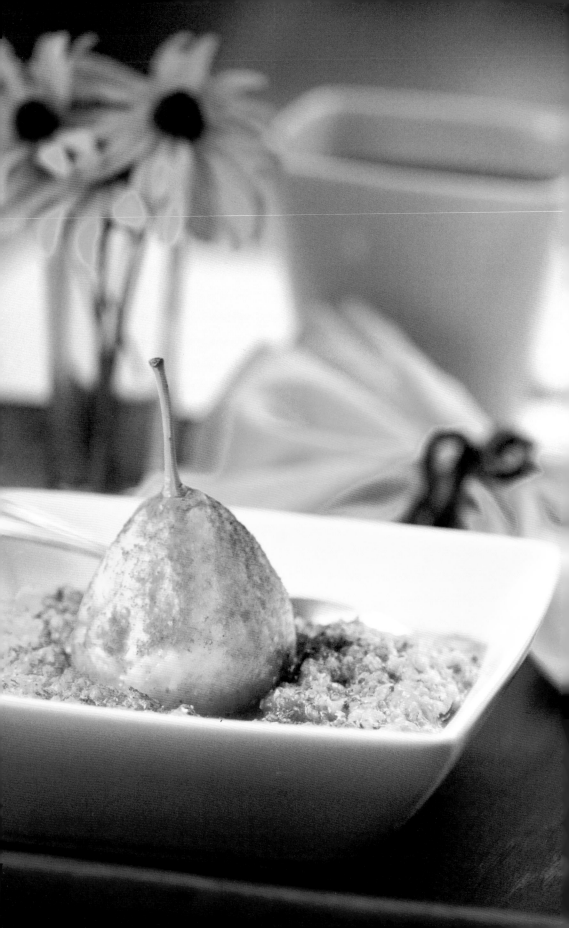

Quinoa Porridge
Start Your Day With Protein and Vitamins.

½ cup quinoa

2 tsp. red quinoa (*optional*)

¼ tsp. ground cinnamon

1½ cups almond milk or coconut milk

½ cup water

2 T. honey or maple syrup

1 tsp. vanilla

Pinch sea salt

1 cup pears, freshly sliced or whole pear, peeled

Nutmeg, freshly ground

Ground cinnamon

Prep: 5 min.   Cook: 25 min.   Serves: 1-2

1. Heat a saucepan over medium heat. Add quinoa and cinnamon. Cook until toasted, stirring frequently, for about 3 minutes.

2. Add almond milk, water, vanilla, honey, sea salt, and pear.

3. Bring to a boil, then reduce heat and cook until porridge is thick and grains are tender, approximately 25 minutes.

4. While cooking, add more water if needed. Stir occasionally, to ensure no burning at the end. Sprinkle with nutmeg and cinnamon, to taste.

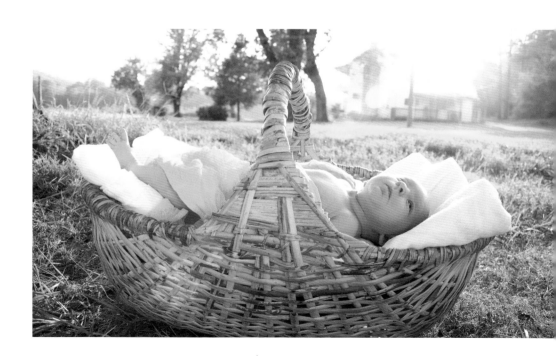

Scrambled Eggs

Easy Energy That You and Your Baby Need

6 large eggs

⅓ cup milk, half-and-half, or water

¼ tsp. sea salt

⅛ tsp. pepper, freshly ground

3 T. butter

⅛ cup green onion, chopped

⅛ cup parsley, chopped

Prep: 5 min. Cook: 10 min.   Serves: 4

1. Beat eggs, milk, salt, and pepper thoroughly with a whisk until well mixed.

2. Heat butter in a 10-inch skillet over medium heat just until butter sizzles. Pour egg mixture into skillet.

3. As you notice the eggs setting on the side and bottom, carefully lift cooked portions with a spatula, so that the uncooked egg portion can flow to bottom. Do not mix.

4. Cook 3 to 4 minutes or until eggs are thickened.

5. Top with green onion and parsley.

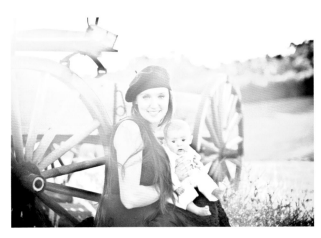

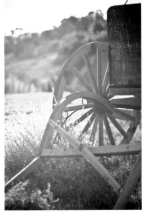

Breakfast

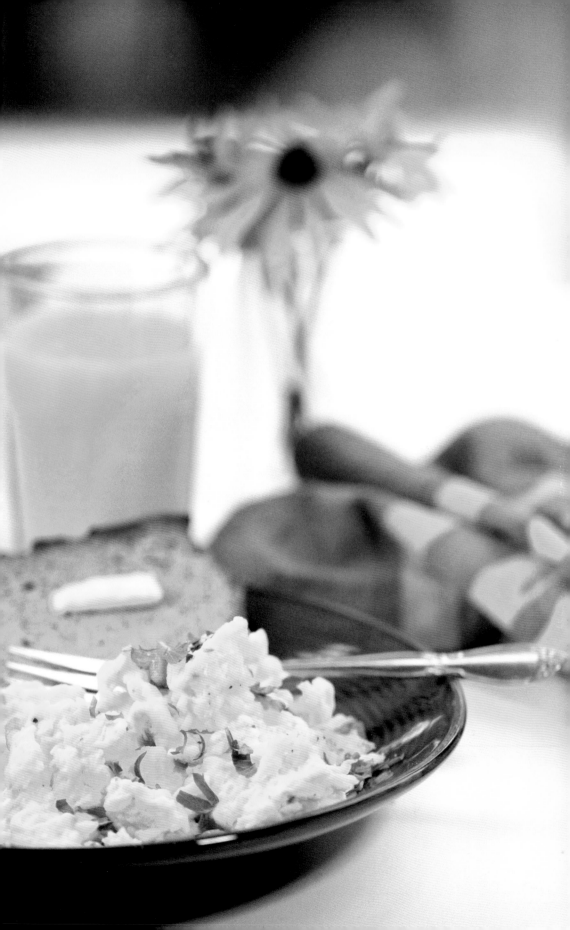

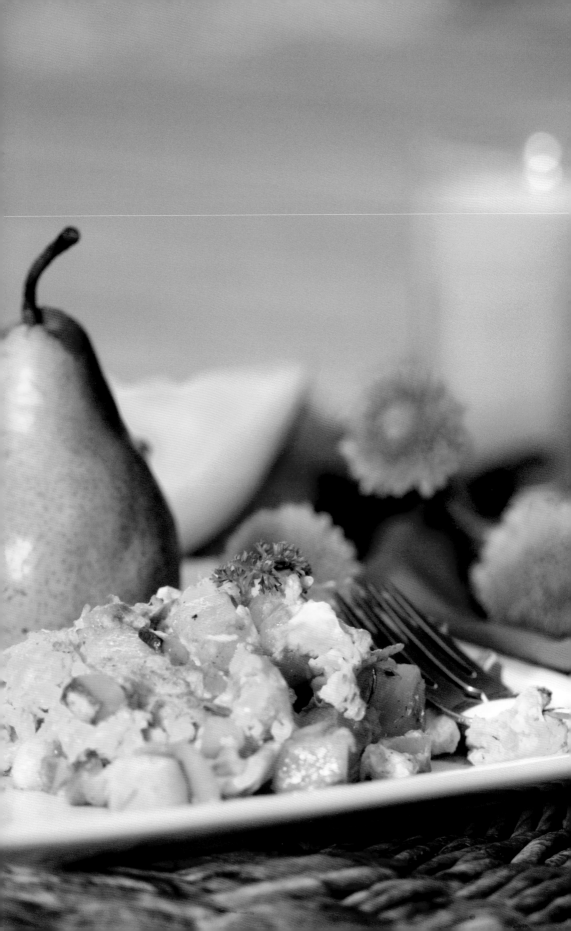

Scrambled Eggs and Potatoes
Sunrise Breakfast; Start Your Day Strong.

6 large eggs

⅓ cup milk, half-and-half, or water

¼ tsp. sea salt

⅛ tsp. pepper, freshly ground

3 T. butter

1 cup potatoes, diced

1 cup onion, diced

1 cup zucchini, diced

1 cup tomato, seeded

½ tsp. rosemary, fresh or dried

Prep: 10 min. Cook: 15 min. Serves: 4 to 6

1. Beat eggs, milk, salt, and pepper thoroughly with a whisk until well combined.

2. Heat butter in a 10-inch skillet over medium-high heat just until butter sizzles.

3. Cook potatoes, onion, zucchini, and tomato in sizzling butter. Stir occasionally, to allow the vegetables to fry on the outside.

4. Pour beaten egg mixture into skillet over cooked mixture.

5. As you notice the eggs setting on the side and bottom, carefully lift cooked portions with a spatula, so that the uncooked egg portion can flow to bottom. Do not mix.

6. Cook 3 to 4 minutes or until eggs are thickened.

Topless Breakfast Quesadilla
What Were You Thinking?

1 peach, peeled and diced

1 pear, peeled and diced

¼ cup almond butter

Cinnamon, to taste

1 T. coconut oil

⅛ cup raw honey

2 tortillas, gluten-free

Prep: 5 min. Cook: 12 min. Serves: 2

1. Spread almond butter on the center of a tortilla.

2. Top with the diced peaches and pears and sprinkle cinnamon on top.

3. Melt coconut oil in a large skillet over medium heat.

4. Place quesadilla in the skillet and cook until golden brown and crisp (about 3-5 minutes).

5. Drizzle honey on top and serve at once.

Breakfast

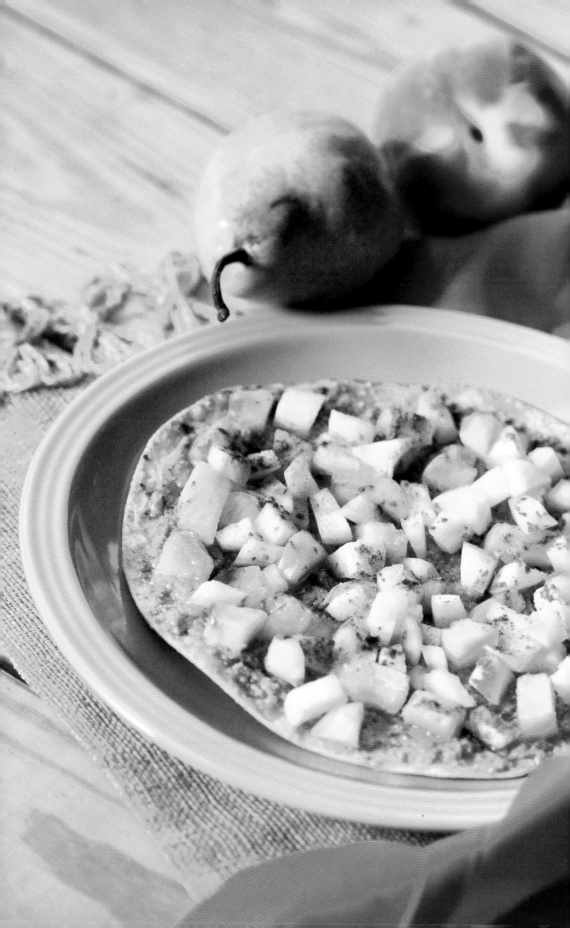

Main Course

🌿 = Gluten-Free/Low-Casein or Casein-Free Recipe*

Making Babies does not stop at conception. Your daily life choices affect your baby. Eating right every once in a while is not good enough. Eat the food that builds a healthy, strong baby.

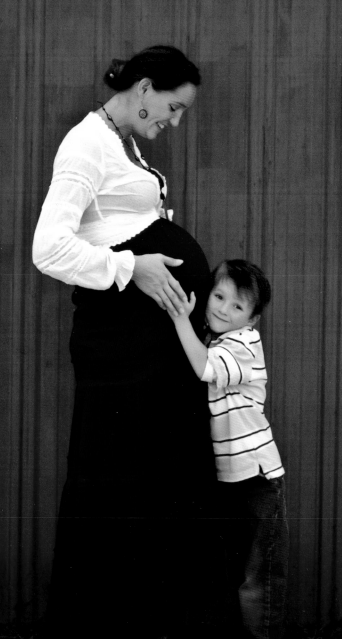

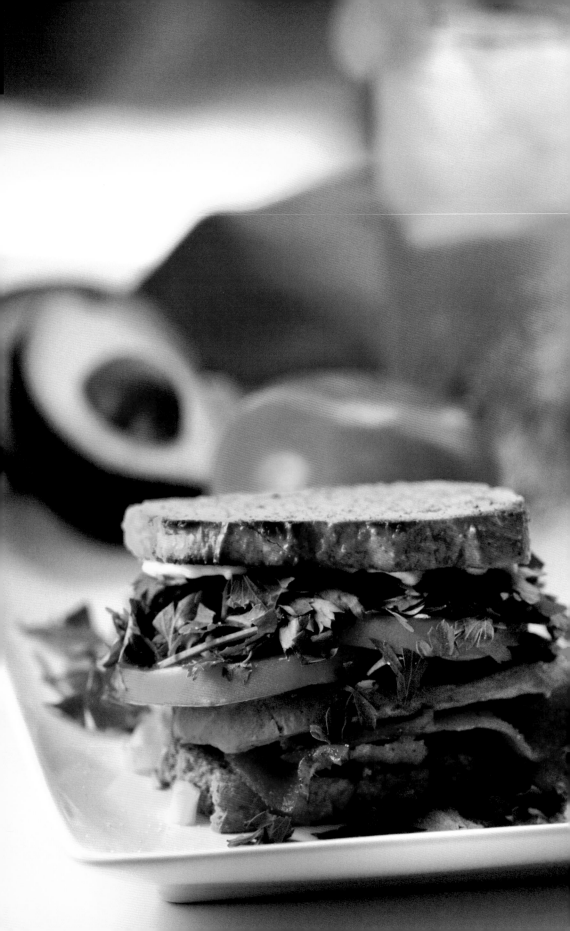

Bacon Sandwiches
Taste, Texture, Smell. This Sandwich Has It All.

1 avocado, sliced

5-6 slices bacon, cooked golden brown

1 green onion, chopped

1 tomato, sliced

¼ cup parsley, chopped

Pinch sea salt

4 slices **Scrumptious Sandwich Bread,** toasted (page 202)

Vegenaise, to taste

Prep: 5 min.   Cook: 15 min.   Serves: 2

1. Layer your sandwich.

2. Garnish with parsley and enjoy.

Don't miss the moments.

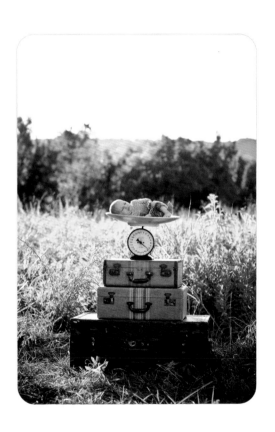

Main Course

Blackened Trout on a Bed of Herbed Quinoa

Wow! What More Can I Say? Love It!

Prep: 10 min.   Cook: 25 min.   Serves: 4

Trout

1 T. paprika

½ tsp. sea salt

½ tsp. garlic powder

½ tsp. basil, dried

¾ tsp. pepper, freshly ground

½ tsp. thyme, dried

1 tsp. onion powder

¼ cup unsalted butter, melted

½ tsp. lemon zest, freshly grated

4 trout (1½ lbs.)

Herbed Quinoa

¾ tsp. sea salt

1 cup quinoa

1¾ cups water

3 tsp. cilantro, freshly chopped

2 tsp. mint, freshly chopped

1 tsp. lemon zest, freshly grated

2 T. butter

Trout

1. Combine first 7 ingredients in a large, shallow dish.

2. Melt butter. Add lemon zest. Dip fish in butter, and then dredge in spice mixture. Place on parchment paper until ready to cook.

3. Heat a large, cast-iron skillet over medium-high heat.

4. Cook fish, 2 at a time, 2 to 3 minutes on each side until fish is blackened and flakes easily with a fork.

5. Serve with fresh lemon wedges.

Herbed Quinoa

1. Put quinoa, salt, and water in a saucepan. Cook on medium-low heat for 20 minutes, or until desired tenderness.

2. Add butter, lemon zest, and fresh herbs. Stir.

Main Course

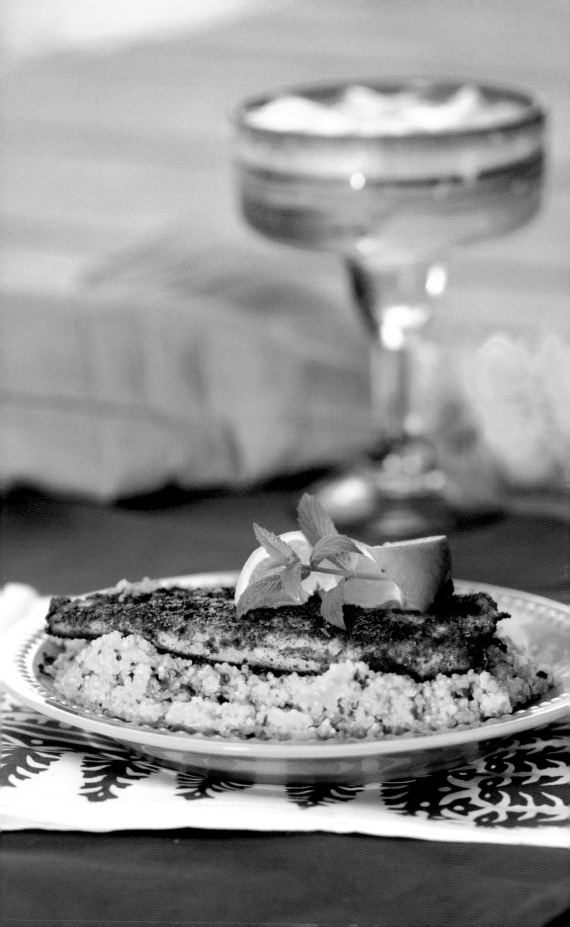

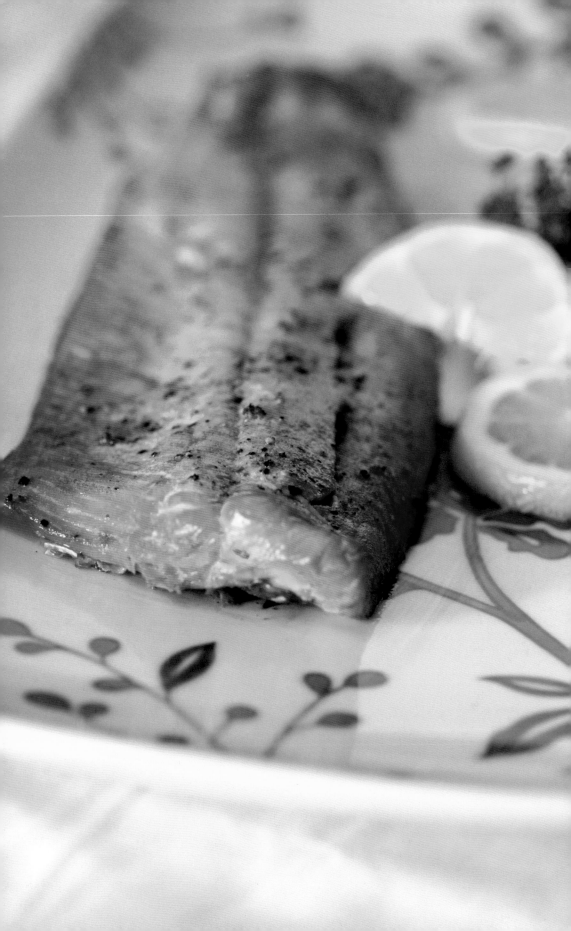

Broiled Fish Steaks

Fish Brains! Oils in Fish Build You and Your Baby's Brain.

4 small salmon, trout, or other medium-firm fish steaks, about ¾-inch thick (1½ lb.)

Sea salt

Pepper, freshly ground

2 T. butter, melted

Prep: 5 min.   Cook: 11 min.   Serves: 4

1. Set oven to broil.

2. Sprinkle both sides of fish with salt and pepper.

3. Brush with half of the melted butter.

4. Place fish on rack in broiler pan. Broil with tops about 4 inches from heat for 5 minutes. Brush with butter. Carefully turn fish; brush with butter. Broil 4 to 6 minutes longer or until fish flakes easily with fork.

Main Course

Chicken Pot Pie

There's Nothing More Comforting on a Cold Day.

1 lb. chicken breasts, boneless, skinless

2 T. grapeseed oil or olive oil

1 small onion, finely chopped

1 stalk celery, finely diced

3 cups mixed veggies, frozen

1 T. sea salt

⅓ cup parsley, finely chopped

1 T. arrowroot powder

1 tsp. garlic powder

Pinch of pepper, freshly ground

1½ cups chicken stock or water

Biscuit Crust

1 cup *Gluten-Free Flour Mix* (page 201)

1 cup almond flour, plus extra for floured surface

1½ tsp. baking powder

1 tsp. sea salt

5 T. butter, cold

⅔ cup coconut milk

Prep: 20 min.   Cook: 50 min.   Serves: 6

1. Rinse the chicken and pat dry. Cut the chicken into ½-inch cubes, then refrigerate.

2. Heat the oil in a large skillet over medium-high heat. Sauté the onion for 8 to 10 minutes, until soft, then lower the heat to medium. Add the celery, mixed veggies, and salt. Cook, covered, for 10 to 15 minutes, until tender.

3. Stir in the chicken, and cook, covered, for 5 minutes, until the chicken is cooked through. Stir in the parsley, and pour into a baking dish.

4. In a small bowl, vigorously whisk the arrowroot powder, garlic, and pepper into the chicken stock until dissolved.

5. Pour over chicken and vegetable mixture.

6. Lay biscuit crust on top, and bake at 400° F for 20 minutes.

Biscuit Crust

1. Mix dry ingredients together. Cut in cold butter and mix in milk

2. Dump dough out on floured surface. Sprinkle with flour and pat down to 1/2 inch. Use a glass cup to cut biscuits out.

Main Course

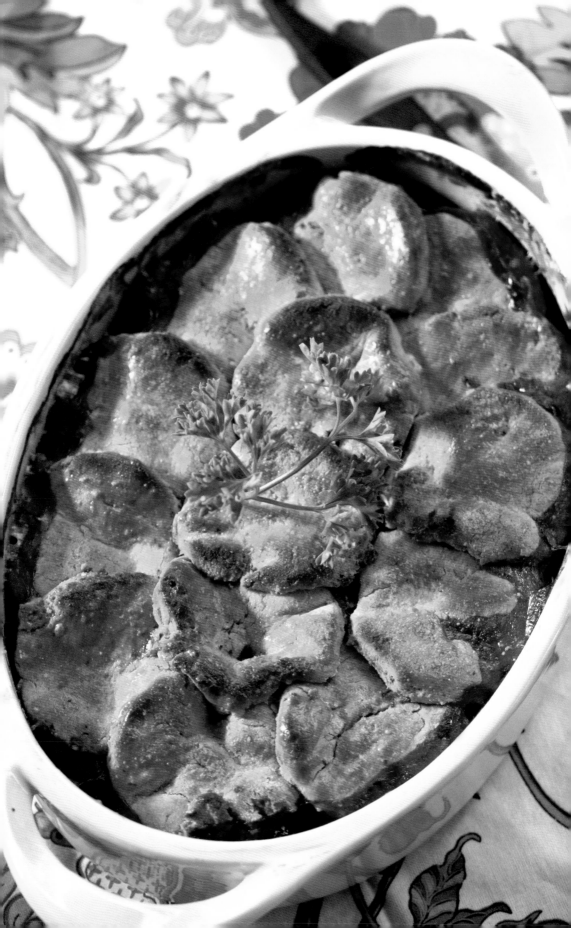

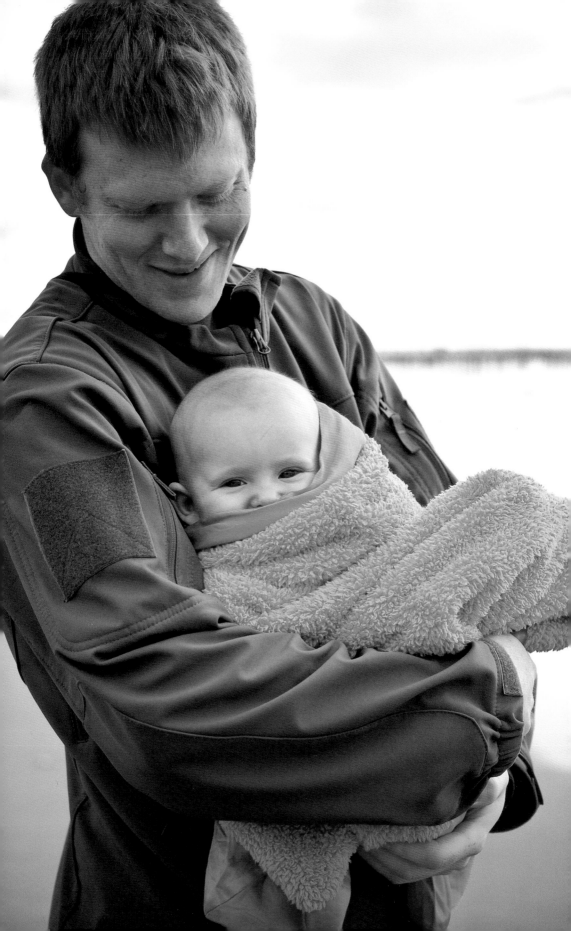

Curried Quinoa

Making Your Baby Smile

1 cup quinoa

3 cups water

1 chicken breast, uncooked and cubed

2 tsp. sea salt

2 tsp. curry powder

2 handfuls baby carrots

1 garlic clove, chopped

¼ cup coconut oil

¼ cup red bell pepper, diced

⅛ cup cilantro, fresh

Prep: 5 min.   Cook: 25 min.   Serves: 2-4

1. In a saucepan, combine first 8 ingredients. Cook on medium-low heat for 25 minutes or until carrots are soft.

2. Serve, topped with red peppers and cilantro.

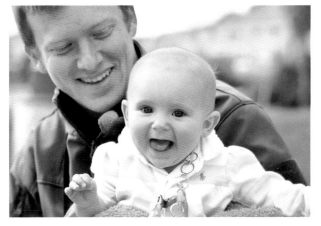
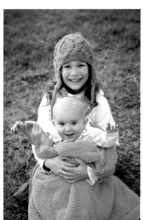

Main Course

Lentil Soup

Cowboy Mush That Makes Barbed-Wire People

½ cup red lentils

½ cup green lentils

½ cup yellow split peas

4 cups water

2 uncooked chicken breasts, cubed

2 tsp. cumin

2½ tsp. sea salt

1 cup cilantro, fresh

¼ cup green onion, chopped

½ cup bean sprouts

Prep: 5 min.   Cook: 20 min.   Serves: 4-6

1. Soak lentils and peas in water for two hours.

2. In a saucepan, combine lentil mixture and next 4 ingredients. Cook on low, covered, for 20 minutes or until lentils and peas are soft.

3. Serve topped with cilantro, green onions, and bean sprouts.

The Warmth of a Daddy's Love

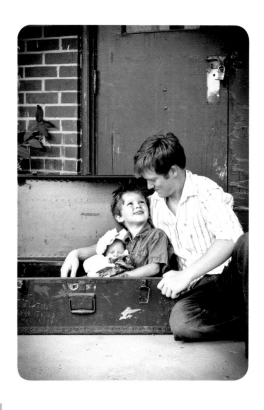

Main Course

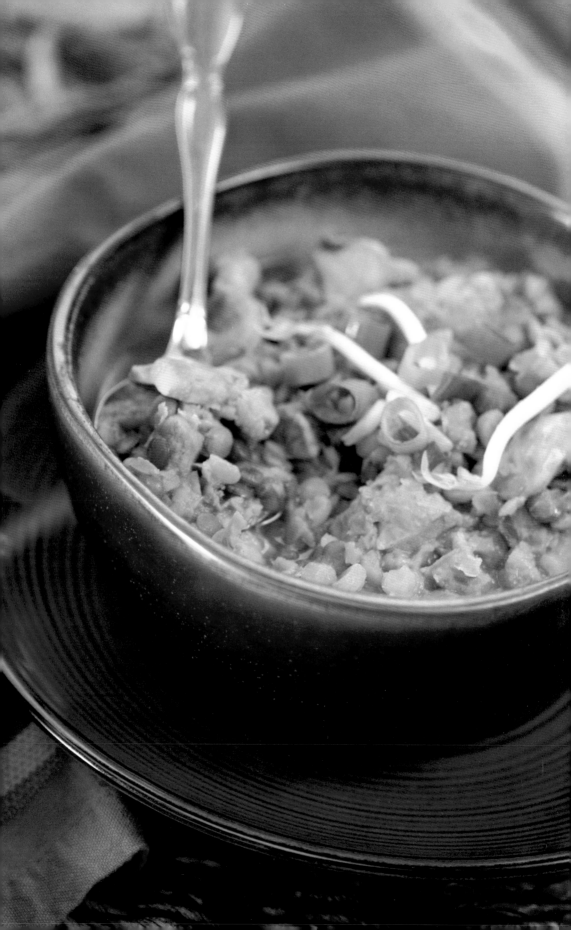

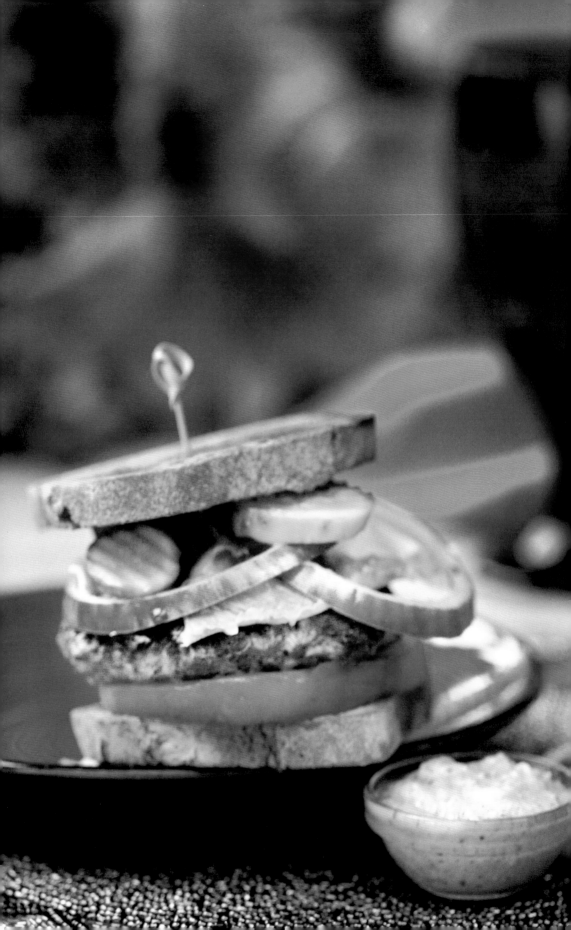

Hamburger
Eat In! It Tastes Better.

2 lbs. ground beef, grass fed

½ tsp. pepper

½ tsp. salt

½ tsp. onion powder

½ tsp. parsley, freshly chopped

1 avocado, sliced

1 tomato, sliced

2 slices of onion

3 leaves of lettuce

8 dill pickles

2 T. mustard

2 T. Vegenaise

4 slices of **Scrumptious Sandwich Bread** (page 202) or other gluten-free bread

Prep: 5 min.   Cook: 8 min.   Serves: 2

1. Wash and slice veggies. Wash lettuce and pat dry.

2. In a bowl, mix first five ingredients together.

3. Pat meat into palm-size patties, about ¾" thick.

4. Fry in pan on stovetop set to medium for 3 minutes. Flip and fry 3 minutes more, or until desired.

5. Toast bread.

6. Layer all ingredients.

7. Enjoy!

Main Course

Herb Roasted Chicken
Sunday Dinner's Best

1 stick (½ cup) butter

¼ cup parsley or rosemary, chopped

3-4 garlic cloves, minced

1 small onion, peeled and quartered

3 tsp. rock sea salt

1 tsp. pepper, freshly ground

5-lb. whole chicken

Fresh parsley or rosemary, as garnish

Prep: 30 min.   Cook: 2½ hours   Serves: 6

1. On stovetop, melt half of the butter. Add garlic and cook for two minutes on medium-high, stirring so it doesn't burn, and allow to brown. Remove from heat and add parsley or rosemary.

2. Remove giblets from cavity of chicken and reserve for another use. Rinse chicken with cold water; pat dry with paper towels. Fold neck skin over back; secure with a wooden pick. Tuck wings under chicken.

3. Stuff chicken cavity with remaining butter and onion. Close cavity with skewers; tie legs together with a string. Place chicken, breast side up, in baking pan. Pour butter-herb mixture over whole chicken. Sprinkle salt over chicken.

4. Insert a meat thermometer into thickest part of thigh, making sure it does not touch bone. Bake at 325° F for 2 hours and 30 minutes, or until thermometer registers 180° F.

5. Cool 15 minutes, garnish, then slice and serve.

Main Course

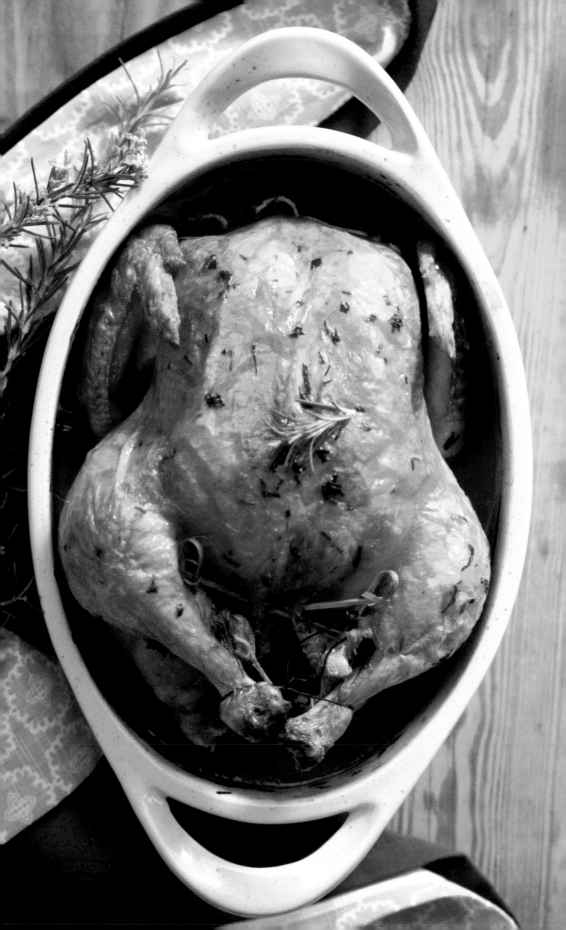

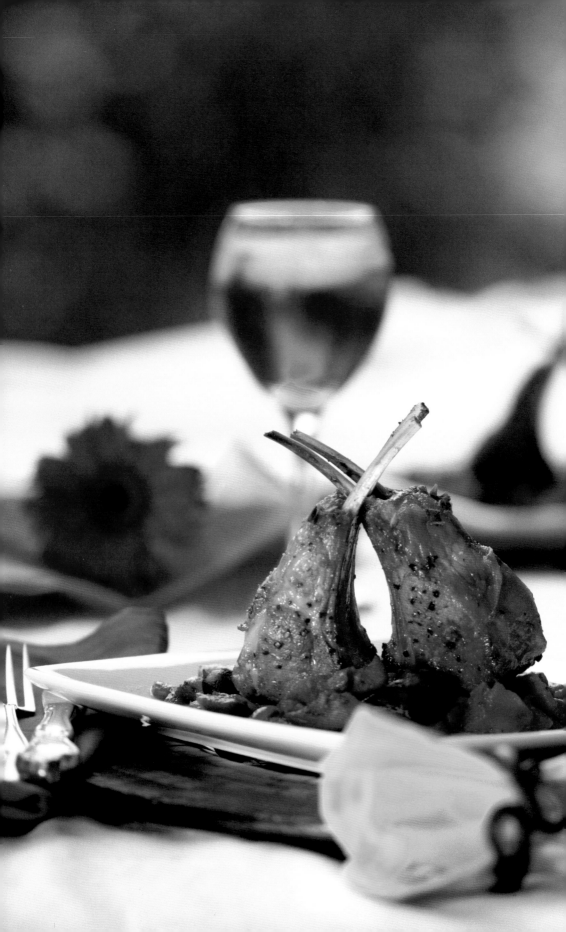

Lamb With Eggplant
So Decadent You Can't Get Enough

1 eggplant, cut in ¾-inch cubes

Sea salt

Pepper, freshly ground

8 lamb chops

3 T. olive oil

1 onion, coarsely chopped

1 garlic clove, finely chopped

14-oz. can chopped tomatoes, in juice

Pinch of raw sugar

16 black olives, pitted and coarsely chopped

1 tsp. fresh herbs such as basil, parsley, or oregano, chopped

2 T. mint, freshly chopped

Prep: 30 min.   Cook: 30 min.   Serves: 4

1. Place a colander on a large plate. Put layers of eggplant cubes in a colander, sprinkling salt over each layer to tenderize. After layering, place another plate over the colander and place a heavy weight on it. Leave for 25 minutes.

2. Preheat the broiler. Rinse the eggplant cubes under cold running water, then dry with paper towels. Season the lamb chops with pepper.

3. Place the lamb chops on the broiler pan and cook under medium heat for 15 minutes until tender, turning once during the cooking time.

4. Meanwhile, heat the olive oil in a saucepan, add the eggplant, onion, and garlic, and fry for 8 minutes until softened and starting to brown.

5. Add the tomatoes and their juice, the raw sugar, olives, chopped herbs, salt, and pepper and simmer for 8 minutes.

6. Serve topped with mint.

Main Course

Miniature Beef Kabobs
Light and Delicious – Lunch With a Punch

Kabobs

1 4-oz. sirloin or rump steak, cut into ½-inch cubes

4 mushrooms, cut into ½-inch cubes, or 8 button mushrooms

½ cup pineapple, cubed

½ cup bell pepper, cubed

½ small onion, cut into ½-inch cubes

Spicy Tomato Marinade

¼ cup olive oil

⅛ cup apple cider vinegar

1 T. parsley, fresh

1 tsp. garlic, freshly crushed

½ tsp. pepper, freshly ground

Small pinch cayenne (*optional*)

Prep: 50 min.   Cook: 5 min.   Serves: 4-6

1. Combine all the marinade ingredients in a large, non-metallic bowl; whisk well.

2. Stir in the meat, mushrooms, and onion. Cover with plastic wrap and let marinate in the refrigerator for 40 minutes.

3. Drain off the marinade and discard. Place alternating pieces of steak and vegetables on skewers, not placing them too closely together.

4. Start up grill or preheat a griddle, pan, or heavy-bottom skillet over high heat. Place the kabobs in the pan and cook, turning frequently, for 5 minutes or until gently browned and cooked through.

5. Pile the kabobs high on platters and serve immediately.

Main Course

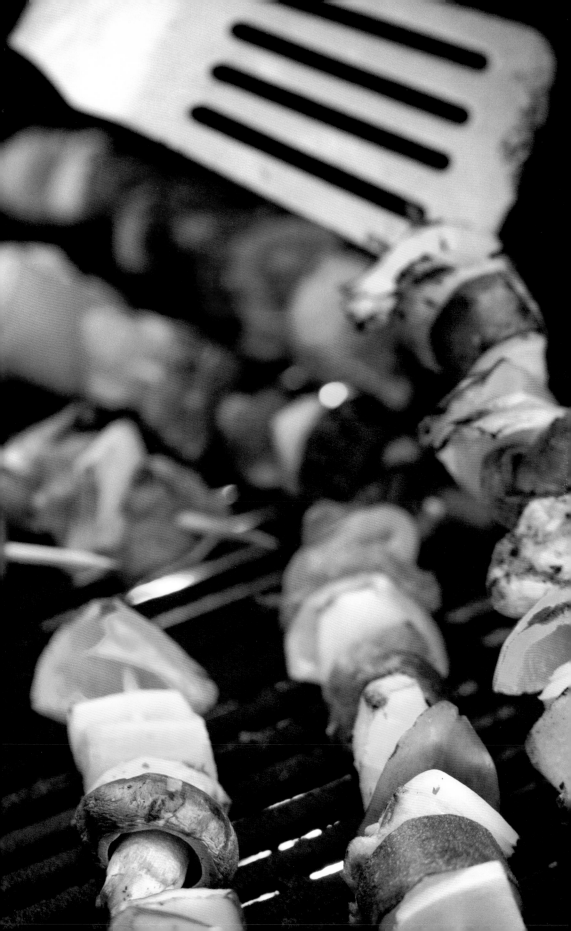

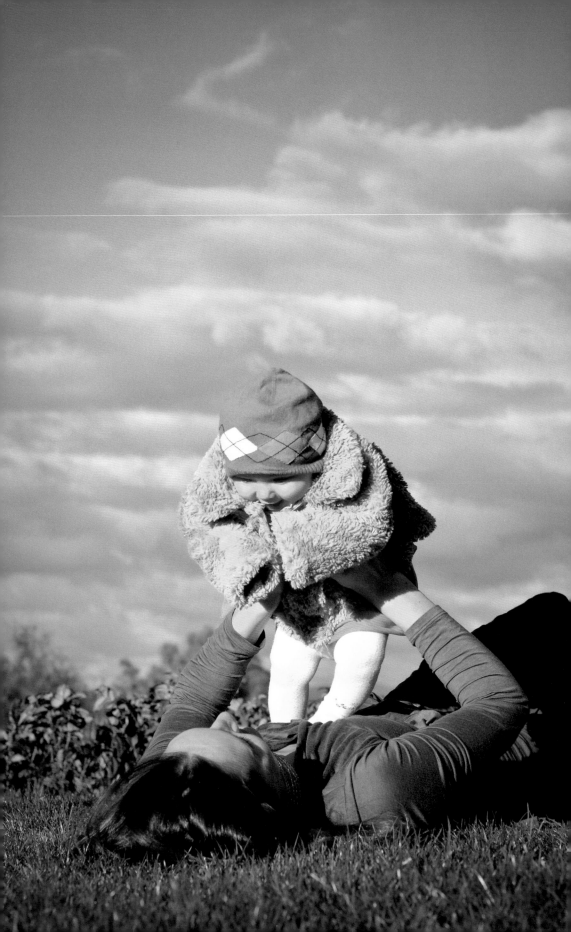

Nourishing Soup
Nutrition for Baby and Me

1 chicken breast, cubed and pan-fried

½ cup quinoa

½ onion, chopped, browned, and puréed

1 garlic clove, minced

1 tsp. parsley, dried

1 cup carrots, chopped

4 cups water

¾ cup cabbage, chopped

2½ tsp. sea salt

Prep: 7 min. Cook: 20 min. Serves: 2

1. In a two-quart saucepan, add all ingredients. Cook on medium-low for 20 minutes, covered.

2. Turn off heat and let stand for five minutes.

3. Enjoy!

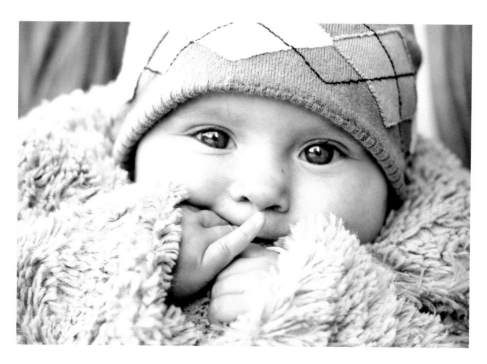

Thai Fish Cakes

I Love the Real Thai Flavors – So Fresh!

Fish Cakes

1 ½ cups crabmeat, freshly cracked, packed, and lightly shredded

1 to 2 Thai chilies, to taste, seeded and finely chopped

2 green onions, finely chopped

½ cup zucchini, finely chopped

⅓ cup carrot, grated

⅓ cup small yellow bell pepper, seeded and finely chopped

½ cup fresh bean sprouts, rinsed

1 tsp. ginger, freshly grated

1 T. cilantro, freshly chopped

1 tsp. basil, freshly chopped

1 T. mint, freshly chopped

2 eggs

1 to 2 T. olive oil

1 tsp. salt

4 T. bread crumbs

Sauce

⅓ cup lime Juice

¼ cup fish sauce

1 T. cilantro, chopped

1 tsp. ginger, grated

1. Mix all the fish cake ingredients together except for the eggs and oil. Whisk the eggs for 1 minute, then stir into the crab mixture. Then, using your hands, press about ¼ cup of the mixture together to form a fish cake.

2. Make the salsa by combining all the ingredients. Spoon into a bowl, then cover and let stand for 30 minutes, allowing the flavors to develop.

3. Heat 1 tablespoon of the oil in a cast-iron pan. Lay fish cakes in hot pan and cook in batches for 2 or 3 minutes on each side over medium heat until lightly browned. Be careful when turning them over. Remove and plate. Repeat until all the fish cakes are cooked, using more oil if necessary. Serve immediately with the sauce and salsa.

Salsa

1 Thai chili, seeded and finely chopped

½ cup cucumber, finely chopped

1 T. cilantro, freshly chopped

1 T. lime juice

1 T. Thai sweet chili sauce

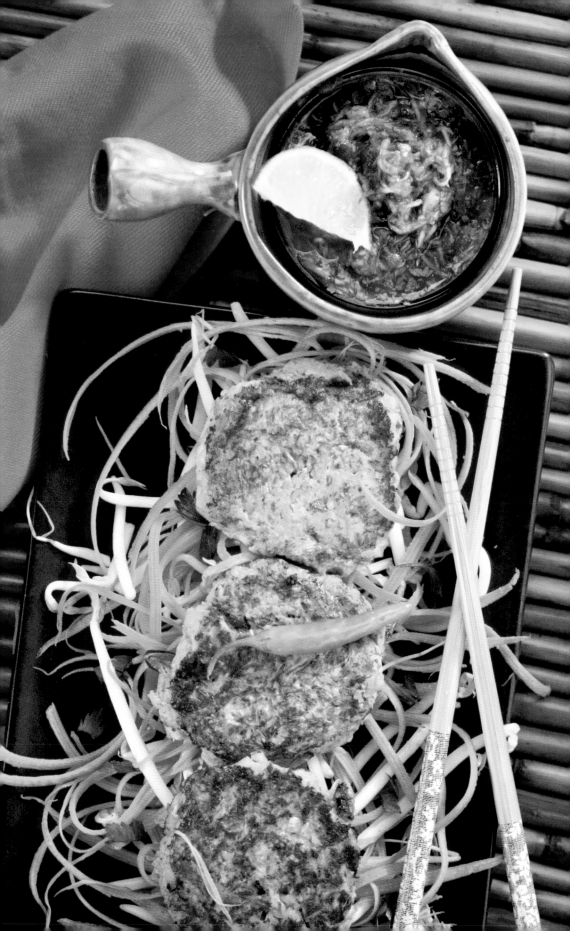

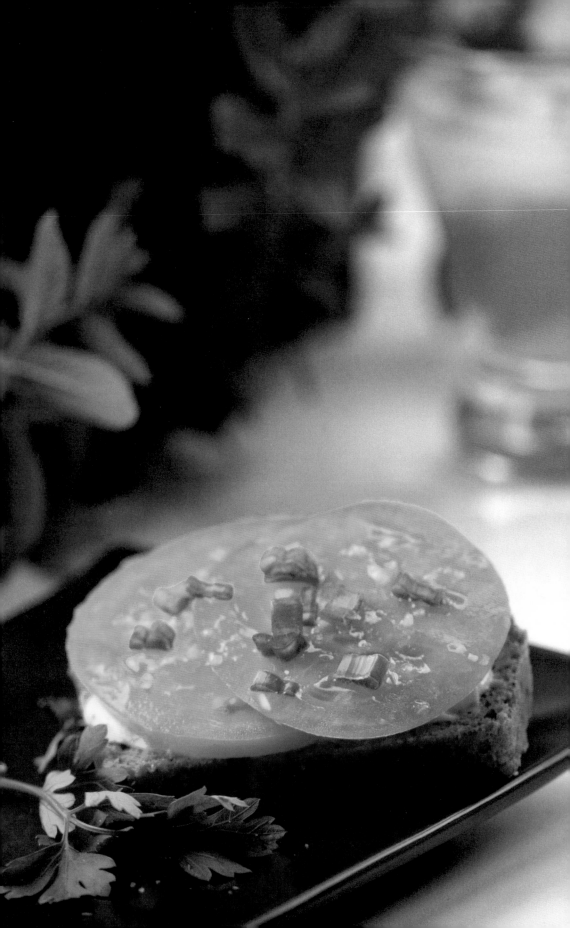

Tomato Sandwich

I Am Thirteen Again Eating This Sandwich.

4 slices **Scrumptious Sandwich Bread** (page 202)

2 T. Vegenaise

2 tomatoes, sliced

1 green onion, chopped

Sea salt, to taste

Parsley, as garnish

Prep: 5 min.   Serves: 4

1. Spread Vegenaise over one side of bread.

2. Lay tomatoes as desired on bread. Top with onions and salt. Garnish with parsley.

Tip From Shoshanna:

This is a great sandwich for a small meal. The bread has nut protein, giving you nutrition and energy.

Main Course

Salads

= Gluten-Free/Low-Casein or Casein-Free Recipe*

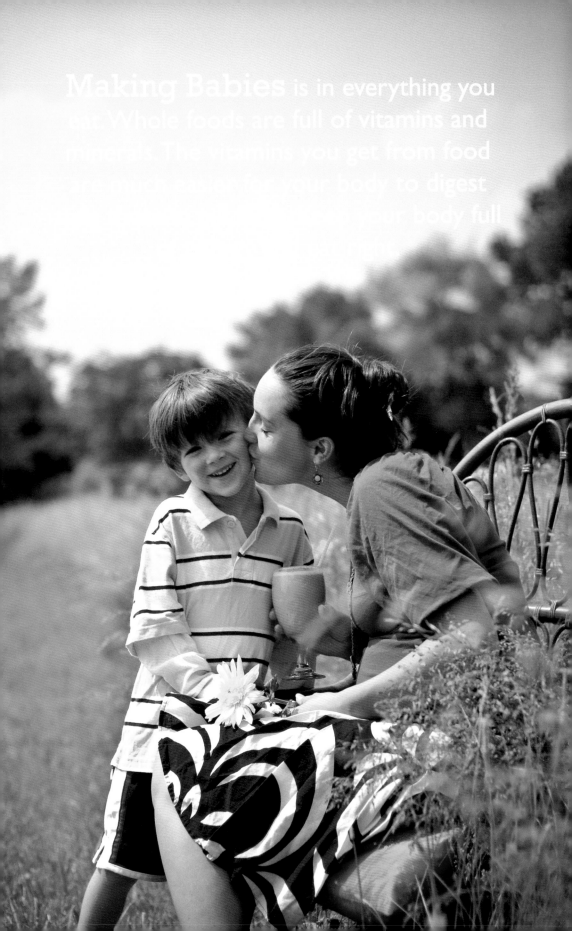

Making Babies is in everything you eat. Whole foods are full of vitamins and minerals. The vitamins you get from food are much easier for your body to digest your body full

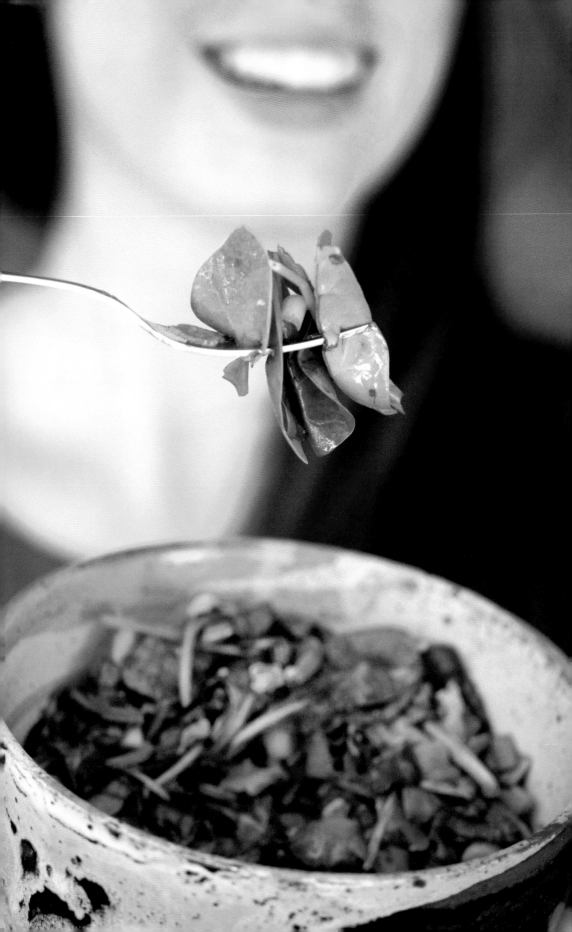

Bacon-Spinach Salad

This Is Some Tasty Iron. Yummy!

8 slices bacon, diced

¼ cup apple cider vinegar, with the mother

5 cups baby spinach

15 medium green onions, chopped

2 tsp. honey

½ tsp. sea salt

¼ tsp. black peppercorns, freshly ground

⅛ cup bleu cheese, crumbled

Prep: 15 min. Cook: 10 min.   Serves: 4

1. Cook bacon in a skillet over medium heat, stirring occasionally, until crisp.

2. Pour off most of the bacon grease. Mix in apple cider vinegar and heat completely; remove from heat.

3. Add spinach and onions to bacon mixture. Top with honey, sea salt, and pepper. Toss until spinach is wilted. Crumble bleu cheese on top.

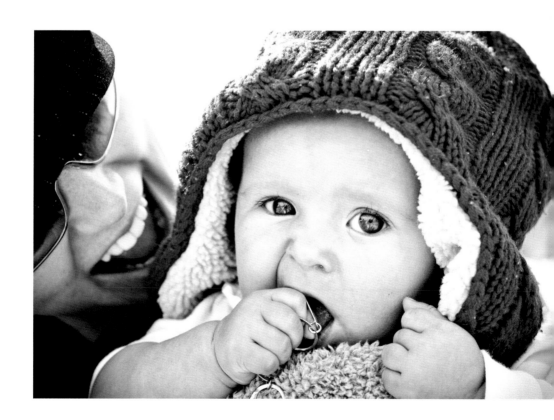

Black Bean Salad

This Is Summer Freshness in Your Mouth.

For a change of taste and pace, replace the traditional potato salad and slaw with this black bean salad.

3 ears corn, fresh

3 to 4 T. lime juice, freshly squeezed

1 T. lime zest, freshly grated

2 T. olive oil

1 T. red wine vinegar

1 tsp. sea salt

½ tsp. pepper, freshly ground

⅛ cup mint, freshly chopped

2 15-oz. cans black beans, rinsed and drained

2 large tomatoes, seeded and chopped

3 jalapeño peppers, seeded and chopped

1 small purple onion, chopped

1 avocado, peeled, pitted, and chopped

¼ cup cilantro, freshly chopped

Prep: 10 min. Cook: 2 hours   Serves: 6-8

1. Roast corn on open flames of gas stovetop or grill, constantly turning until evenly roasted, about five minutes. Cut corn from cob.

2. Whisk together the next 7 ingredients in a large bowl.

3. Add corn, beans, and remaining ingredients; toss to thoroughly coat.

4. Cover and chill for at least 2 hours.

Salads

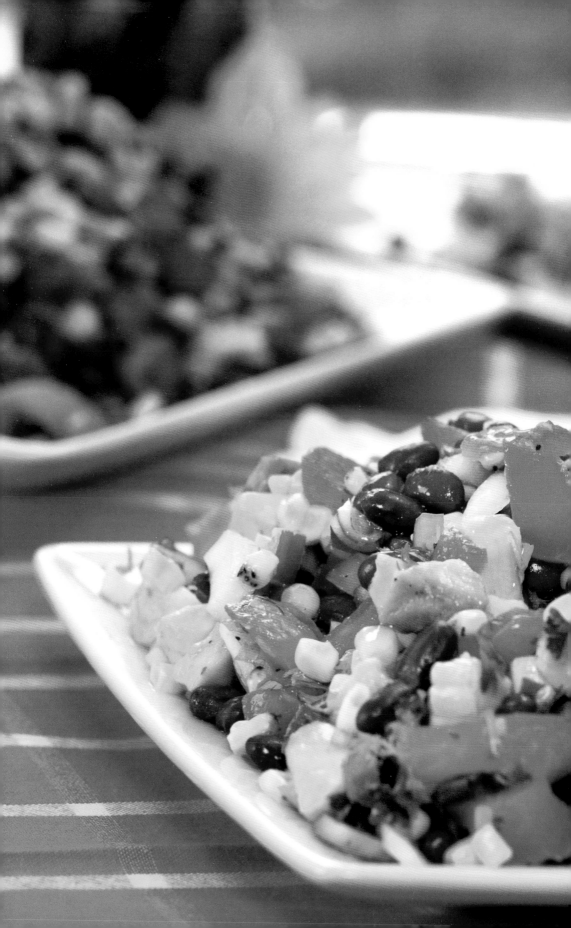

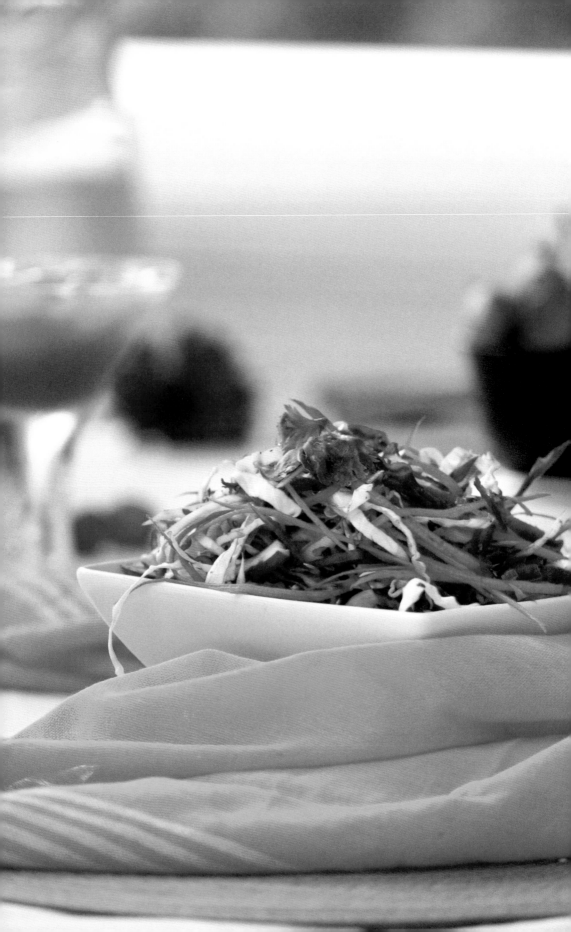

Costa Rica Slaw

Cabbage Is Good for Your Man!!!

½ head green cabbage, thinly sliced and chopped

½ head red cabbage, thinly sliced and chopped

1 medium carrot, peeled and grated

1 raw beet, peeled and grated

½ cup fresh cilantro, chopped

¼ cup olive oil

2 T. apple cider vinegar

1 tsp. raw honey

1 tsp. sea salt

½ tsp. pepper, freshly ground

½ cup mint, freshly chopped

Prep: 15 min.   Serves: 8

1. Combine the cabbage, carrot, beet, and cilantro in a large bowl.

2. Whisk together the olive oil, vinegar, honey, salt and pepper in a small bowl.

3. Spread dressing over the salad, toss, and serve.

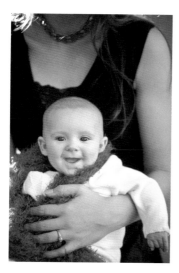

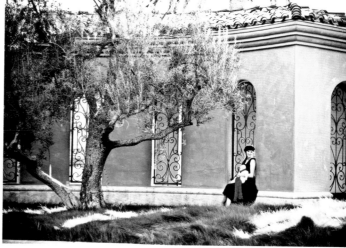

Curry-Mango Chicken Salad
Spicy and Sweet – Kind of Like Me!

2 chicken breasts, boneless and skinless

2 quarts water

½ tsp. pepper, fresh cracked

2½ tsp. curry powder

1¾ tsp. sea salt

Dash of coriander

Pinch or two of cayenne pepper (*optional*)

4 T. Vegenaise

1 cup pecans, chopped

1 cup mangoes, diced

¼ cup cranberries

⅓ cup celery, diced

Prep: 30 min.   Chill: 1 hr.   Serves: 6

1. Boil chicken breasts in water, covered, for 20 minutes or until thoroughly cooked. Remove chicken and let cool. Save broth for soup or another use.

2. Cube cooled chicken. Chill in refrigerator for one hour.

3. Mix pepper, curry powder, salt, coriander, cayenne, and Vegenaise together.

4. Pour over chicken and the rest of the ingredients and lightly toss. Serve in romaine lettuce as lettuce wraps or as sandwiches on gluten-free bread.

Making babies is art.

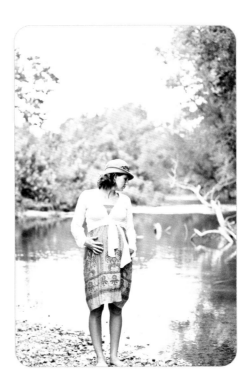

Salads

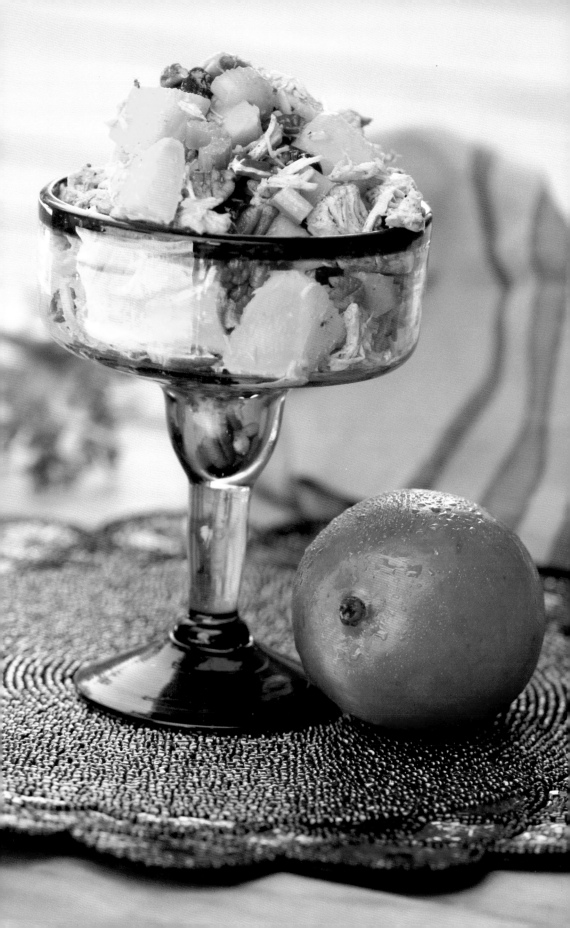

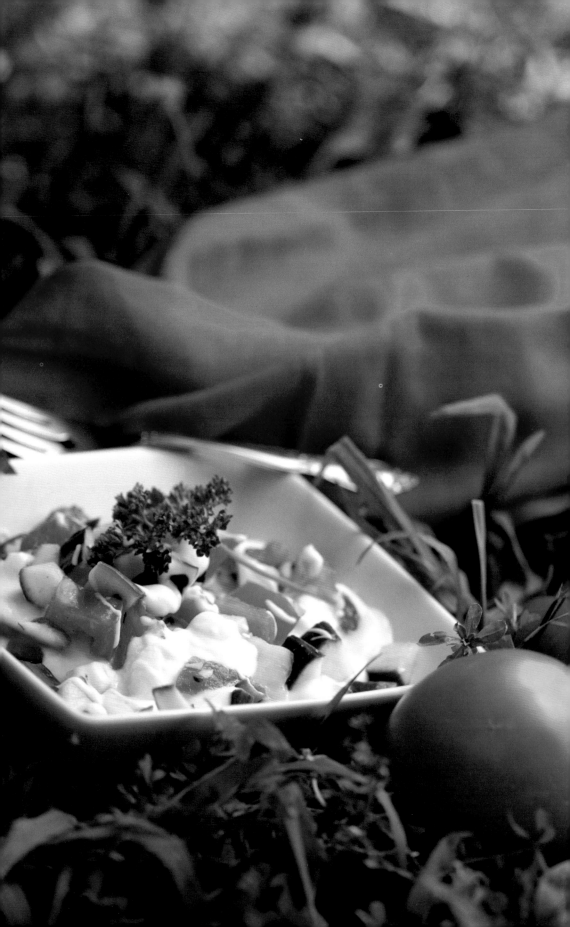

Cucumbers and Tomatoes in Yogurt

Summer Is Here When You Eat This.

1 medium cucumber

1 T. green onion, chopped

½ tsp. sea salt

¾ cup tomatoes, chopped

1 T. cilantro or parsley, freshly chopped

¼ tsp. ground cumin

dash of pepper, freshly ground

½ garlic clove, minced

½ cup plain yogurt

Prep: 20 min. Chill: 40 min. Yield: 2 cups

1. Cut cucumber lengthwise; scoop out seeds. Chop cucumber.

2. Mix cucumber, onion, and salt; let stand 15 minutes. Stir in tomato.

3. Mix remaining ingredients except yogurt; toss with cucumber mixture. Cover and refrigerate for 40 minutes to blend flavors.

4. Drain completely. Just before serving, stir in yogurt.

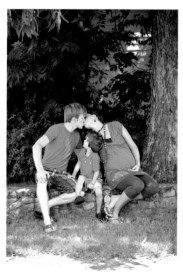

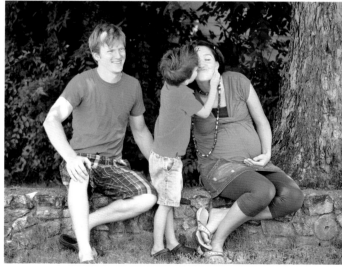

Salads

House Salad

Happy, Healthy and More Energy!

8 cups mixed salad greens of choice

2 cups mixed fresh vegetables of choice, chopped

½ small purple onion, sliced thinly

3 cups chicken, cooked and coarsely chopped or cooked ham, cubed

1 cup mozzarella cheese, cubed

1 large avocado, peeled and sliced

6 slices bacon, cooked and crumbled

3 cups croutons

1 recipe **Cashew Ranch Dressing** (page 300)

Croutons

3 cups bread of choice, cubed

1 T. parsley, freshly chopped

3 garlic cloves, chopped

1 tsp. sea salt

⅛ cup olive oil

Prep: 15 min.   Serves: 6

1. Toss together first 3 ingredients.

2. Top with chicken, cheese, and avocado slices. Sprinkle with bacon and croutons.

3. Serve with ranch dressing.

Croutons

1. Mix together all ingredients exept olive oil. Drizzle olive oil over mixture.

2. Bake at 375° F for 10 minutes.

Salads

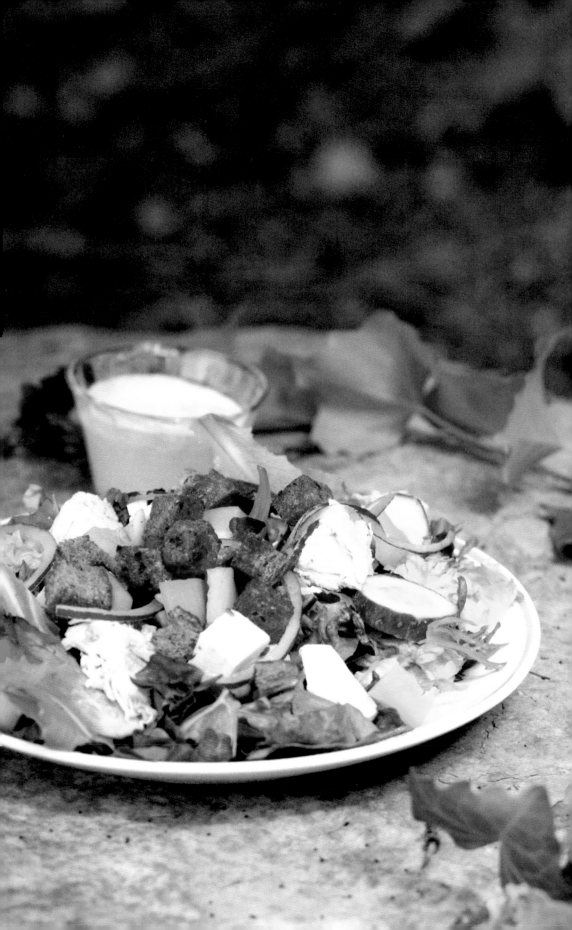

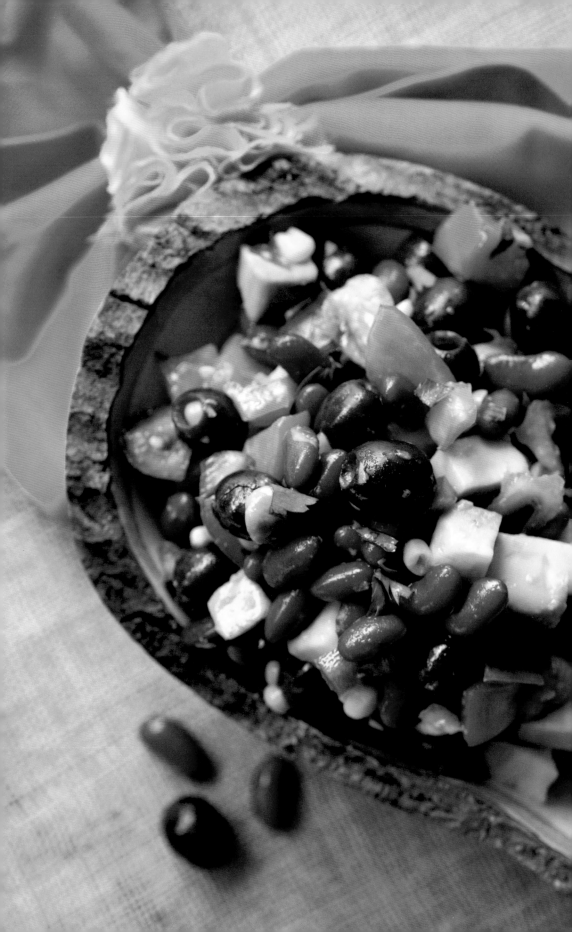

Eat Outdoors Salad
Go on a Picnic With Your Man.

Salad

1½ cup dark red
kidney beans (15-oz. can),
cooked

1 cup avocado, chopped

1 cup tomatoes, chopped

½ cup bell peppers, diced

1 cup black olives

1 fresh cob of corn

1 T. parsley, freshly chopped

Dressing

¼ cup olive oil

½ cup lime juice

1½ tsp. sea salt

½ tsp. rosemary

½ tsp. peppercorns, freshly
cracked

1½ tsp. lime zest, freshly
grated

Prep: 10 min. Cook: 5 min.   Serves: 6

1. Roast cob of corn over open flames on a stovetop or grill, continually turning corn until roasted (about 5 minutes). Cool and cut corn off cob.

2. Combine all ingredients in a salad bowl.

Dressing

1. Combine all dressing ingredients in a jar and shake until well combined.

2. Pour over salad, then toss and serve.

Salads

Go to Greece Salad

Salad

5 cups spinach, torn into bite-size pieces

4 cups Boston lettuce, torn into bite-size pieces

½ cup feta cheese, crumbled

¼ cup chives, sliced

24 olives, pitted

3 medium tomatoes, cut into wedges

1 medium cucumber, sliced

1 recipe **Lemon Dressing** (page 294)

Prep: 20 min. Serves: 8

Salad

1. Combine all salad ingredients in a salad bowl.

2. Pour dressing over salad, toss, and serve.

Salads

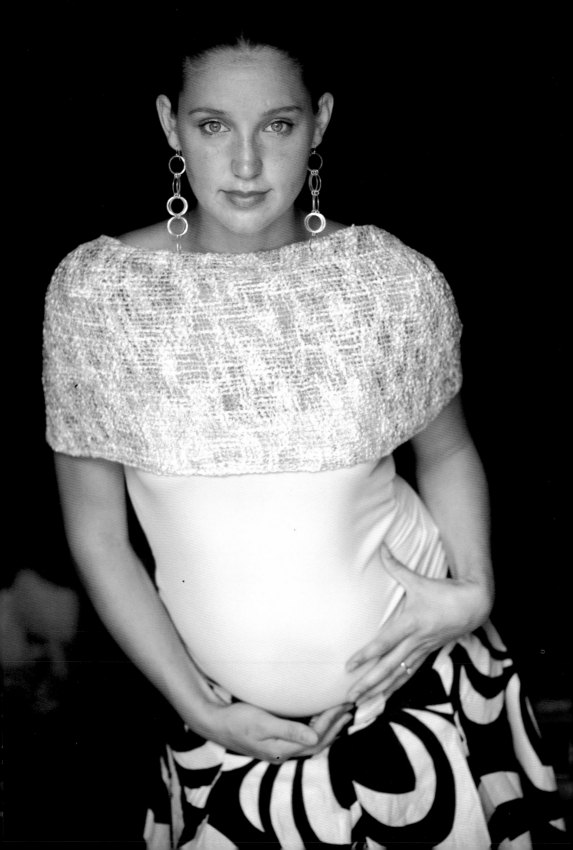

Lemon Dressing
Fresh Lemon Zest Makes Me Happy.

¼ cup grapeseed oil or olive oil

2 T. lemon juice, freshly squeezed

1 tsp. lemon zest, freshly grated

½ tsp. honey

1 ½ tsp. Dijon mustard

¼ tsp. sea salt

⅛ tsp. peppercorns, freshly ground

Prep: 10 min.   Yield: 1/3 cup

1. Shake all ingredients together in tightly covered jar until combined well.

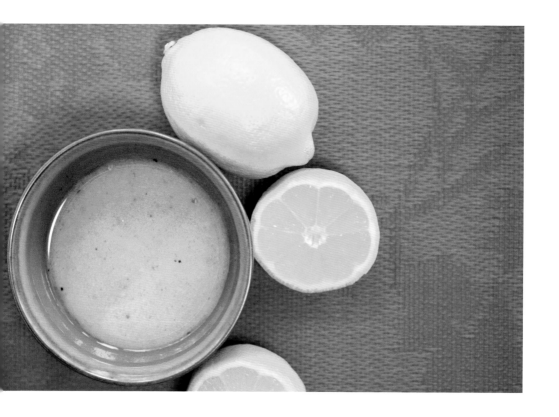

Lime-Cilantro Dressing
A Wonderful Taste of Mexico

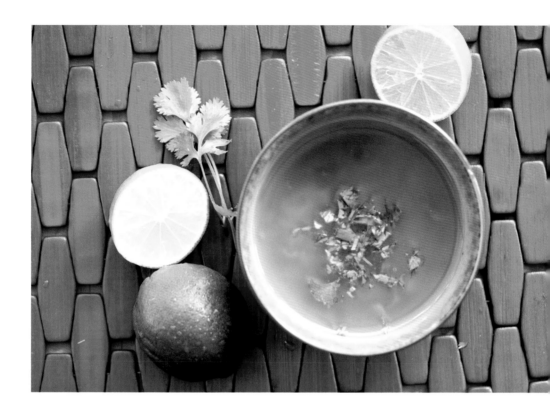

½ cup olive oil or grapeseed Oil

⅓ cup lime juice, freshly squeezed

1 tsp. lime zest, freshly grated

3 T. cilantro, freshly chopped

1½ tsp. ground cumin

1 tsp. sea salt

⅛ tsp. peppercorns, freshly ground

3 garlic cloves, minced

Prep: 10 min. Yield: 1 cup

Shake all ingredients in tightly covered jar until combined well.

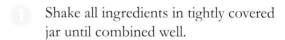

Salads

Lettuce Wraps
These Are Simply Wonderful.

Filling

3 T. coconut oil

3½ lbs. ground turkey

⅛ cup + 2 tsp. Bragg's Liquid Aminos

½ tsp. pepper, freshly ground

2 T. onion powder

1 tsp. sea salt

1 cup parsley

1½ cups cilantro

½ cup basil, chopped

½ cup mint, chopped

1 cup green onions, chopped

2 tomatoes, diced

2-5 garlic cloves, minced

1 cup bean sprouts

Asian Cucumbers

1 cucumber

1 tsp. honey

¼ cup water

1 tsp. sea salt

¼ cup apple cider vinegar (with the mother)

1 tsp. sesame seeds

Sauce

½ cup lime juice

3 T. fish sauce

2 T. cilantro, chopped

1 red Thai pepper, diced

Other Toppings

1 cup carrots, shredded

1 lime, sliced

Leafy or romaine lettuce

Prep: 15 min. Cook: 10 min. Serves: 6-8

Filling

1. Put oil in a pan. Cook turkey. Add Bragg's Liquid Aminos and pepper.

2. In a bowl, add cooked meat, onion powder, and next 8 ingredients. Mix together. Lightly stir in bean sprouts.

Asian Cucumbers

1. Peel stripes, lengthwise around cucumber. Cut cucumber in half, lengthwise and de-seed it with a spoon. Slice cucumber thinly. Combine honey, water, salt, and vinegar and pour over cucumbers. Let cucumbers sit for 30 to 45 minutes. Pour liquid off and add sesame seeds.

Sauce

1. Mix all ingredients.

Serve filling with Asian cucumbers, sauce, carrots, and lime on side. Use lettuce as wraps, soft-taco style.

Salads

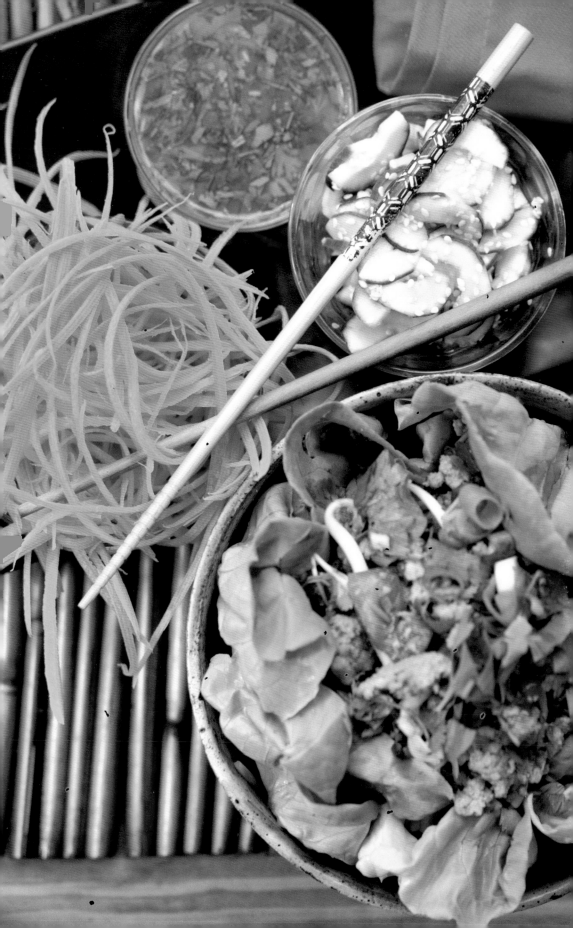

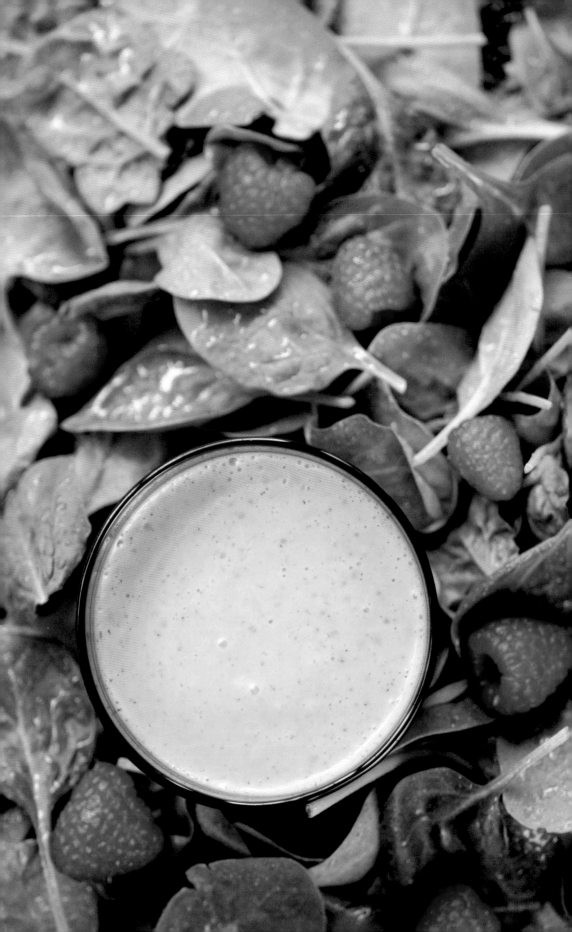

Raspberry Vinaigrette
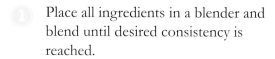
Better for You Than Anything You Can Buy

¾ cup olive oil

¼ cup apple cider vinegar, **Berry Herbal Brew** (page 12) or raspberry vinegar

1 tsp. sea salt

2 T. raw honey

1 tsp. dried basil

½ cup red raspberries, fresh or frozen

¼ cup water

Prep: 5 min. Yield: 1½ cups

1. Place all ingredients in a blender and blend until desired consistency is reached.

Store extra dressing in the refrigerator for up to 2 weeks.

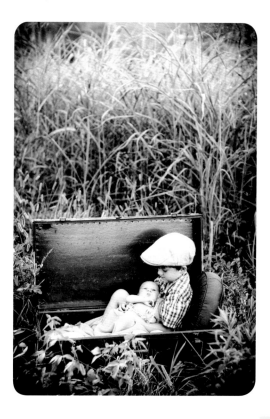

Jeremiah James takes good care of Penelope Jane.

Salads

Cashew Ranch Dressing

This Is One of My Husband's Favorites.

¾ cup cashews

½ cup water, boiling

2 T. lemon juice

¼ cup apple cider vinegar

3 T. olive oil

½ tsp. sea salt

1 T. garlic powder

1 T. onion powder

3 T. basil, freshly minced

3 T. dill, freshly minced

Prep: 2 hours Yield: 1 cup

1. Pour boiling water over cashews and soak 2 hours or overnight in the refrigerator. Drain water from cashews.

2. Combine all ingredients in a blender or food processor and blend until it reaches a smooth texture. You can also use this as a delicious dip.

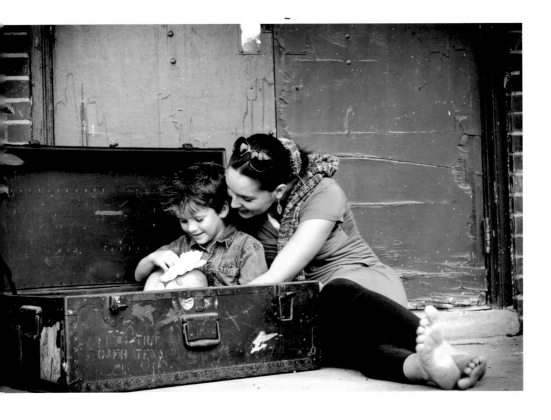

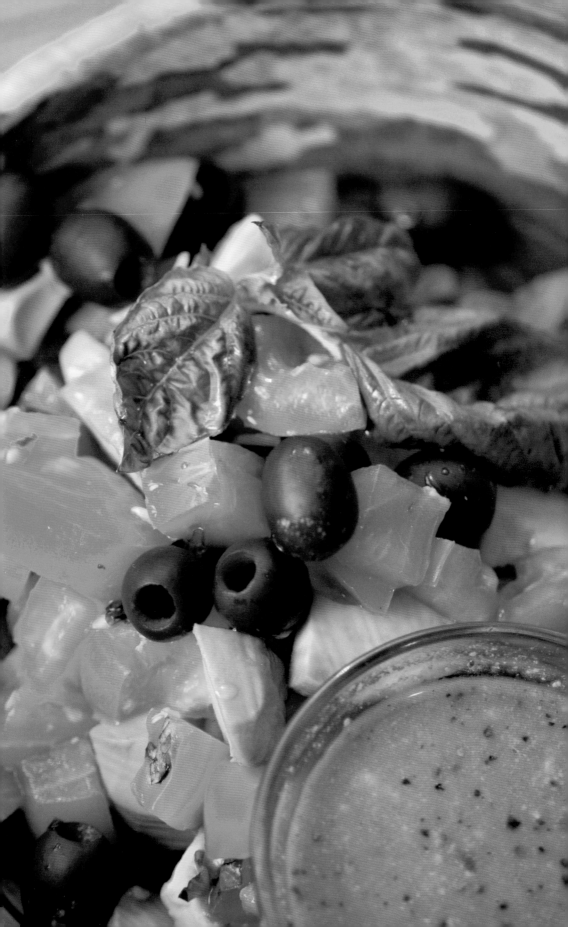

Tomato-Avocado Salad
Avocados Are Great for Your Baby's Brain.

Salad

2 beefsteak tomatoes

2 avocados, pitted, peeled, and sliced

1 handful fresh basil leaves, torn into pieces

20 black olives

Fresh crusty bread, to serve on the side, (*optional*)

Mozzarella cheese (*optional*)

Dressing

4 T. olive oil

1½ T. red wine vinegar

1 tsp. coarse grain mustard

Sea salt

Pepper, freshly ground

Prep: 8 min. Serves: 4

Salad

1. Cut tomatoes into thick wedges and place on a large platter.

2. Arrange the sliced avocado with the tomatoes.

3. Drizzle dressing over salad.

4. Sprinkle the basil and olives over salad and serve at once with fresh, crusty bread.

Dressing

1. Whisk together all ingredients.

Salads

Sauces and Condiments

🌿 = Gluten-Free/Low-Casein or Casein-Free Recipe*

Making Babies organically is not easy when it comes to condiments and sauces. They are so full of corn syrup, dyes and preservatives it is crazy. Now you can make some delicious recipes and feed both of your bodies organically.

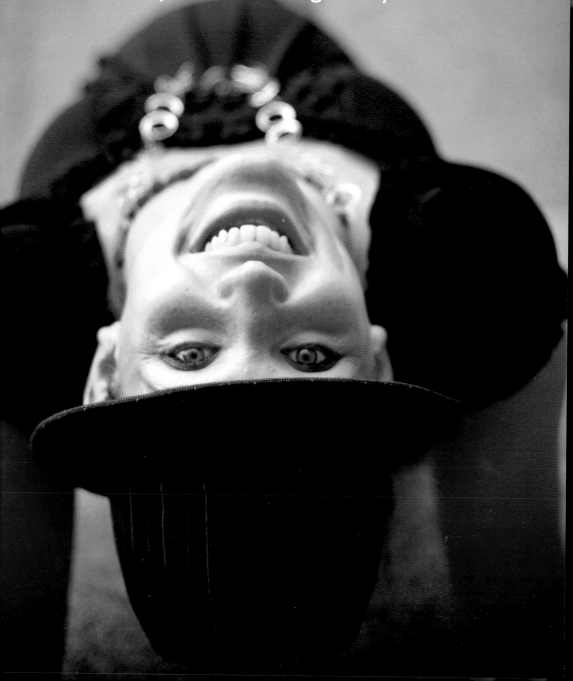

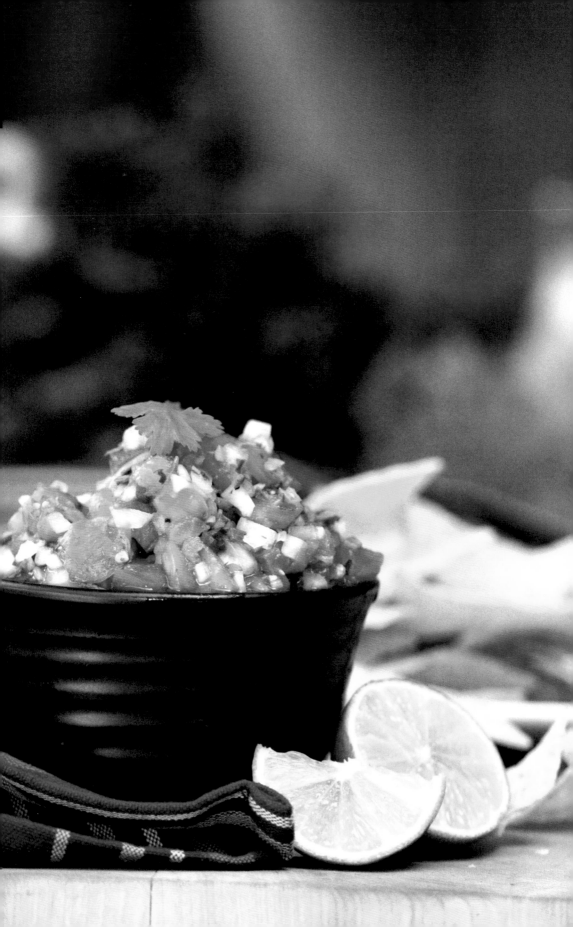

Fresh Tomato-Cilantro Salsa
A Perfect Blend of Flavors

5 firm, vine-ripened tomatoes, diced

⅓ medium onion, finely chopped

⅓ bunch cilantro, chopped

½ jalapeño chili pepper, diced

1 garlic clove, minced

1 lime, juiced

¼ tsp. ground cumin

½ tsp. sea salt

½ tsp. pepper, freshly ground

Prep: 10 min.   Yield: 2 cups

1. Combine the tomato, onion, cilantro, jalapeño, and garlic in a medium bowl.

2. Stir in the lime juice, cumin, salt, and pepper to taste.

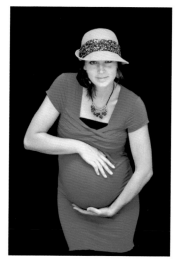

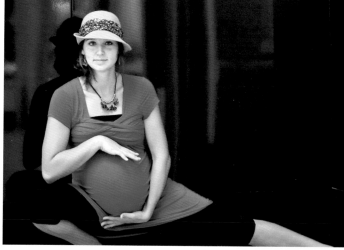

Guacamole
Great on Veggies, Chips, Sandwiches and More

2 avocados, pitted and peeled

1 lime, juiced

¼ tsp. lime zest

4 T. firm tomato, diced

1 T. cilantro, chopped

2 tsp. onion, diced

½ garlic clove, minced

½ tsp. jalapeño chili pepper, minced

Sea salt

Pepper, freshly ground

Prep: 10 min.   Yield: 1 cup

1. Coarsely mash the avocado in a bowl.

2. Add the rest of the ingredients and gently stir to combine.

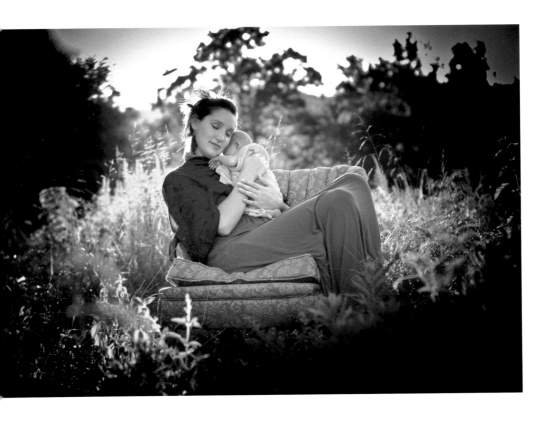

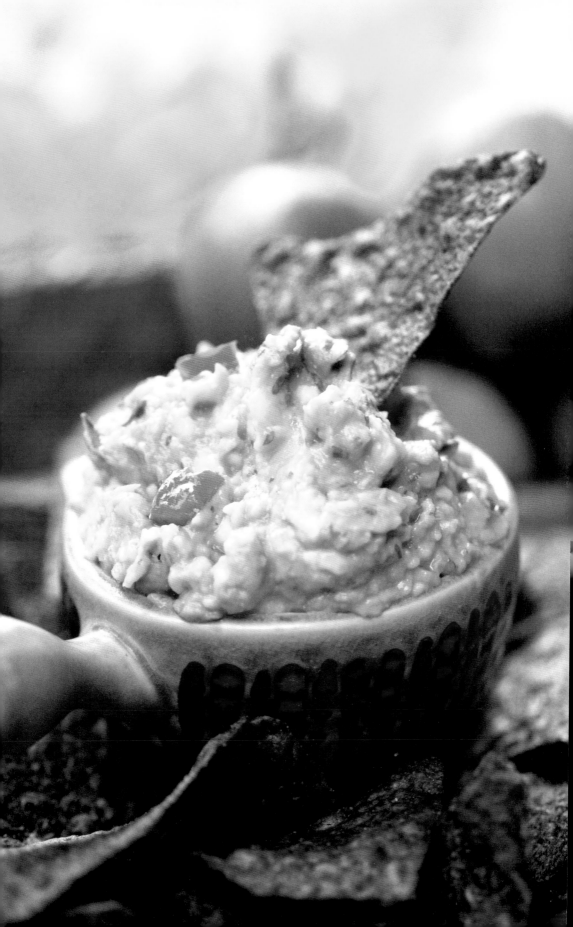

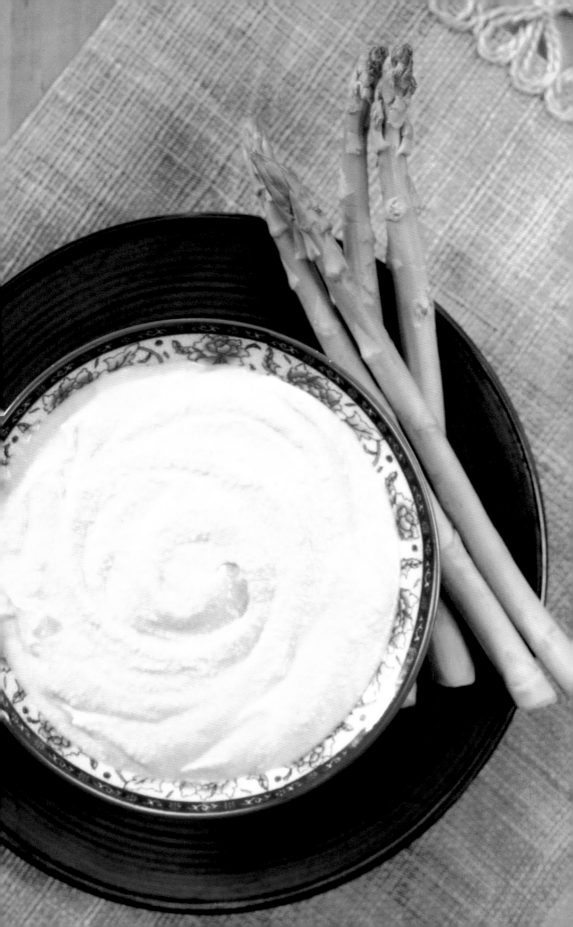

Hummus

Eat Good Food and Make a Healthy Baby.

This hummus is multi-purpose and can be used as a dip, spread, salad addition, or as a sandwich filling.

15-oz. can garbanzo beans (chickpeas), drained and liquid reserved

½ cup sesame seeds

1 garlic clove, halved

3 T. lemon juice

1 tsp. sea salt

Parsley, freshly chopped

Prep: 8 min.   Yield: 2 cups

1. Place reserved bean liquid, sesame seeds, and garlic in a food processor. Cover and blend on high speed until mixed.

2. Add beans, lemon juice, and salt. Cover and blend on high speed, stopping blender occasionally to scrape sides, until it becomes a smoothie consistency.

3. Spoon into serving dish. Garnish with parsley. Serve with fresh, raw vegetables.

Hummus With Crudités
Perfect for an Afternoon Snack

6 oz. lentils or garbanzo beans, cooked

½ cup tahini (Omit if using lentils.)

2 garlic cloves

½ cup lemon juice

Sea salt

3 T. water

1 T. olive oil

Pinch of cayenne pepper

¼ cup cilantro, diced (*optional*)

1 tsp. jalapeño peppers, diced (*optional*)

Prep: 5 min. Cook: 20 min. Serves: 4

1. Drain and rinse garbanzos. Place them in a food processor with tahini, garlic, and lemon juice. Season to taste with sea salt. Process, gradually adding water, until smooth and creamy.

2. Scrape chickpea mixture into a serving bowl and make a hollow in the center. Pour olive oil into the hollow and sprinkle with cayenne, cilantro and jalapeños.

3. Serve hummus with your choice of crudités, such as raw vegetables or pita bread.

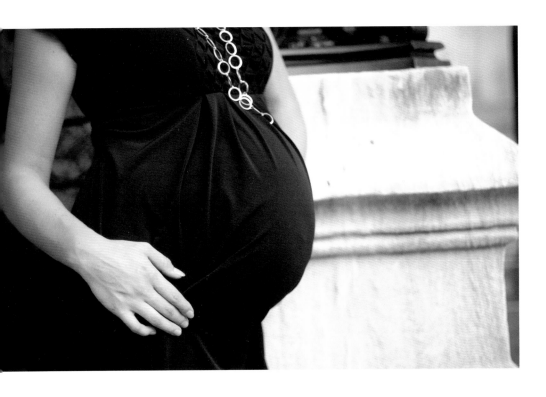

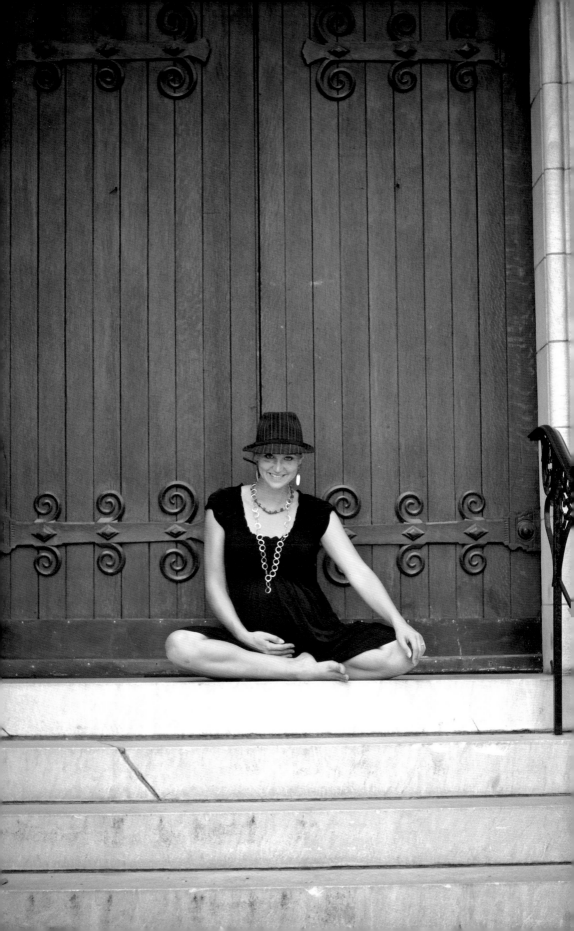

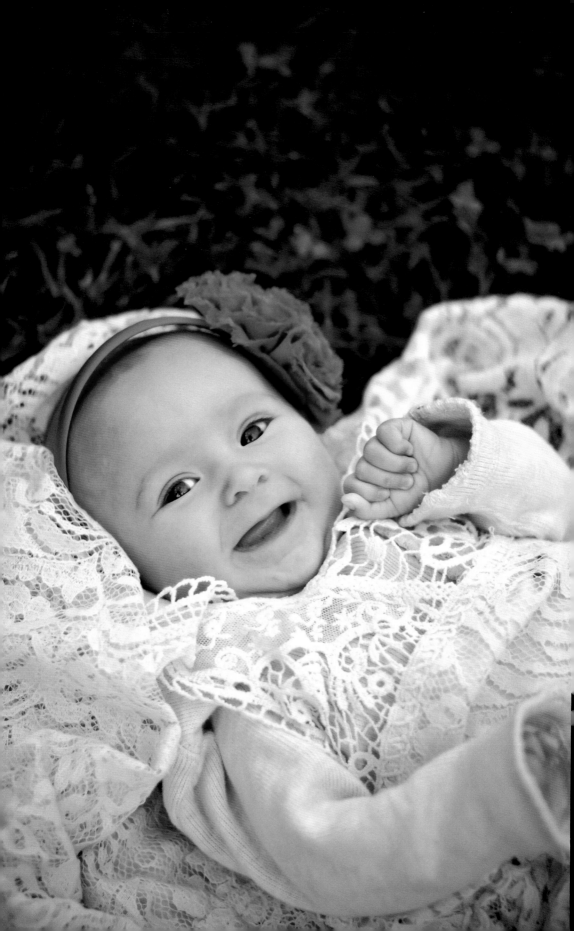

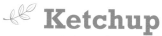

Ketchup

Ketchup That Brings You Up

½ cup sun-dried tomatoes

¼ cup raisins

about 1-2 cups water

½ cup apple cider vinegar (with the mother)

¼ cup onion powder

1 T. sea salt

½ cup extra water (*optional*)

Prep: 7 min. Yield: 1¾ cup

1. Soak sun-dried tomatoes and raisins in about 1-2 cups water for four hours.

2. Drain sun-dried tomatoes and raisins and purée all ingredients in a high-powered blender.

Store in refrigerator up to 10 days.

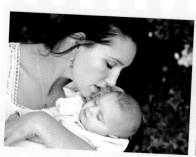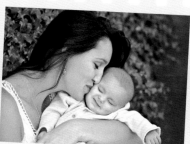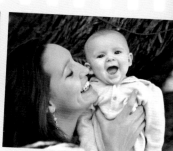

Babies are little people watching and learning from everything we do.

Sauces and Condiments

Original Pesto
Great for Your Heart

Pesto can be used in a variety of ways, whether with pasta, salad, meats, vegetables, or as a spread on sandwiches. Absolutely delicious.

2 cups firmly packed fresh basil leaves

¾ cup Parmesan cheese, grated

¼ cup pine nuts

½ cup olive oil or grapeseed oil

3 garlic cloves

½ tsp. sea salt

Prep: 10 min.   Yield: 1¼ cups

1. Place all ingredients in a blender or food processor. Cover and blend on medium speed for 2½ minutes or until smooth. Stop occasionally to scrape sides.

2. Use pesto immediately, cover and refrigerate for up to 5 days, or freeze for up to 1 month.

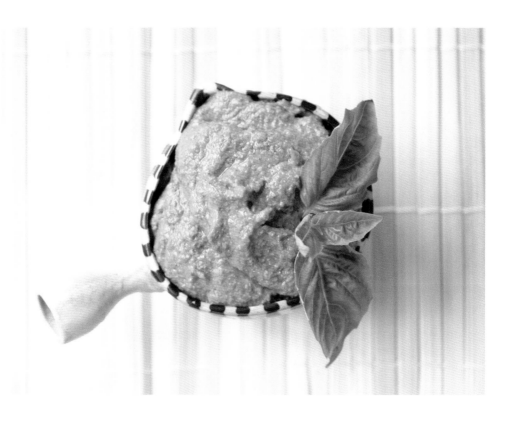

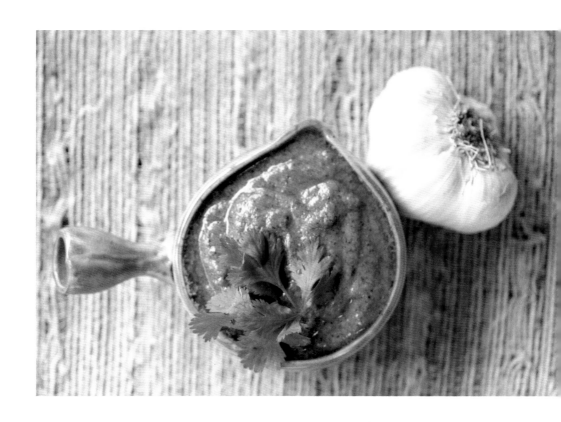

 # Pesto From Cilantro

Delicious Food With a Purpose

1 cup fresh cilantro leaves

1 large garlic clove

6 T. coconut oil, melted in a warm pan

2 T. lemon juice, freshly squeezed

1 cup walnuts

½ tsp. sea salt

Prep: 7 min.   Yield: 1¼ cups

Combine all ingredients in a blender or food processor; then serve as a dip or over chicken.

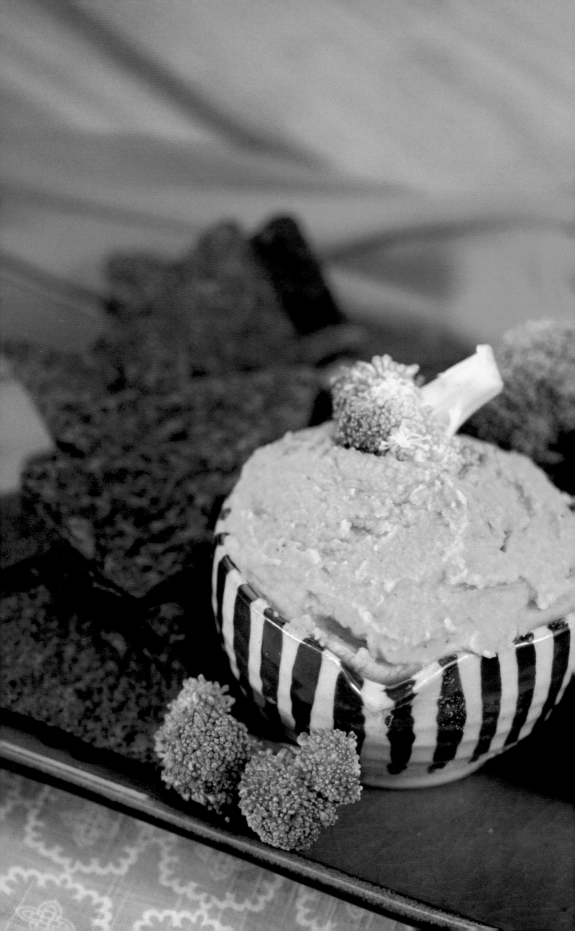

Red Lentil Dip

Simply Delicious and Healthy

2 tsp. olive oil

3 T. cilantro, chopped

2½ tsp. ground cumin

2 tsp. ginger, freshly grated

1 garlic clove, minced

1 cup red lentils, rinsed

1½ cups water

1 T. lemon juice, freshly squeezed

1 tsp. sea salt

Prep: 5 min.   Cook: 25 min.   Yield: 3 cups

1. Heat oil in a saucepan over medium-high heat. Add cilantro, cumin, ginger, and garlic. Sauté until the garlic just begins to brown.

2. Stir in the lentils and 1½ cups water and bring to a boil. Reduce the heat to medium-low, cover, and cook, stirring occasionally until the lentils are soft and the water is absorbed, approximately 15 minutes. Add an additional ¼ cup of water if the lentils don't become soft enough to mash.

3. Blend the lentils and stir in the lemon juice and salt.

4. Serve according to temperature preference.

Great with anything from veggies to crackers.

Vegetable Broth

Broth Gives You a Warmth, Inside and Out.

6 cups vegetables, coarsley chopped, such as: bell peppers, carrots, celery, leeks, mushroom stems, potatoes, spinach, zucchini

1 medium onion, coarsely chopped

½ cup parsley sprigs

8 cups cold water

Basil leaves, 2 T. freshly chopped or 2 tsp. dried

Thyme leaves, 2 T. freshly chopped or 2 tsp. dried

1 tsp. sea salt

¼ tsp. black pepper, freshly ground

4 garlic cloves, finely chopped

2 bay leaves

Prep: 20 min. Cook: 1 hr. 15 min. Yield: 8 cups

1. Heat all ingredients to boiling in a 4-quart stockpot; reduce heat. Cover and simmer 1 hour and 15 minutes, stirring occasionally.

2. Cool for 10 minutes. Strain broth through cheesecloth-lined sieve; discard vegetables and seasonings. Use broth on same day, or cover and refrigerate up to 24 hours or freeze for up to 6 months.

Sauces and Condiments

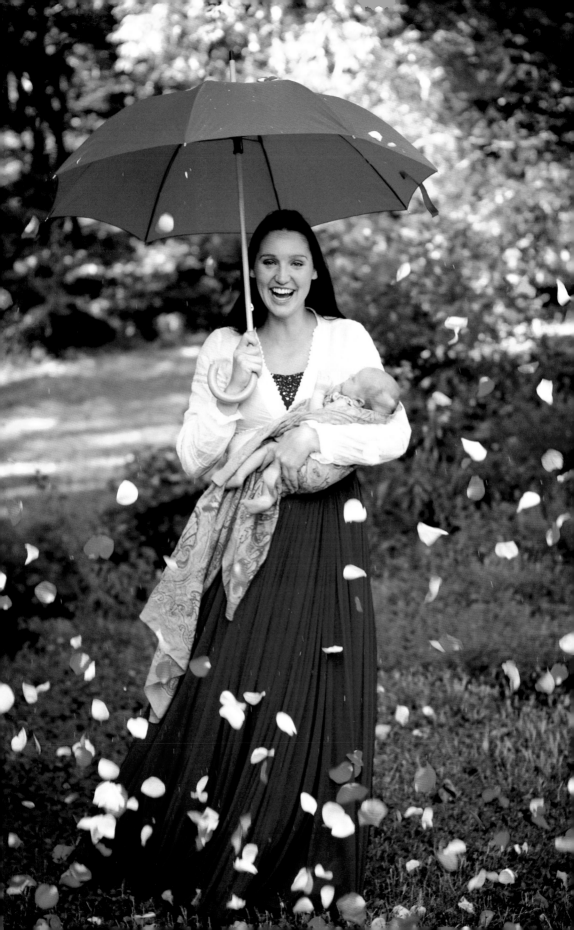

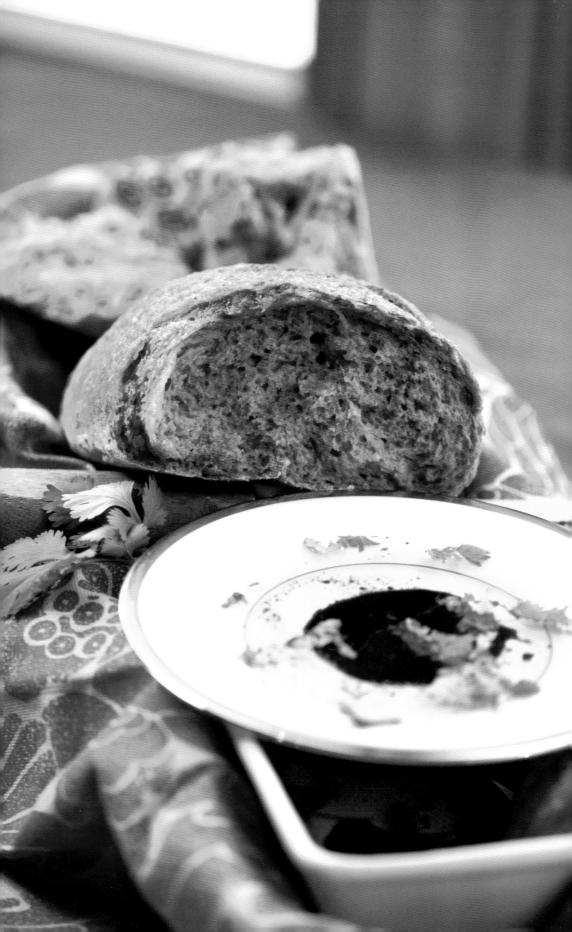

Vegetable or Bread Dip

½ cup extra virgin olive oil

¼ cup balsamic vinegar

⅛ cup fresh herbs, chopped

Prep: 3 min. Yield: 3/4 cups

1. Whisk together all ingredients, until combined.

2. Serve with bread or veggies of choice.

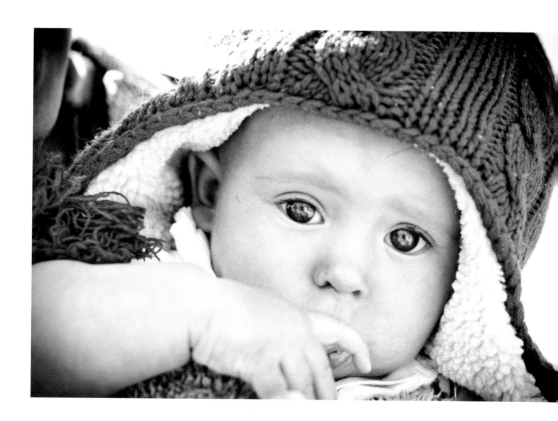

Vegetables and Side Dishes

Making Babies starts before
conception and goes through your
growing baby's life. You are building a baby.
That means cells, organs, blood, and life.
You are building something inside of you
that scientists can only dream of doing.

🌿 = Gluten-Free/Low-Casein or Casein-Free Recipe*

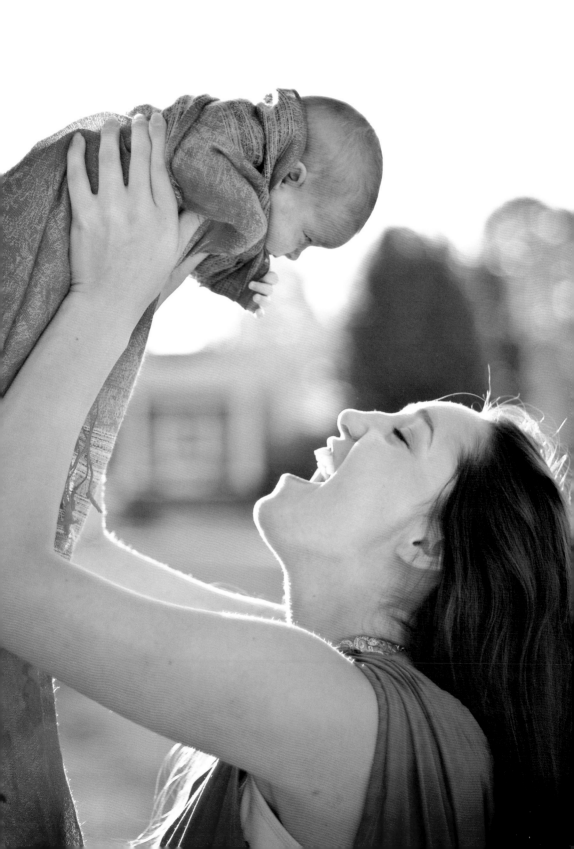

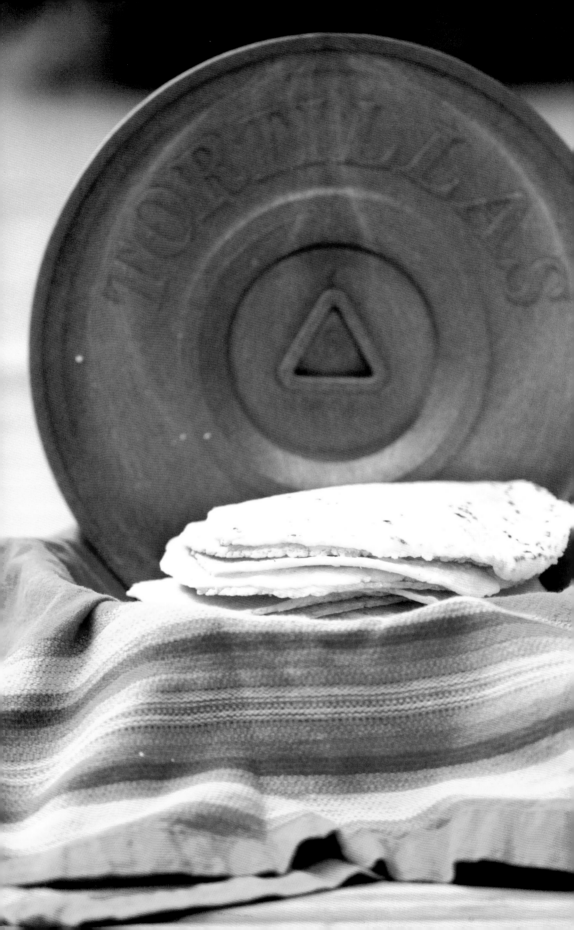

Fresh Corn Tortillas
Much Better Than Store-Bought!

2 cups corn masa flour

1 tsp. sea salt

1½ cups water, plus more if needed

Prep: 20 min.   Cook: 20 min.   Yield: 16 tortillas

1. Combine the masa flour and salt in a medium bowl, then add the water.

2. Using your hands, mix for about 2 minutes, or until the mixture forms a soft dough. Add more water if needed, 1 tablespoon at a time. The dough should be soft but not sticky, dry, or crumbly.

3. Divide and shape the dough into 16 equal balls.

4. Heat a pan or griddle over medium-high heat.

5. Cover each side of a tortilla press with plastic wrap and press each dough ball until it is 5 to 6 inches in diameter. Turn the flattened tortilla a quarter turn and press it again. Repeat this process until you've pressed the tortilla a total of four times, resulting in an evenly shaped tortilla. Also, you can roll out your tortilla with a rolling pin, in a similar fashion as the tortilla press.

6. Cook each tortilla on the heated griddle for about 1 minute on each side, or until cooked, but not crisp - causing it to easily break.

7. Store the cooked tortillas in a clean kitchen towel on a plate or a tortilla warmer to keep moist and warm until serving.

Hazlenut-Parmesan Asparagus

Asparagus Is So Good for You and Baby.

2 cups water

2 lbs. asparagus spears

2 T. butter

3 cups mushrooms, sliced

1 ½ tsp. basil leaves, freshly chopped or ½ tsp. basil leaves, dried.

¼ tsp. sea salt

¼ tsp. fresh pepper, coarsely ground

¼ cup Parmesan cheese, shredded

¼ cup hazelnuts, chopped

Prep: 15 min. Cook: 10 min. Serves: 8

1. Heat water to boiling in a 12-inch skillet. Add asparagus. Bring water back to a boil, then reduce heat to medium.

2. Cover and cook 5 minutes or until crisp-tender. Drain; set aside.

3. Melt butter in skillet over medium-high heat. Stir in mushrooms. Cook 2 minutes, stirring frequently until mushrooms are light brown.

4. Stir asparagus, basil, salt, and pepper into mushrooms until vegetables are coated with seasonings and asparagus is heated through. Sprinkle with Parmesan and hazelnuts.

Vegetables and Side Dishes

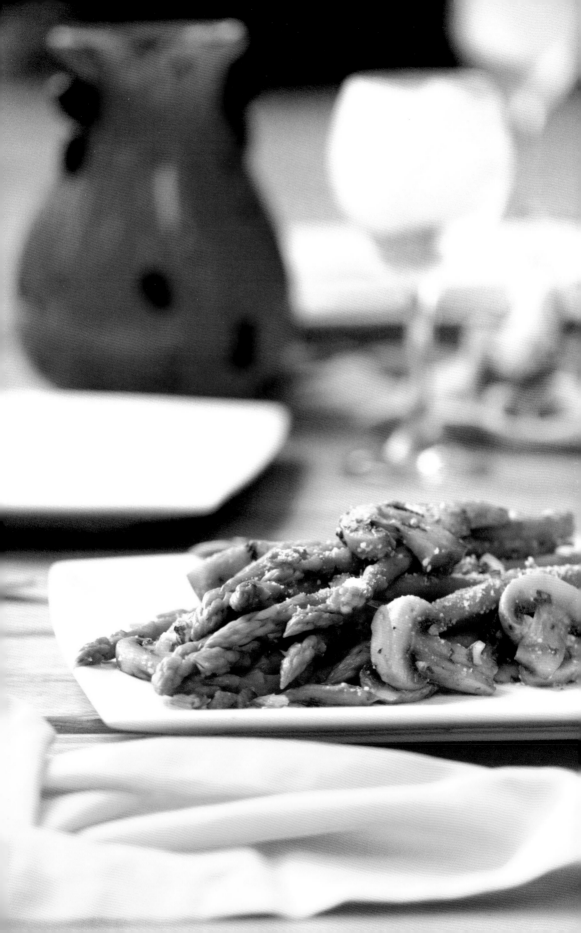

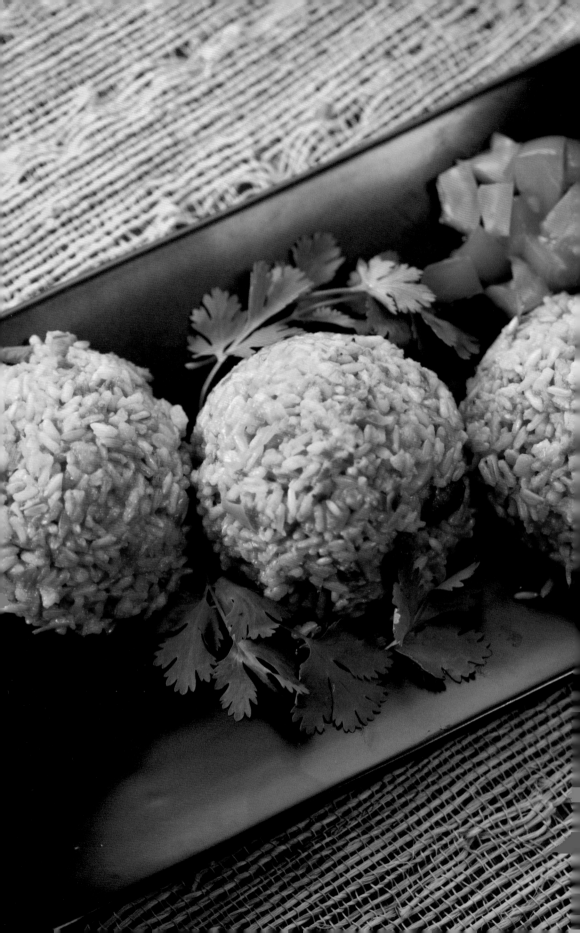

Mexican Rice

A Great Recipe for Cooking Good Food at Home

Recipes for Mexican rice can vary from cook to cook, but most agree on one thing: toast the rice in olive oil before adding a few spices and canned tomatoes (with the liquid).

1 cup brown rice

¼ cup olive oil

½ medium onion, diced

½ bell pepper, diced

1 garlic clove, minced

¾ cup tomatoes, freshly diced, or canned tomatoes, diced, no salt added (about half of a 14½-oz. can)

1¾ cups **Chicken Broth** (page 38) or **Vegetable Broth** (page 320)

1 tsp. sea salt

½ tsp. cumin

¼ tsp. turmeric

½ cup cilantro, chopped

Prep: 15 min. Cook: 45 min.   Serves: 6

1. Rinse the rice in cold water through a colander until the water runs clear.

2. Heat ⅛ cup of olive oil in a large saucepan over medium heat. Sauté onions, peppers, and garlic until tender, not mushy. Place in a separate dish.

3. Heat remaining olive oil. Add the rice and sauté until slightly toasted.

4. Add the sautéed vegetables, tomatoes, broth, salt, cumin, and turmeric to the rice, and stir to combine.

5. Cover, bring to a boil, and reduce the heat. Simmer for about 30-40 minutes without lifting the lid, until the rice is tender and the liquid is absorbed. Fluff with a fork, top with cilantro, and serve.

Vegetables and Side Dishes

Mixed Vegetable Bruschetta
A Great Way to Eat More Veggies

2 garlic cloves

3 T. olive oil

1 red bell pepper, halved and seeded

1 orange bell pepper, halved and seeded

4 thick slices baguette or ciabatta bread

1 fennel bulb, sliced

½ onion, sliced

2 zucchini, sliced diagonally

2 tomatoes, thinly sliced

Sea salt

Pepper, freshly ground

Fresh sage leaves, to garnish *(optional)*

4 T. **Original Pesto** (page 316)

Prep: 8 min. Cook: 10 min.   Serves: 4

1. Crush garlic in oil. Brush a grill pan with oil and preheat. Cut each bell pepper half lengthwise into 4 strips. Toast the bread slices in a toaster.

2. When the grill is hot, add the bell peppers and fennel and cook for 5 minutes, then add the onion and zucchini and cook for 5 more minutes until all the vegetables are tender but still with a slight crisp. Be sure not to have any vegetables topping one another.

3. Spread pesto on toast and lay the tomato halves on top. Place on warm plates. Place the grilled vegetables on top of the toast, drizzle with olive oil, and season with salt and pepper to taste. Garnish with sage leaves and serve immediately.

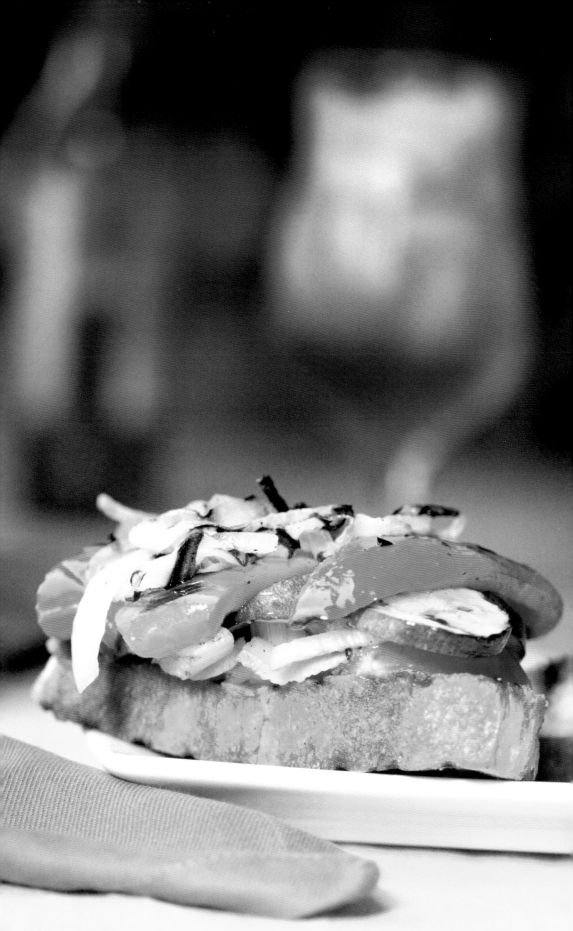

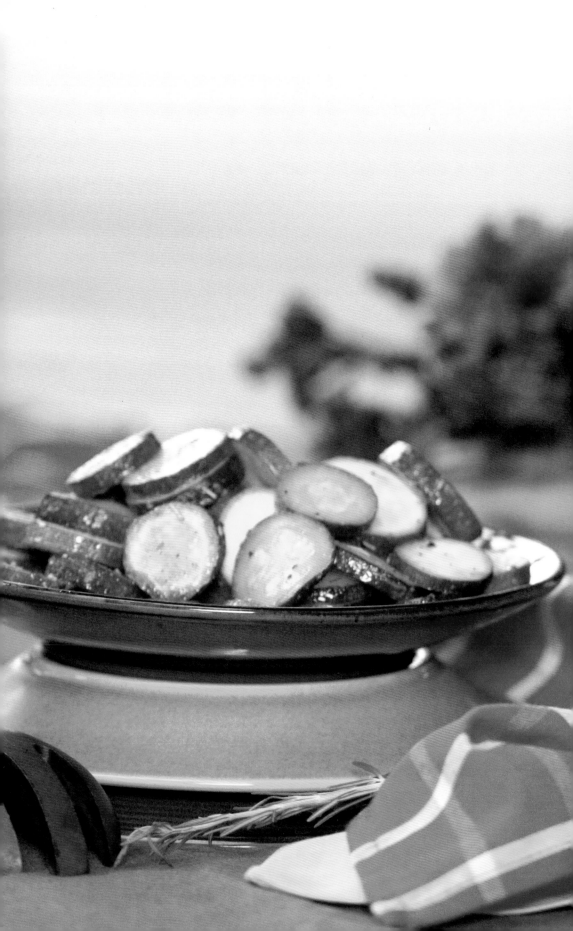

Rosemary Vegetables
These Flavors Work Really Well Together.

2 zucchini

2 T. butter

½ tsp. sea salt

½ tsp. onion powder

¼ tsp. rosemary, fresh or dried

¼ tsp. garlic, freshly minced

¼ tsp. pepper, freshly ground

1 T. water

Prep: 3 min. Cook: 8 min.   Serves: 4

1. Cut zucchini into ½-inch wide slices.

2. Combine all ingredients in a pan and heat on medium-high for 5 to 8 minutes or to desired tenderness.

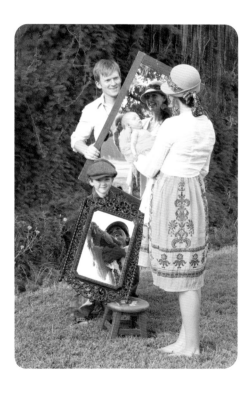

Our children are our reflections. Be something worth duplicating.

Sautéed Garlic and Mushrooms
High in Vitamin C and Great With Steak

2 T. butter

2 T. olive oil

2 garlic cloves, minced

½ tsp. sea salt

¼ tsp. pepper, freshly ground

1 lb. mushrooms, sliced

Chopped fresh parsley, if desired

Prep: 15 min. Cook: 5 min.   Serves: 4

1. Heat all ingredients except mushrooms and parsley in a 12-inch skillet over medium-high heat until butter is melted.

2. Stir in mushrooms.

3. Cook for 5 minutes, stirring frequently, until mushrooms are light brown. Sprinkle with fresh parsley.

Vegetables and Side Dishes

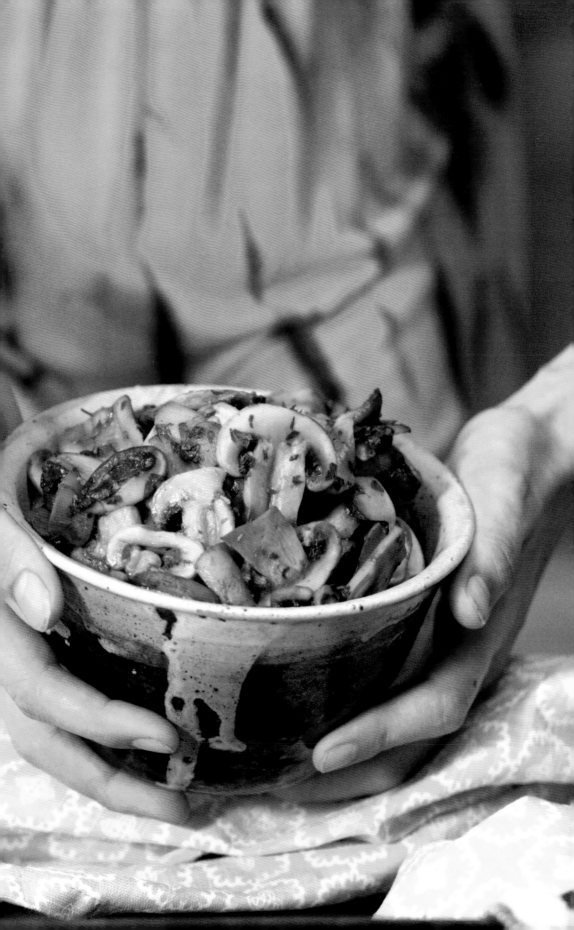

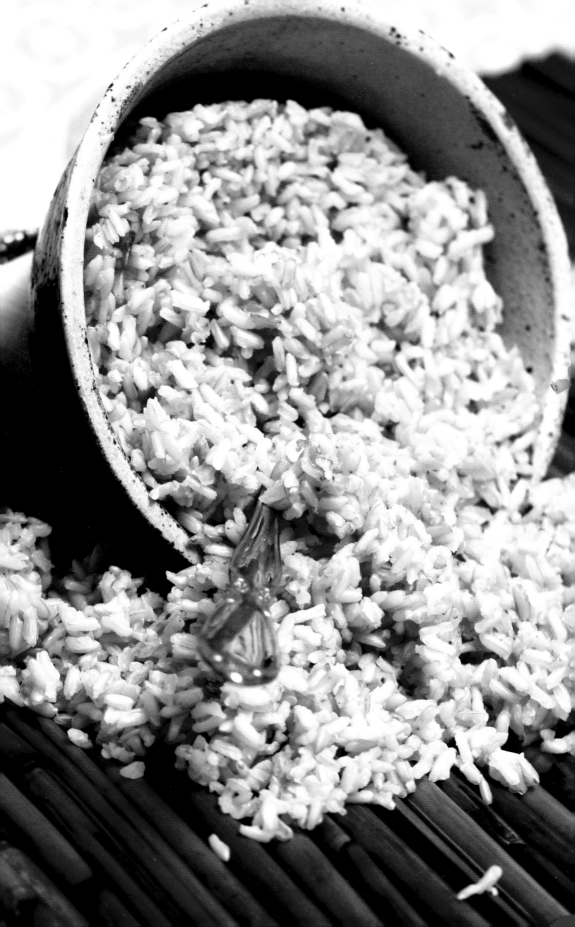

Simple and Basic Brown Rice
Dry Cooking the Rice First Gives It a Toasted Flavor.

1 cup brown rice

2½ cups water or broth

1 tsp. sea salt

Prep: 5 min. Cook: 50 min.   Serves: 4

1. To remove starch, rinse the rice thoroughly under cold water until water runs clear.

2. Dry sauté the rice in a skillet over medium heat until the grains are opaque. Meanwhile, combine the water and salt in a saucepan and bring to a boil over high heat.

3. Add the sautéed rice to the boiling water, reduce the heat to low and cover. Simmer for 45 minutes, or until the rice is tender and the liquid is completely absorbed.

4. Remove pan from heat and let sit covered for 10 minutes longer. Fluff the rice and serve.

For a richer flavor, replace the water with chicken broth.

Vegetables and Side Dishes

Simple Vegetables
A Wonderful Way to Eat Your Summer Veggies

12 pattypan squash, about 1 inch in diameter, sliced

2 medium red bell peppers, cut into 6 pieces

1 large red onion, cut into ½-inch slices

Salt, to taste

Pepper, freshly ground, to taste (*optional*)

Marinade

1 tsp. sea salt

½ tsp. pepper, freshly ground

¼-½ cup olive oil or butter

1 tsp. oregano or parsley, freshly chopped

Prep: 10 min. Marinate: 1 hour Grill: 15 min.
Serves: 6

1. Place squash, bell peppers, and onion in a large rectangular baking dish. Pour marinade over vegetables. Cover and marinate 1 hour.

2. Heat coals or gas grill for direct heat, or heat grill pan on stove top.

3. Remove vegetables from marinade; reserve marinade. Cover and grill vegetables over medium heat for 12-15 minutes, turning and brushing vegetables with marinade 2 or 3 times, until tender. Sprinkle with salt and pepper to taste.

Vegetables and Side Dishes

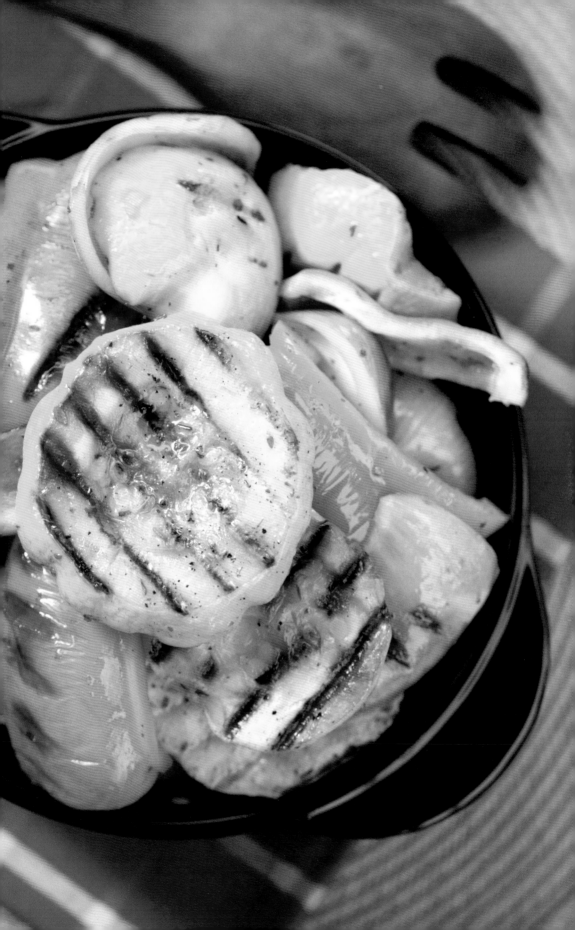

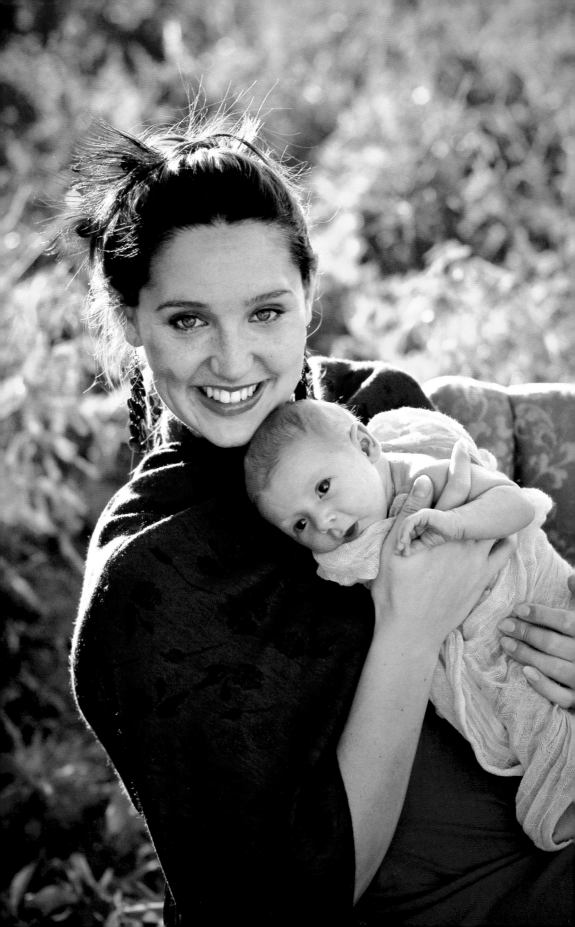

Did You Know?

Did you know that it is important that you learn about your own health? You know your body better than anyone else. What you eat and what you do, can make a world of difference. Be in charge of your own nutritional health. Learn and live well!

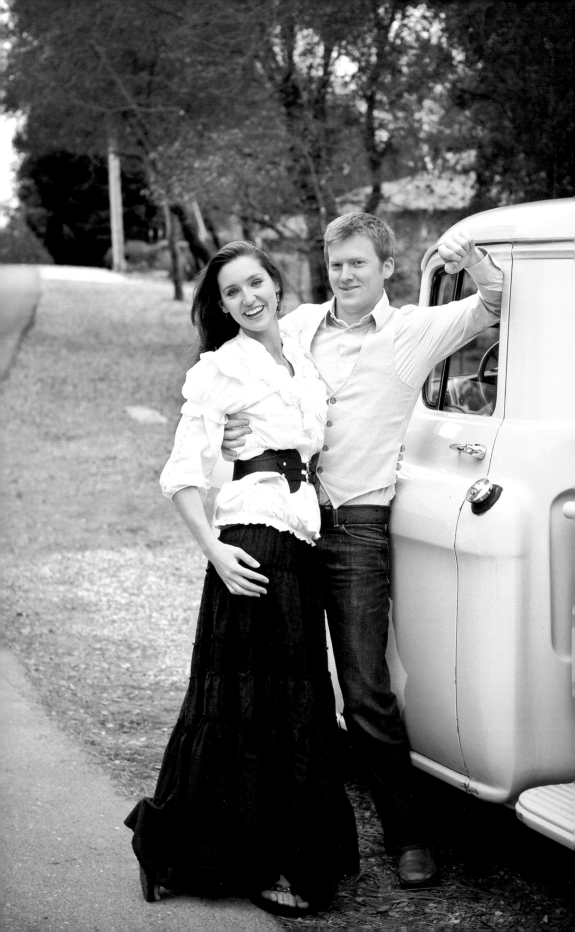

Fertility

When it comes to fertility, there are a few things that you should remember:

1. Drink water and unsweetened herb teas.
You need to stay hydrated. This will continually clean your body's filter, giving you a better chance of conception.

Herb teas that I like for fertility and through pregnancy are: peppermint, spearmint, lemongrass, ginger, red raspberry leaf, nettle, chamomile, and red rooibos. Also some of my favorite tea mixes from my store are: Mama's Red Raspberry Brew, Sleep Tight Tea, Rise and Shine, Double-E Immune Booster, and Very Berry. They are yummy and they make me feel great!

2. Eat right.
Your food fuels your body. Just as in a car, bad fuels can run your body down. The food you eat can hurt or help your chances of conception. Stay away from processed food, preservatives, and fried things. Eat whole foods, non-GMO, and organic as much as possible.

3. Exercise.
Exercise helps balance your body, levels out your hormones, de-stresses you, and gives you happy endorphins. You might be ready to make babies all night long.

4. Get plenty of sleep.
Sleep is very important. Plan on a good 8 hours or more every night. Your body needs rest to recharge, so drink a cup of chamomile tea and go to sleep.

5. Take vitamins.
Vitamins help complete your nutritional health. It is important to have all your vitamins, because your baby will need them, starting at conception. Vitamins can make a really big difference in your pregnancy, from getting pregnant to the health of your baby. Make sure you are taking folic acid, B-vitamins, and omega fatty acids. You can also talk to your nutritionist about prenatal vitamins.

Did You Know?

Relax. Don't Stress.

Stress is not good for you or your baby. It can even affect conception. So relax and take your B-vitamins. Get your sleep. Take some time for yourself to enjoy life. Make some decadently healthy food and have a date with your sexy man.

Being stressed and uptight is not going to make anything better. It will only hurt you and those around you. It is also good to practice relaxing and breathing. Relax your whole body. Sink down into your chair. Breathe deep down in your abdomen. Relax your shoulders. Relax those tight back muscles. Breathe. Relax your face and all your face muscles. Let all the stress run out of your body. Practice makes perfect. Practice relaxing, not stressing.

Music for Baby

It has been tossed about that a baby listening to music while in the womb will be more intelligent. Well, I do not know if that is true, but I do it anyway. I danced, sang, and listened to music while I was pregnant. Both of my children came out with a beat in their foot. Penelope loves music and loves to dance. Research has shown that if a baby listens to music in the womb she will recognize it up to one year, suggesting that the developing brain is capable of storing and recovering memories over a long period of time.

Did You Know?

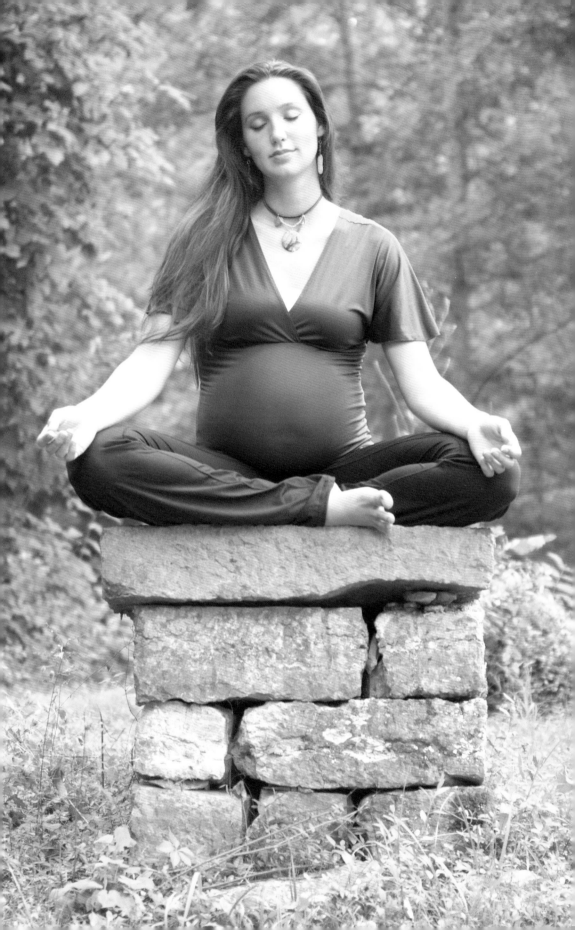

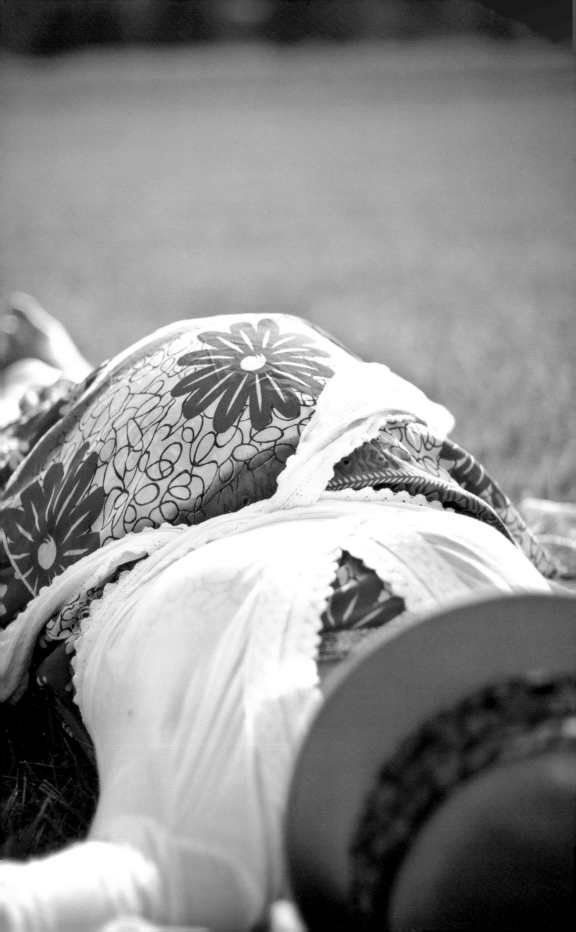

Vitamins & Minerals

The food you eat every day needs to feed your body vitamins and minerals. You get vitamins and minerals from the whole foods you eat. Your body can digest vitamins and minerals more easily in food form rather than pill form, yet it is not always easy to get all the vitamins you need from food. There are some vitamins I like to take that are very important to the health of my baby and me.

Vitamin D, omega fatty acids, folic acid, and all B-vitamins are on the top of my list. Small amounts of vitamins A, K, and E are good, especially for breastfeeding.

Vitamin D

Give your child a beautiful smile! Your body needs vitamin D to help build your baby's bones and teeth. A vitamin D deficiency during pregnancy can cause growth retardation, abnormal bone growth, skeletal deformities, and delayed physical development in your baby, and preeclampsia and a higher likelihood of needing a C-section for you.

Omega Fatty Acids

Do you want a smart baby? Researchers found that new mothers with higher blood levels of the omega-3 fatty acid (DHA) had infants that were advanced in levels of attention spans well into their second year. During the first six months of life, these infants were two months ahead of those babies whose mothers had lower DHA levels.

Folic Acid

Have a healthy baby! When a woman has enough folic acid in her body before and during pregnancy, it can prevent major birth defects such as spina bifida, anencephaly, and others. I take 800 mcg or micrograms of folic acid every day.

If you have or someone in your family has had a birth defect of the brain or spine, you may want to talk to your nutritionist about taking 4,000 mcg of folic acid to lower your risk of having a baby with these birth defects.

Did You Know?

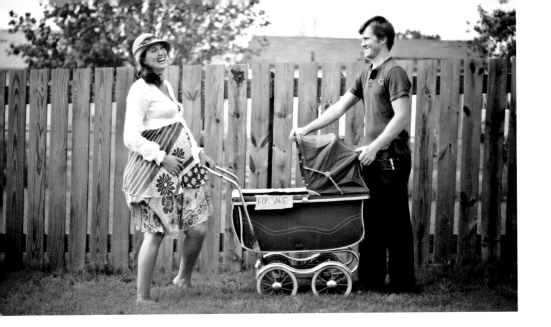

B Vitamins

Forgetful mama? Take your Bs. Bs build your brain and your baby's brain. Bs help form new red blood cells, antibodies, and neurotransmitters, and are vital to your baby's developing brain and nervous system. They also help your body metabolize protein, fats, and carbohydrates.

Feeling sick? Taking vitamin B6 can relieve nausea or vomiting from morning sickness.

Vitamin A

Vitamin A is important for your baby's growth. Your baby needs it for the development of his heart, lungs, kidneys, eyes, bones, and more. Vitamin A also helps with fat metabolism, postpartum tissue repair, fighting infections, and much more. Vitamin A is found in animal products such as eggs, milk, and liver, as well as in fruits, vegetables, and herbs. I like to get my vitamin A by drinking Red Raspberry Brew. It has alfalfa in it, and alfalfa is full of vitamin A. I drink no more than one glass a day in my first trimester. Second trimester, I drink a little more. Starting at five months, I drink four cups a day, refreshing and preparing my body for birth. I love it!

Vitamin K

Many people use vitamin K for scars, stretch marks, swelling, high cholesterol, spider veins, bruises, and burns. It is also used topically for skin conditions. I like to get my K vitamin in leafy green vegetables, such as spinach, broccoli, and brussels sprouts.

Did You Know?

Vitamin E

High doses (more than 400 IU per day) of vitamin E were once recommended to expecting mothers, but they found that it can cause bad problems in mother and baby. Most recommended doses now are around 20 to 30 IU, but most of us can get all the E vitamins we need in the foods we eat. I like to get mine by eating raw sunflower seeds, almonds, spinach, olives, papaya, leafy greens, and blueberries.

Minerals

Calcium is very important. I like to drink egg shell water or liquid cal-mag also called Liquid Calcium Magnesium Citrate. If you do not get enough calcium, then you may get bad leg cramps, especially at the end of your pregnancy. Take your calcium. You and your baby need it.

I get most of my minerals from Celtic Sea Salt. It is full of natural minerals that you and your baby need. I eat it on my food. It is raw, unprocessed sea salt. We carry Celtic Sea Salt at Bulk Herb Store.

Not all salts are the same. Processed salt will make you hold water and your hands and feet will swell. It will also raise your blood pressure. Stay away from table salt and all processed salts. (See Salt Vs. Salt on page 365.)

Iron

You need lots of iron. Your body almost doubles in blood in the first few months of pregnancy. Your blood carries oxygen to your baby. Lack of iron equals less oxygen for your baby. Also, lack of iron will make you tired. Iron in pill form is hard for your body to digest and can cause constipation and other problems. I like to eat my iron in whole foods. I eat spinach, kale, parsley, and cilantro in my daily diet. Adding citrus (lemon, lime, orange) with your greens helps break the iron down better for your body's absorption.

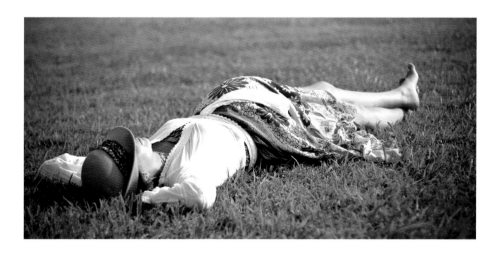

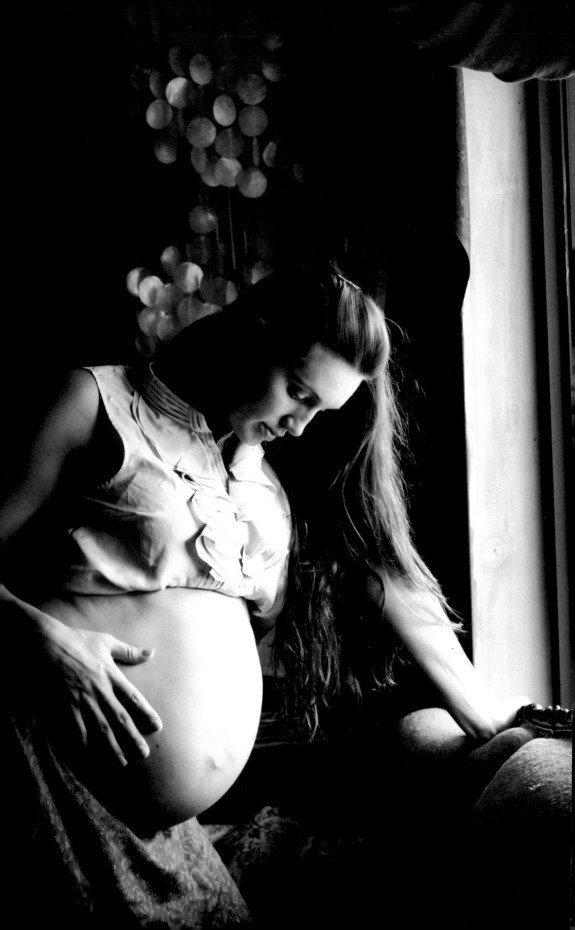

Vitamins Your Baby Needs

Folic acid and vitamin B12 to make red blood cells.

Vitamin C to produce collagen.

Vitamin D and calcium for bone building.

DHA omega-3 fatty acids, riboflavin, and zinc for brain development.

Iron for oxygen, boosting the baby's brain, and giving overall health to your baby.

Vitamin B1 or thiamin helps build your baby a healthy nervous system, muscles, and heart.

Building Your Baby's Brain

When a baby is born and his mother has high levels of omega fatty acids in her blood, it is found that her baby will be 2 or 3 months ahead of other babies for the first six months of life. Fats make up sixty percent of the brain and the nerves that run every system in the body. The cells of the human brain need essential fatty acids to grow and function.

Did You Know?

Morning Sickness

Exercise

Exercise is very important. It helps to balance all those crazy hormones that are making you sick. I like to swim. It helped me so much when I was pregnant with my first child. Swimming was something I could do every day while living in the city. Not crazy over-arm swimming, but stay-moving exercise swimming. Walking, dancing, prego exercises are also good. Even if you do not feel like it, get up and go exercise. It will make you feel better!

Eat right

You will feel so much better eating good foods in small portions often. Your baby needs most of your body's resources to build. Eating processed food and too much food is too hard for your body to deal with. Eat what your body needs, even if it is not always what you want. Think about how each food does something good or bad to you and your baby. Eating right will make you feel better.

B6 vitamin

Studies show that vitamin B6 (also known as pyridoxine) helps relieve queasiness. To ease nausea and vomiting, I like to take 10 to 25 mg, three times a day. To reach this amount, I take B6 supplements.

Ginger and Peppermint

Ginger and peppermint help with digestion and nausea. Whether fresh or in a tea or tincture, there are many ways you can use them. My favorite ways to use them are: in a **Ginger Tincture** (see page 46), in peppermint tea, and as peppermint essential oil, breathing it in and rubbing it on my temples.

Sleep

Sleep is so important. Your body is on overtime and needs a lot of rest to recharge. It is constantly working hard to make your little baby's body stronger. You can let it, by sleeping. If you do not get enough sleep, you can get very morning sick, and it is not good for you and baby. Go take a nap!

Water

Stay hydrated. Your body needs water to flush your filters out that are working so hard. If you get dehydrated, it can cause some very bad nausea. Dehydration can be very serious for you and your baby. Drink to health.

Regular

Don't get constipated. Constipation can really get you sick fast. Take fiber, such as **Nutritional Fiber** (page 71) if you need it, but keep yourself regular.

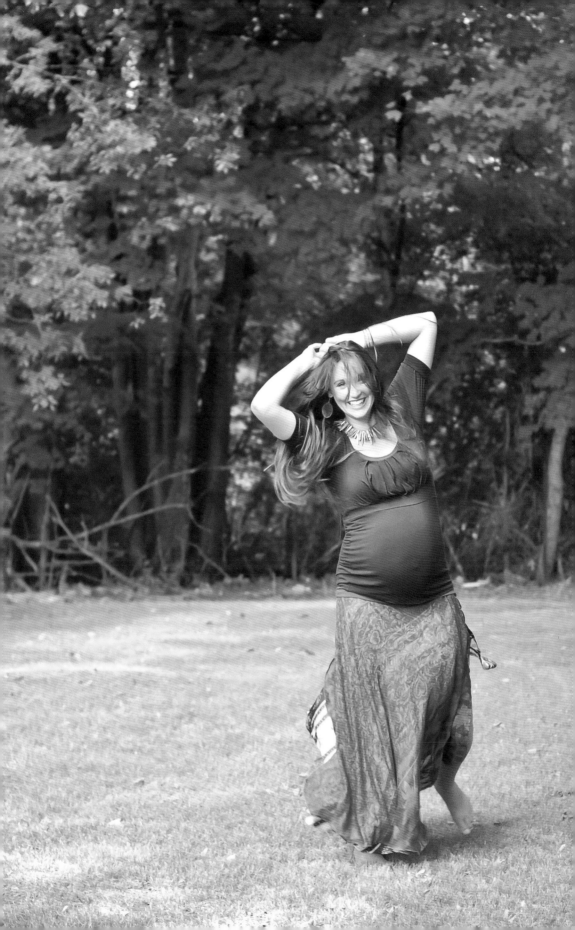

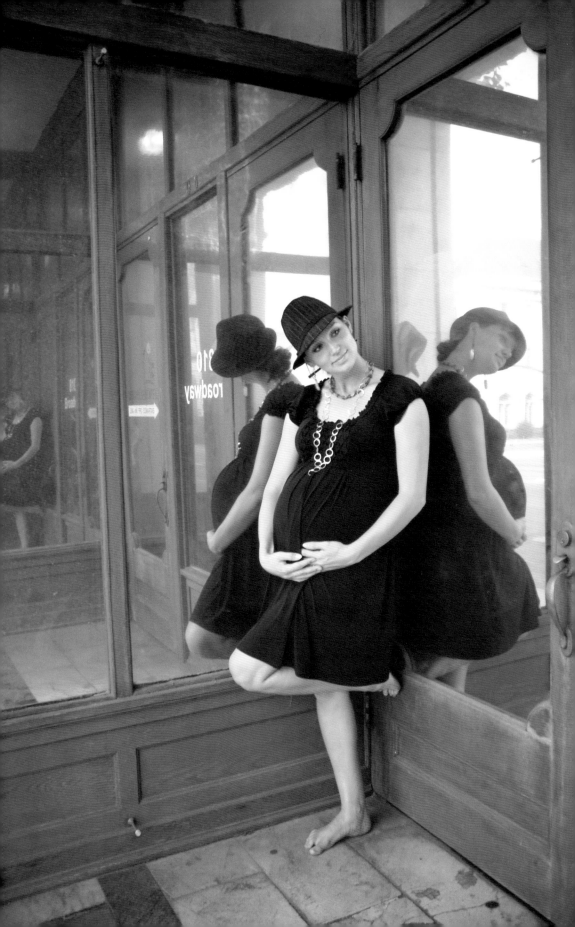

Tips for Morning Sickness

1. Eat something high in protein before going to bed.

2. Eat two saltine crackers before your head leaves the pillow.

3. Have sips of ice water when your stomach gets the urge to purge.

4. Stay hydrated.

5. Ginger in teas, tinctures, cookies, even just the spice can be helpful in preventing nausea. Don't exceed 1,000 mg of ginger a day.

6. Acupressure bands can be worn like bracelets and can curb nausea.

7. Smaller, frequent meals definitely help.

8. Drinking or just inhaling peppermint tea helps.

9. Try almond butter, a handful of almonds, or another protein snack before rising from your bed.

10. A teaspoon of apple cider vinegar in a cup of warm water has been said to be effective.

11. Eat small amounts throughout the day to avoid becoming too full, or alternately, too hungry.

12. Only take iron-free prenatal vitamins. Get your iron from plant sources.

13. Red raspberry leaf tea has been used by many pregnant women to ease morning sickness. Speak to your doctor or midwife before taking.

14. Vitamin B6 also provides relief for many pregnant women; don't take more than 25mg a day.

15. Foods you might be able to hold down if you are morning sick: raw vegetables, salad with fresh lemon, not dressing, bland soup or broth, plain fruits and vegetables, ginger, peppermint tea, plain popcorn, saltine crackers, graham crackers, dry toast, oatmeal, quinoa, celery sticks, carrot sticks, apples, raisins, prunes, tart or sour pickles, brown rice, unseasoned mashed potatoes with butter or milk only, plain baked potatoes, water, fruit juices, frozen fruit juice bars, seltzer water, regular (non-diet) ginger ale, herbal teas (spearmint, peppermint, chamomile, raspberry), ginger root tea.

Did You Know?

Mama's Got Energy

The food you eat is the fuel your body is burning. Pregnancy and nursing take a lot out of you. You need to eat right. It is more important than ever before. Sugars and starches can get you down, but protein is a must. It will keep you going.

Don't get constipated. That will drag you down.

Drink water and stay hydrated.

Low iron levels can really make you tired. If you do not have enough iron, you and your baby are not getting enough oxygen. I do not take iron in pill form, because it can cause morning sickness and constipation. You can get iron in green things such as kale, spinach, turnip greens, and such. Adding citrus with it (lemon, oranges, etc.) helps break the iron down better for your body to absorb more easily. I also like to make an iron infusion or tincture to take. (See pages 34 and 99.)

Exercise keeps your endorphin levels high, making you feel better and giving you energy. Try to get at least an hour of exercise a day.

Eat 6 Small Meals a Day

Try eating 5 or 6 small meals a day rather than 3 larger ones. Your body is getting crowded with a baby, so there is not a lot of room for big meals. You will feel so much better eating small portions. It is very important that you eat what you and your baby need – not what you always want. You and your baby will feel better and be healthier. Processed food and too much food is too hard for your body to deal with, giving you indigestion. Think about what you eat, because it fuels your body and builds your baby. Make sure you are still eating balanced meals. Eating right will make you feel better.

Don't get constipated; but if you do struggle with this, change your eating habits immediately and remember, do not spend a lot of time on the toilet trying to push it out. Excessive pushing can cause hemorrhoids.

Did You Know?

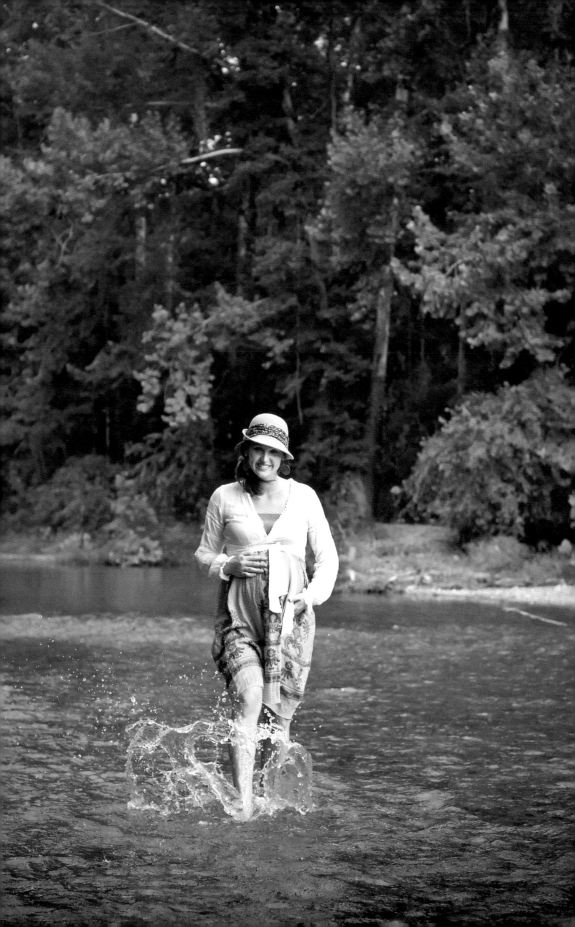

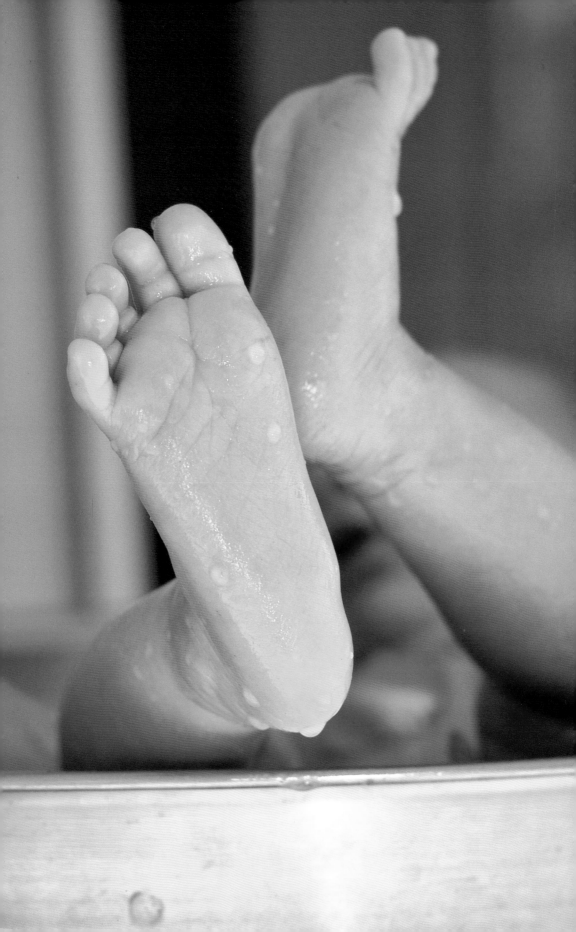

Colicky Baby

It's estimated that up to 40% of all infants have colic. It commonly starts 3 to 6 weeks after birth and ends by the time the baby is 3 months old. A mother's diet can help ease it or cut it out altogether. Here are a few things that sometimes bother your baby, even though you breastfeed: milk products (not mother's milk), wheat, peanuts, soy, sugars, garlic, and cabbage. If your baby has colic, holding your baby close to you so he can breathe in your smells will comfort him. You can try rocking, swaying, swinging, or gently bouncing on an exercise ball; all of these are comforting and also help babies calm down or pass gas.

Calm for Baby

When your baby is crying, run through a mental checklist: Is she hungry? Does she need her diaper changed? Is she tired, hot, cold, or gassy? If all of those things are taken care of and she is still crying, take her outside. Babies love being outside and moving about. The wind, birds, colors, and light flickering through the trees will calm a baby better than a rocking chair. If you want something calming that is indoors, you can always try noise from a running shower, sink, faucet, or fan.

Did You Know?

Babies Need Touch

Studies have been done that show touch and massage have a positive effect on infant weight gain and survival rates. Babies that are picked up, hugged, kissed, cradled, stroked, and massaged are shown to gain weight faster, be more alert, crawl and walk earlier, sleep better, and have increased feelings of security, trust, and comfort. Nurturing your baby's needs through touch will help your baby feel more relaxed and cry only when she has needs; it is also great for mama by helping to balance hormones and strengthening the bond between mama and baby. Nursing is a big part of touch. Penelope and I love our times throughout the day, when we go in and lie on my bed. I nurse and stroke her; she smiles up at me with delight every time. Half of the time James (Dad) comes in and lays there with us. She keeps one hand on him while she is nursing. She loves it, and so do we!

Pregnancy and Sleep

Sleep on your left side, with your knees bent and a pillow between your legs. This will increase the amount of blood and nutrients that reach your baby. I like to put another pillow under my belly and one on my back. That way if I do roll over in the night, I never lie flat on my back. Sleeping on your back can bring about all kinds of problems: backaches, difficulty breathing and digesting, hemorrhoids, and lowered circulation to your heart and your baby. If you are experiencing heartburn during the night, you can also try sleeping in a propped-up, sitting position.

Did You Know?

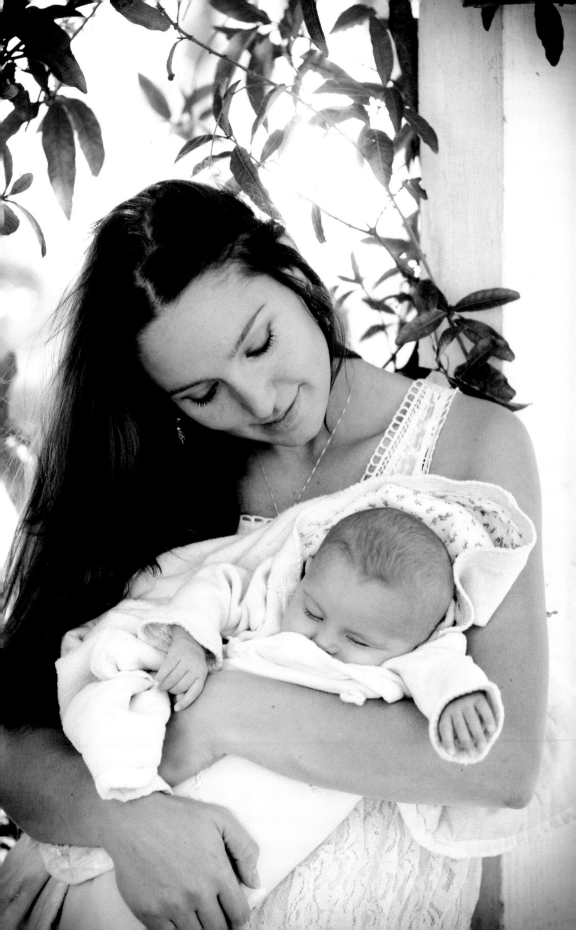

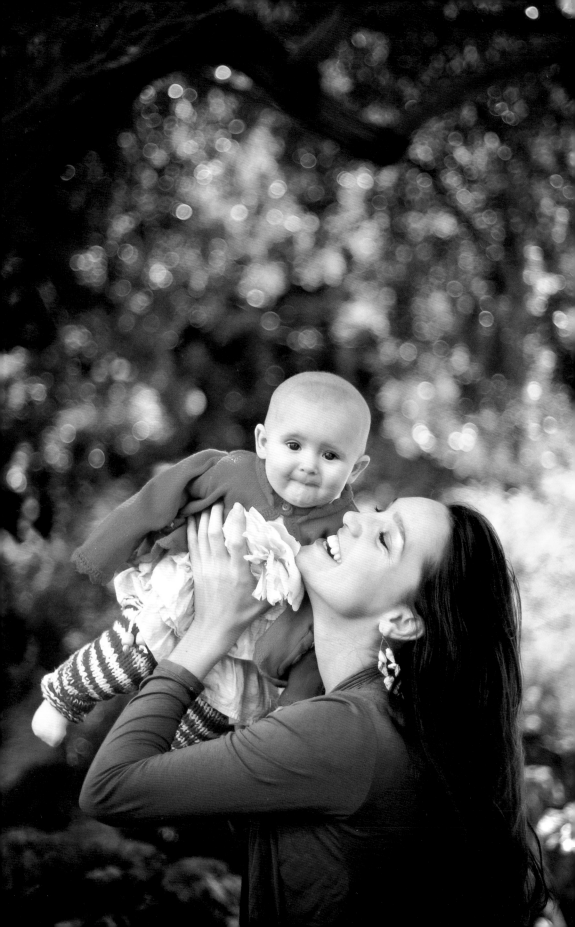

Postpartum Depression

Postpartum depression is real. Some of you may ask what it is. Some call it the "baby blues," but whatever you call it, it can lead to feelings of anxiety, tearfulness, irritation, and restlessness. PPD can start one or two weeks after delivery. You may have some of the following symptoms:

- Agitation or irritability
- Changes in appetite
- Feelings of worthlessness or guilt
- Feeling withdrawn or unconnected
- Lack of pleasure or interest in most or all activities
- No concentration
- Low energy
- Problems doing tasks at home or work
- Negative feeling
- Significant anxiety
- Trouble sleeping

What can you do? Take your vitamins. Get your sleep. Get your exercise. Eat healthy foods. Cut preservatives and sugars out of your diet. Nurse your baby. Spend time each day cuddling and loving on your baby. This will help to level your hormones and get you out of it. Also, make sure you get out of the house at least once every day, even if it is just for three minutes to get the mail. Fresh air and getting away from four walls is a big help! Keep your chin up! It won't last forever.

Salt vs. Salt

Salt that has been processed (chemicals) and refined (chemicals) is BAD for you. Salt that is raw and unprocessed is GOOD for you. It contains many vitamins and minerals and studies show that GOOD salt does not raise your blood pressure like BAD salt does. I like to use Celtic Sea Salt - good salt that is GREAT for you.

No Preservatives

Processed foods contain additives such as flavorings that change a food's taste, colorings that change the way it looks, preservatives that extend its shelf life, and dietary additives, such as vitamins, minerals, fatty acids, and other supplements. Basically, anything in a package is processed and has some form of preservative. Eat as many whole foods (raw foods that you cook) as you can. Eliminate preservatives. I know you cannot eliminate them all, but keep this on the forefront of your mind so as a life style you eat whole foods.

Exercises for Mama

Exercise is hard to fit in with your new life as a mama. Cleaning, cooking, nursing, burping, and changing diapers keep you quite busy. That is why I use life's everyday chores to work out. While nursing or burping my baby, I sit on an exercise ball, bouncing by clenching my butt cheeks together. While sweeping, I look like an ostrich strutting around. Keep your back straight, abs tight, and knees bent while you sweep. That is a picture your neighbor will never forget! Wash some dishes with rock-tight muscles. Exercise your kegel muscle or keep those abs and legs tight and clench that butt together. You are going to get in shape so quickly you will love it! I also do leg lifts in bed while putting Penelope to sleep. You have got to try it! It gives you energy and gets you back in shape. You will be astonished how quickly you will shed those baby pounds.

Cool fact: Did you know that your body uses 300 calories a day when you are breastfeeding? That does not mean you need to eat more. It is just God's way of letting you lose that baby fat.

Most women can start exercise at 6 weeks, but you need to check with your doctor first.

Did You Know?

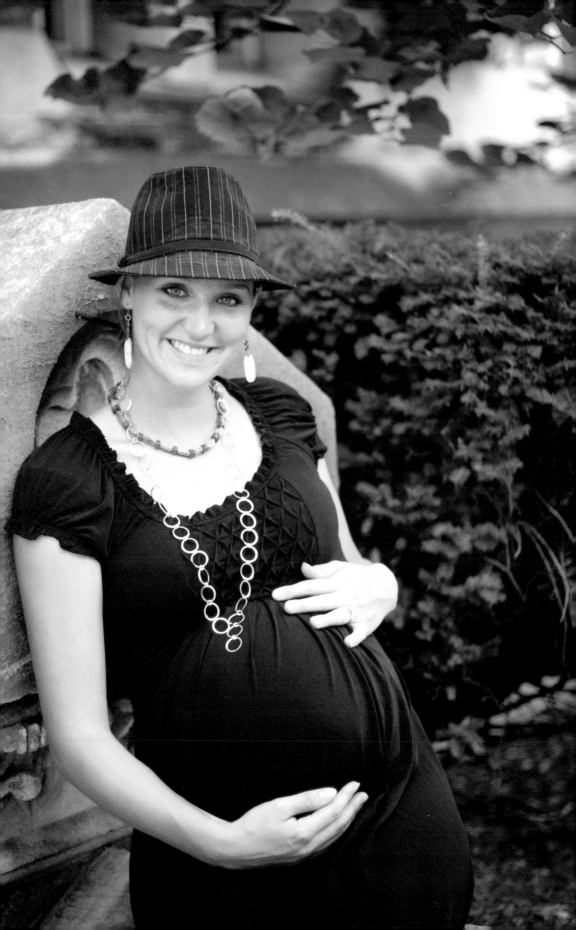

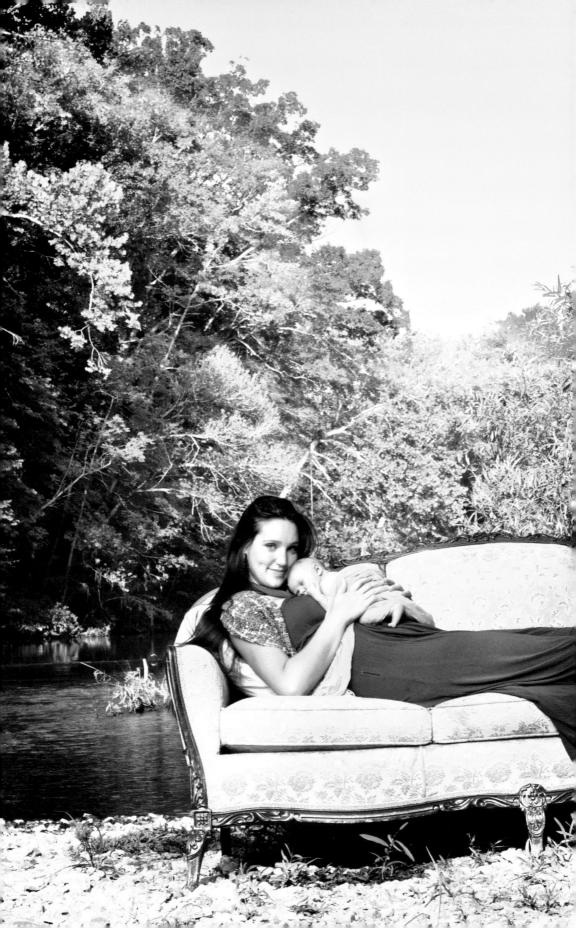

Cal-Mag

Your baby is building bones, muscles, and teeth, and needs lots of calcium and magnesium. Calcium also plays an important role in the development of your baby's heart. If you are not taking enough calcium and magnesium, then your body takes it from your bones and muscles. Both of these minerals are critical to ensuring the good health of mother and baby during pregnancy.

Toward the end of your pregnancy you may get cramps in your legs. Liquid cal-mag really helps. I took it every night before bed while I was pregnant. It helped me sleep, protected my bones, and kept me from getting cramps. When I did forget to take it, I got cramps. Ouch!

Also, calcium plays an important role in the development of your baby's heart. For mom, calcium can help to prevent osteoporosis. (Your baby will leech calcium from your bones if you are not ingesting enough to support development.)

Blood Types

There are three main blood types A, B, and O. Babies inherit their blood type from one of their parents. For example, if you have blood that is O-negative, and the baby's father has type A, then your baby could have type A, and your body could make antibodies that would attack your next baby's blood. Bottom line, if you are having a baby at home, make sure that you talk to a midwife or doctor about your blood type to avoid danger to you and your baby.

Did You Know?

Nursing

Nursing is so good for babies; I do not know where to start. There is nothing close to breastmilk in any formula. Breastmilk is living food that gives life to babies. I am not kidding. Breastmilk is full of our probiotics, healthy fats, carbohydrates (healthy sugars), proteins, vitamins, minerals, enzymes, and healthy bacteria. Breastmilk provides your baby with important antibodies that help fight against many infections and protect against many diseases. It was designed by God to provide your little one with everything he needs. It is the perfect formula for the development of your baby's body.

Moms who breastfeed have a much lower risk of breast cancer, ovarian cancer, and bleeding after birth. I could go on and on. IT IS AWESOME!!!

See Mama's Milk Tea on page 462.

Foremilk and Hindmilk

For the first few days after your baby is born, you have colostrum. This builds your baby's immune system and gets her off to a great start. Then your milk comes in. You think your boobs might burst. They won't, but you could have milk Super-Soaker fights with your husband! At this point you will probably have too much milk and need to pump a little before you nurse. You have foremilk and hindmilk. As your baby starts to nurse, she gets foremilk. After a little while of nursing, it turns into hindmilk. Both are important. That is why you need to nurse one breast until it is drained before you start the next. My babies rarely nurse more than one breast at a sitting. As your baby is going through a growth spurt, she will want more than one breast.

If you want to increase the volume of your milk you can stimulate your nipples and breasts between nursing sessions. Babies are usually hungry every four hours, but some days they will want to eat all day long. GROWING BABIES!!!

Did You Know?

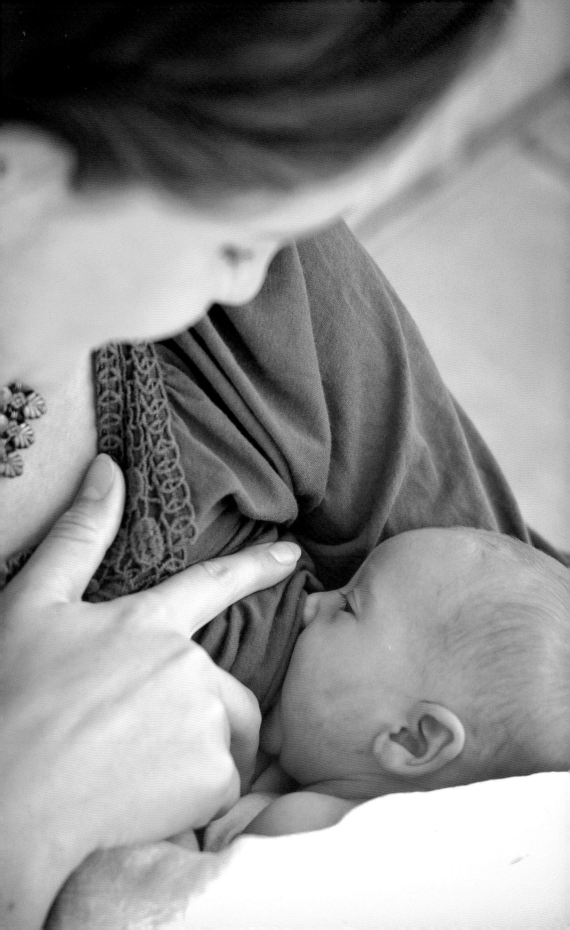

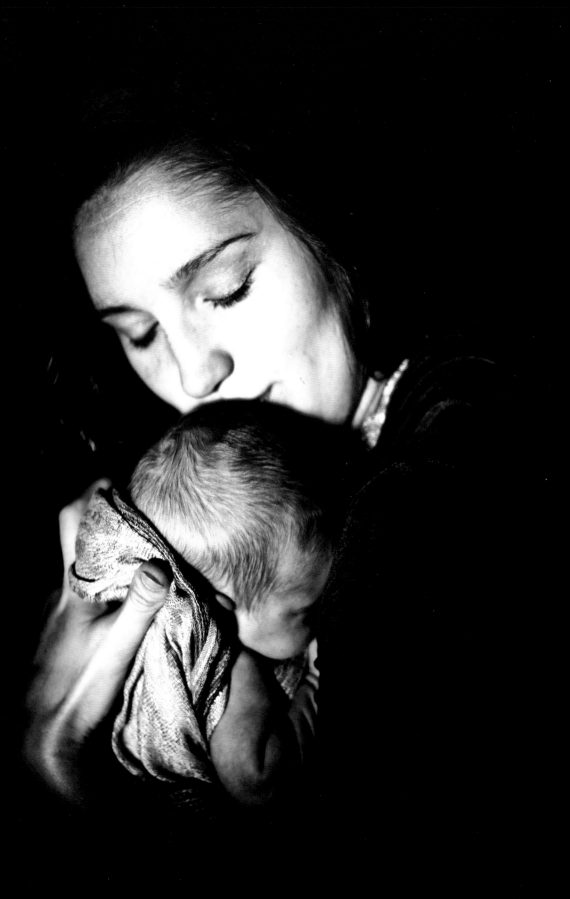

Labor and Birth

Going through labor and birth is like an athlete winning a gold medal. It is the greatest, biggest, hardest, best thing you will ever do. It is not easy, but it is worth it! I loved my births! They were fun!! Yes, it is a lot of work, but the natural high you get from a job well done is out of this world. It is the biggest workout of your life. Prepare for it. Plan for it. Practice for it. When it comes, relax and enjoy the workout.

There are three stages of labor.

1. Stage one. You are excited, walking and dancing, but you know you are in labor.

2. Stage two. You are concentrating and surprised it hurts this much. At the end of stage 2 you do not think you can take much more.

3. Stage three. You are pushing. You are tired. You are excited - your baby is almost here!!

Here are a few things that are great to have in labor.

- Fun music to dance to during the first stage of labor
- Hot sock for your lower back (Learn how to make one on page 392.)
- Ice chips and someone to feed them to you silently.
- Two hands that are strong and can massage in silence.
- Someone who has trained with you to help you relax and talk you through each contraction. (Husband, best friend)
- Young coconuts, to keep you hydrated and feeling great!
- Straws, so someone else can hold your drink.

This might sound a little crazy to you, but you need to teach yourself to relax even when everything around you is in chaos. It makes such a difference in birthing. You will appear to be asleep through most of your labor if you practice this well. You will teach your body not to fight the contractions, but let them do their work. If you fight them your body will have to work twice as hard. So relax! Here are some relaxing techniques to practice. It is nice to have someone to coach you through it, but you can do it by yourself.

Relax! Breathe deep down in your abdomen.
Breathe! Let all the air out. Breathe! Relax!
Relax your arms, shoulders, and hands.
Let all the tension leave your face. Relax. Breathe deep.
Relax your eyes and all the muscles of your face.
Relax! Let your body droop into the pillow. Relax.
Sink down into your bed. Relax. Breathe.
Breathe deep down in your abdomen. Relax!

Jaundice

Before your baby is born he lives off of your body's nutrients through your placenta. Then the little guy comes into the world. His body has to start doing all the work by itself. He is using his liver for the first time, and sometimes it takes a little while for his liver to take over its tasks. There is a natural waste in everyone's blood called bilirubin, which the liver normally removes and then flushes out through stools. If it does not get flushed out, it builds up pigment that makes the eyes and skin turn yellowish. This is called jaundice. Jaundice can cause brain damage, deafness, seizures, weak muscle tone, and even death.

Jaundice occurs in about 60 percent of all newborns. Here are some of the symptoms.

- Yellowish skin and corners of eyes
- Is hard to wake
- Sucks or nurses poorly
- Appears floppy or stiff (or alternates between both)
- Arches the neck or back backwards
- Develops a high-pitched cry or fever
- Has unusual eye movement

What can you do? From the very first day, make sure your baby gets sun. I sun my babies at least 15 minutes every day. I strip them down to their God-given birthday suit to soak up the sun. We sit on the porch if it is really warm. Sometimes we sit in the car if it is windy. If it is cold we sit by the window with the most sunlight coming in, but we always make sure we get sun. This works GREAT!!! (Talk to your doctor or midwife, as too much sun exposure can be harmful.)

Nurse more frequently. Make sure she gets lots of fluid.

Talk to your doctor if your baby starts showing signs of jaundice after seven days or if it lasts longer than 14 days.

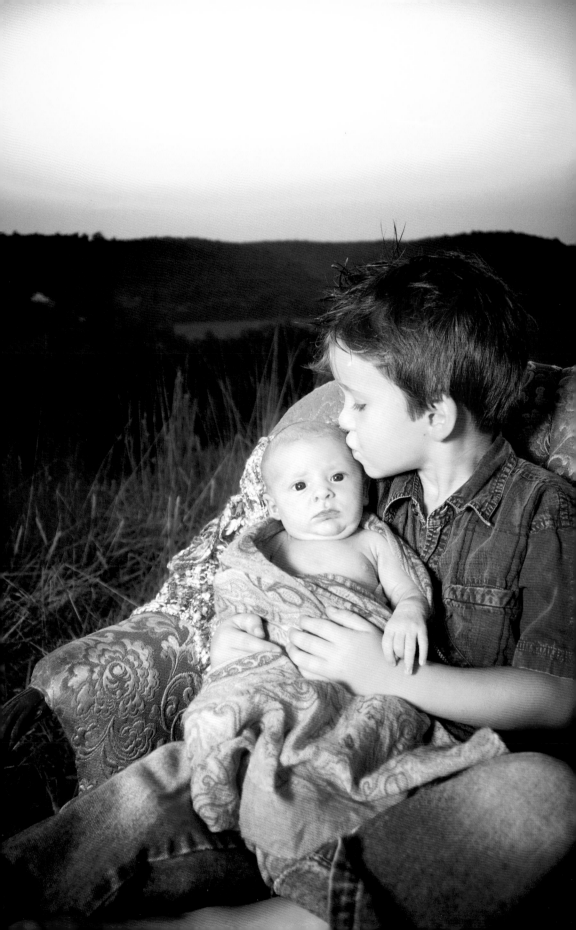

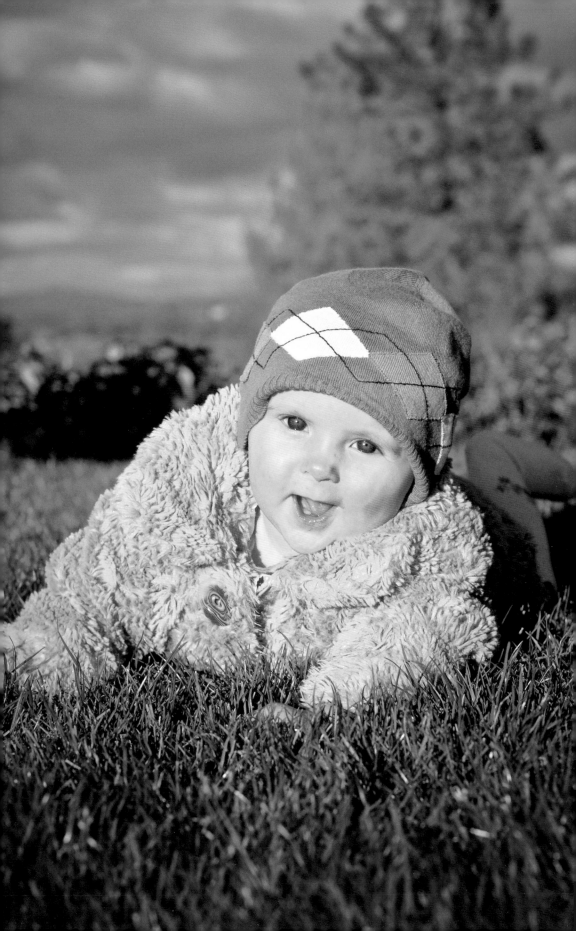

Non-GMO and Organic

Most of our main vegetables are genetically modified organisms (GMO). GMO foods are made by changing DNA and mixing animal DNA with plant DNA, creating new strains of seeds. The problem is, when you start trying to make something out of the original, it is always just a knock-off. "In the beginning God created" great food. We just keep screwing it up. GMO foods are not good for a growing baby or a body that wants to live healthy and long. They can cause all kinds of health problems. You can get seeds that are non-GMO and grow good food, or be careful when buying food. I know you cannot always avoid eating GMO foods, but make it a life choice to try. GMO foods are also full of chemicals. This is another thing that gets us sick and keeps us down. It is always best to go organic when you can.

Mercury in Fish

Mercury is bad for you and your baby. It can be quite serious. Lots of fish contain high levels of mercury. Avoid eating fish with high levels of mercury. Here are some that you can eat.

Lowest mercury:
Anchovies, butterfish, catfish, clam, crab (domestic), crawfish, crayfish, flounder, haddock, hake, herring, mackeral (North Atlantic), mullet, oysters, perch (ocean), salmon (canned or fresh), sardines, scallops, shrimp, squid (calamari), tilapia, trout (freshwater), whitefish, and whiting

Low mercury:
Bass (striped, black), carp, cod (Alaskan), halibut (Pacific and Atlantic), lobster, mahi mahi, monkfish, perch (freshwater), snapper, sea trout (weakfish), tuna (canned, chunk light), and tuna (skipjack)

Did You Know?

Circumcision

Baby boys are born with a hood of skin covering the end of their penis. Circumcision is removing the hood of skin and revealing the end of the penis. Approximately 55% to 65% of all newborn boys are circumcised in the United States each year. We chose to have our son circumcised because it will be easier for him to keep himself clean and he will have a lower risk of infections and disease.

A friend of mine married a man who was not circumcised. Intimacy was continually getting his penis infected. At 32 years old he had to go in and get circumcised. It takes a lot longer for a man to heal up than a baby.

If you decide to have your son circumcised, it is best to have it performed during the first 10 days. We chose to have our son circumcised on the eighth day, because studies show that your baby's level of vitamin K is highest on that day (vitamin K helps blood clotting). Circumcision after the newborn period can be a more complicated procedure and usually requires general anesthesia.

Diapers

Do you know what your baby is wearing? Disposable diapers not labeled as "unbleached" or "bleached with peroxide" contain dioxin. What is dioxin? It is a by-product of bleaching paper. Dioxin can cause damage to the central nervous system, kidneys, and liver. That is not a healthy thing to have wrapped around your baby's bottom. You can buy disposable diapers that are dioxin-free or use cloth diapers.

Did You Know?

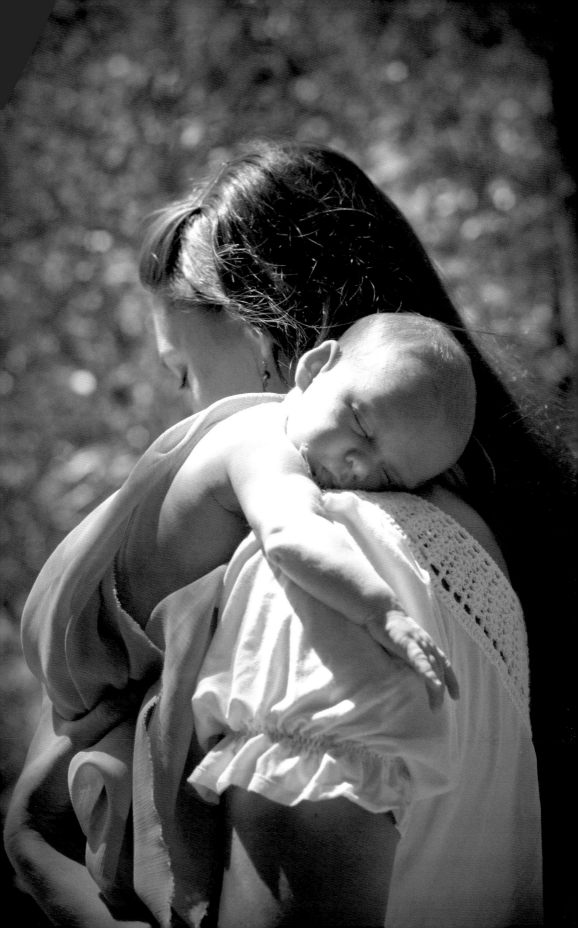

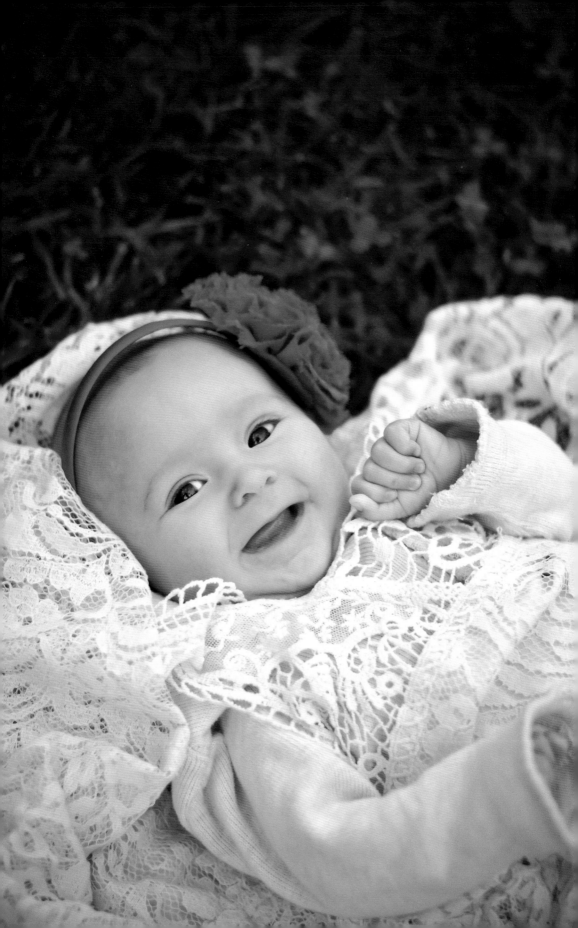

Foods for Fertility

Go organic and non-GMO everywhere you can. Some good foods for fertility are: beans, peas, lentils, raw nuts, almonds, walnuts, pumpkin seeds, quinoa, fruits and vegetables, cabbage, beets, carrots, asparagus, artichokes, sweet potatoes, blackberries, blueberries, kiwi, papaya, pomegranates, oranges, avocados, leafy greens, kale, spinach, oysters and shellfish, coconut oil, olive oil, flax oil, omegas, healthy fats, turmeric, milk thistle, red raspberry, alfalfa leaf, and nettle leaf.

Aloe

The aloe vera plant is an amazing herb. It grows skin and heals things back together faster than anything I have ever seen. It is a wonderful carrier herb that you can mix with other herbs that you want to penetrate the skin. The problem is that because it is such a great carrier, it can also carry chemicals and toxins into your body. Your skin is your biggest organ. What goes on, goes in. If you have a product with aloe, or make a product with aloe, make sure it is all organic. If you are using it to clear a diaper rash, make sure you use nontoxic diapers. Organic cloth is best.

Heartburn

Heartburn can happen a lot in pregnancy. Your body is stuffed full of baby, and there is not a lot of room for anything else. To avoid it, I eat small meals. I do not eat fried, highly greasy, or packaged foods. If I do get heartburn, a spoonful of raw honey or apple cider vinegar, "with the mother," helps soothe my throat and balance the pH of my stomach, which stops the heartburn.

Did You Know?

Good Fat Vs. Bad Fat

Good fat vs. bad fat is a big thing. Fats are very important to our diet. We need them to stay healthy and strong, and build a baby. Good fats help our sugar and insulin metabolism and therefore, contribute to our goals of healthy living, weight loss, and weight maintenance. Not all fats are equal – there are good fats and bad fats.

Good fats are in a lot of raw and unprocessed foods such as nuts, milk, butter, coconuts, avocados, seeds, olive oil, and fruits. There are also good fats in fish and grass-fed organic or wild animals.

Bad fat is in fried foods, processed foods, animal fats that are homogenized or full of antibiotics and hormones, and genetically modified foods.

Reflections

Did you know that more is caught than taught? Children are constantly reflecting the people they are around. If you want a sweet, snuggly, happy baby, then be that for them. I always make sure I am close by when my kids wake up. The moment I hear my baby waking, I start making sweet noises of love and affection. I go and pick her up or lie down beside her, snuggle, kiss, hug, tickle, and play peek-a-boo. This happy time sets a mood for your baby. It gives her security, confindence, and builds a stronger bond that makes her happier.

Did You Know?

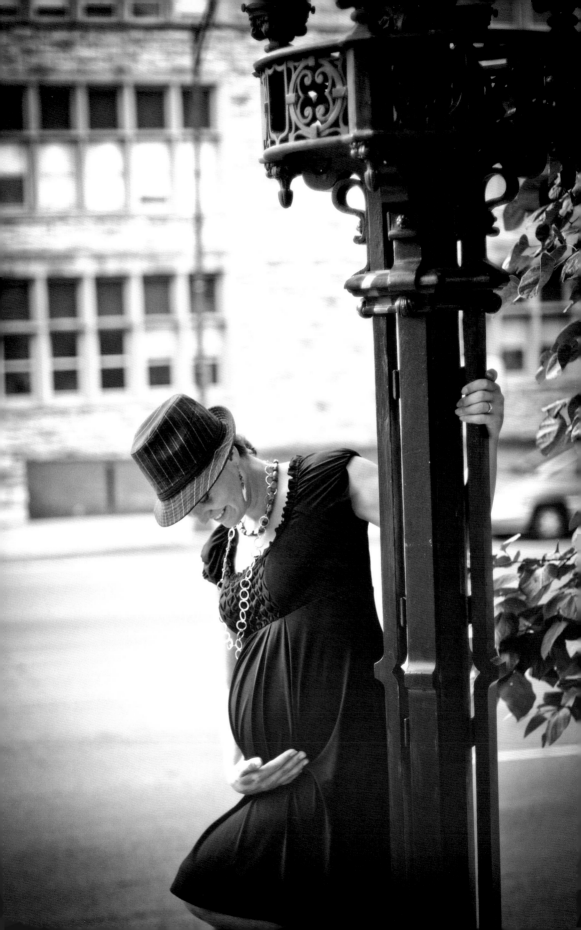

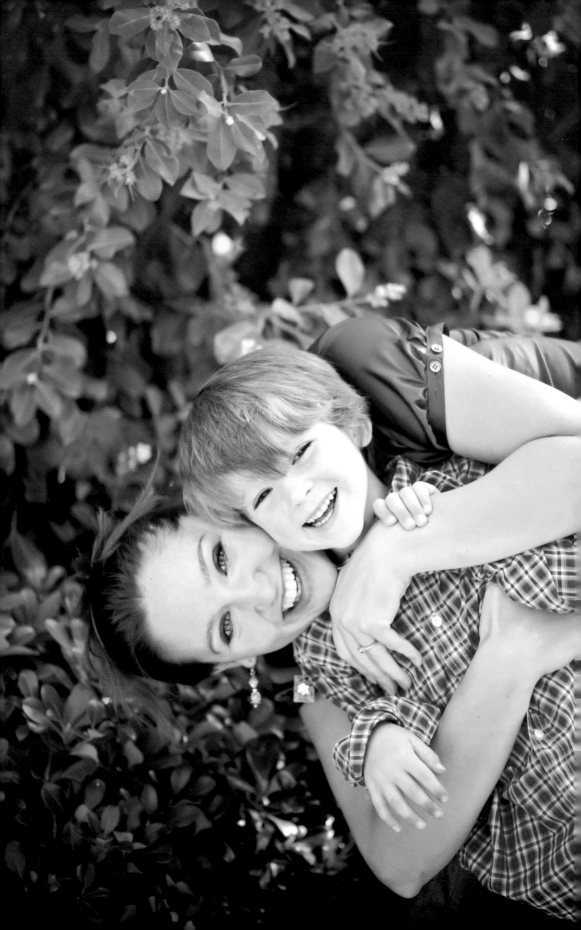

Herbs Work

Herbs work! They do great things! They work so well, you need to be careful with them. I always start very small and work up to how much I want to take. I pay close attention to how I am feeling, so I know what they are doing. Just because you find something that works well, does not mean more is better. Please be responsible when using herbs and talk to your nutritionist or midwife, or research it yourself.

New Zealand Colostrum

100% New Zealand Colostrum is not homogenized. You can get it without hormones, antibiotics, and pesticides. It is rich in nutrients, enhancing the growth of cells, muscles, tissue, bone, and cartilage. This stuff is awesome!

Boy vs. Girl

The man's sperm carries the boy chromosome (Y) and the girl chromosome (X).

The Y chromosome is weaker, faster, and short-lived. Because the Y chromosome is weaker, it lives better in an alkaline environment. If you are more acidic, you might tend to have more girls. You can help alkalize your body with diet, herbs, and a pinch of baking soda in your daily drinking water. Because the Y chromosome is fast but has a short life span, if you want to increase your chances of having a boy, wait until right before your ovulation and then have sex.

The X chromosome is stronger, slower, and lives longer. Because it is stronger, it can live in an acidic environment, whereas the Y has a hard time. If you want to increase your chances of having a girl, have sex 5 days before ovulation and then not again. Because the X lives longer, it will be the only one around when you ovulate, thus increasing your chance of having a girl.

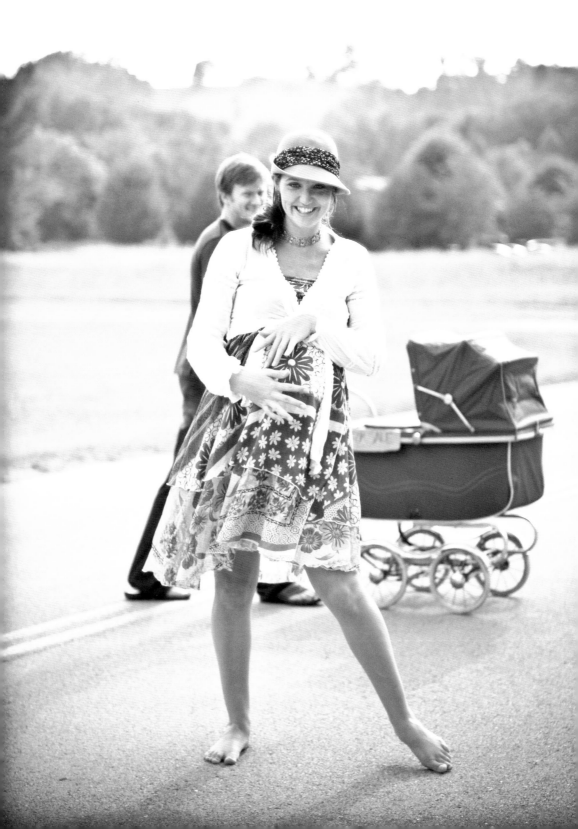

Grandma's Remedies

Old-fashioned remedies are left behind in this modern world. I love their simplicity and usefulness. My grandmas always had one for every situation.

Grandma's Rocking Chair
by Shoshanna Easling

Rocking in my grandma's chair
that my grandma gave to me

Once she rocked my mom there
With wildflowers in the air

Rocking with a lullabye
Sleeping baby, do not cry

Now I'm rocking you each night
tucking you in, oh, so tight

Grandma's gone to Jesus now
Hanging out above the clouds

Mama reflects Grandma now
Grandma would be very proud

I reflect my mama too
Just like I was meant to do

Mommy's best I want to be
for my Miss Penelope

Someday she will be like me
like my grandma I can see

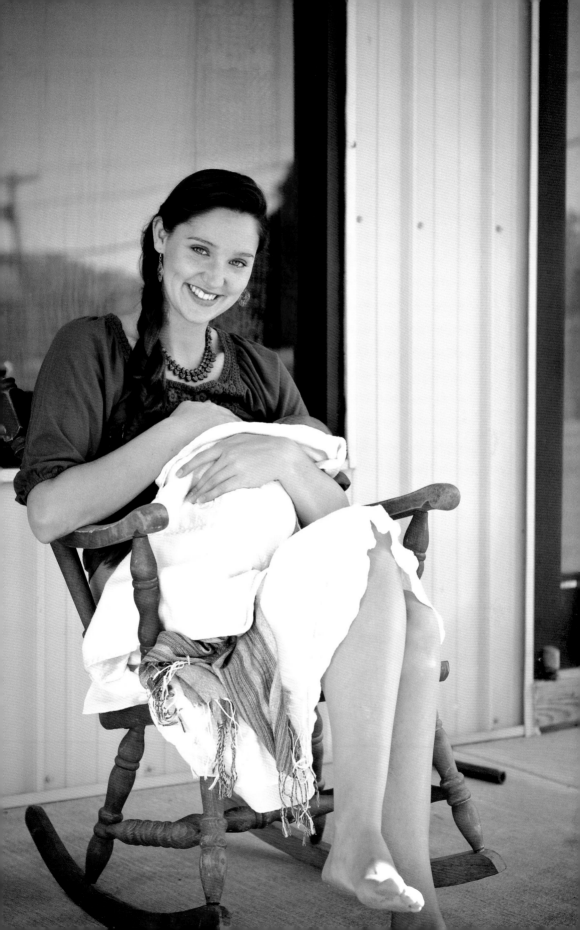

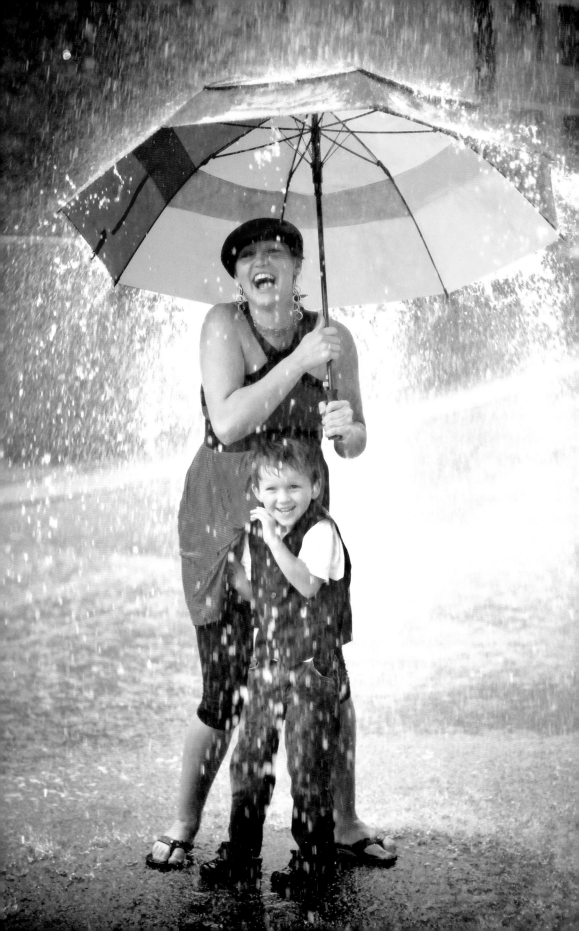

Morning Sick No More
Feeling Great Every Day

1 cup **Chicken Broth** (page 38) or **Vegetable Broth** (page 320)

2 saltine crackers

¼ tsp. parsley, chopped, (*optional*)

10 to 20 mg vitamin B6, 3 times a day

1. Heat broth over low heat for 3 minutes or until hot. Pour into a bowl; garnish with parsley. Eat the broth and crackers. Take a dose of B6 with water or the broth.

2. Take a shower. Do not use anything with a scent. Just water is fine.

3. Walk, swim, dance - do some exercise that you love for 30 minutes.

4. Eat a few bites every few hours. Do not eat big meals. Eat more small ones.

Relaxing and Nourishing Tea
Breathe. Relax. Enjoy a Warm Cup of Tea.

This tea helps relax those tight, cramping muscles and nourishes your sore body. It has a sweet, flowery taste and a warm color. It is simply wonderful!

½ cup rose hips

2 cups hibiscus petals

2 cups rose petals

½ cup lavender flowers, whole

3 cups lemon balm, leaf

3 cups chamomile flowers, whole

1 cup passion flower, herb

Prep: 5 min.   Yield: 12 cups tea mixture

1. Mix all ingredients together. Store in an airtight glass jar or zip-top bag in a cabinet.

2. To make a cup of hot tea, add 1 or 2 teaspoons of the premixed herbs to 1 cup of boiling water. Let it steep for 5 to 10 minutes, strain, and add honey (raw is best) to taste.

Sore Feet Soak

This Is a Great End to the Day.

1 cup sea salt

1 cup epsom salt

1 cup baking soda

2 gallons hot/warm water

10 drops of lavender
essential oil (*optional*)

1. Place all ingredients into a large bowl and stir. Soak feet 20 to 30 minutes. Towel dry and prop feet up.

2. Take two tablespoons liquid cal-mag.

3. Eat two stalks of celery.

Hot Sock

Everyone Needs a Hot Sock!

Growing up we always made hot socks to use on an ache or just to warm the bed.

1 athletic sock, clean and
thick so that grains cannot
fall through

Dried beans, rice, or flax

Dried herbs of your
choice, such as lavender,
rose, eucalyptus, or
peppermint

1. Fill sock with beans, rice, or flax and herbs. Fill it as full as you want, but leave space for the filling to move around.

2. Tie the end off with a string or rubber band, making sure it is well secured. You do not want it coming open and the contents going all over the place.

3. To heat, place in baking dish and heat in oven at 200° F for 20 minutes, or in the microwave for 1 minute. If you are using a microwave, make sure your rubber band does not have metal on it.

4. You can also make it a cold sock by putting it in the freezer for 45 minutes.

Grandma's Remedies

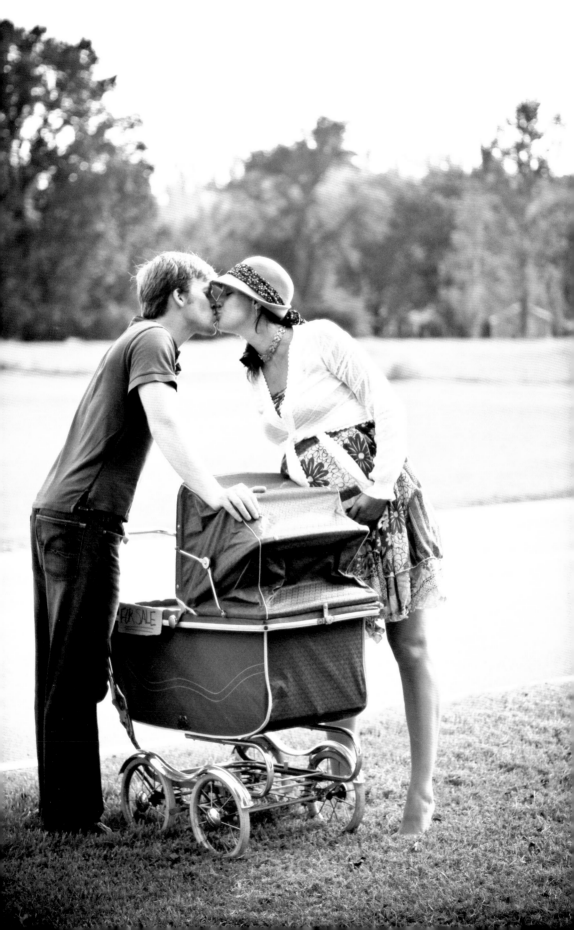

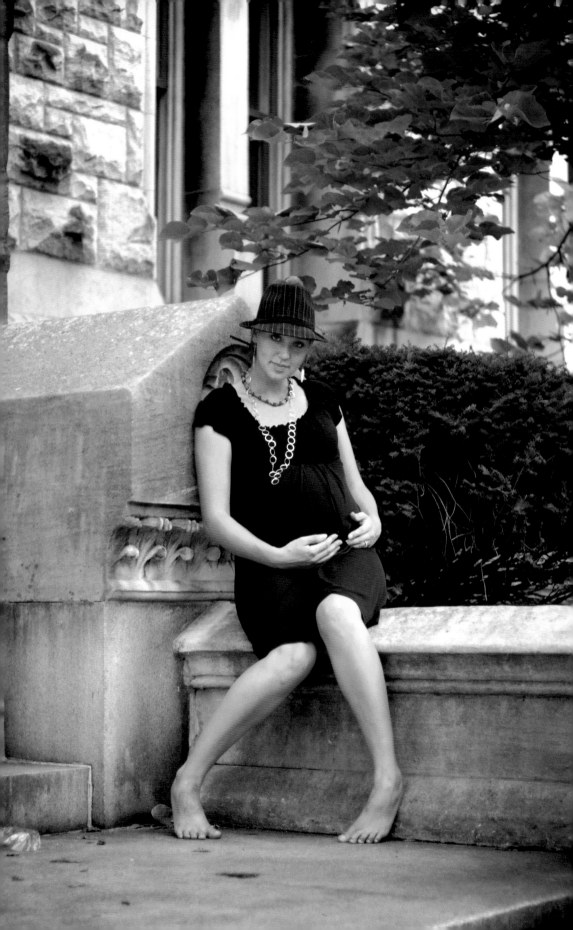

Horsetail Tincture
Beautiful Skin That Shines

Helps with skin's elasticity, hair, and nails.

Horsetail/shavegrass, dried, cut, and sifted

Vodka

Prep: 5 min.   Soak: 6 weeks   Yield: 1-3 cups

1. Fill a quart- or pint-size glass canning jar ⅔ full with horsetail/shavegrass.

2. Pour in vodka, filling up the jar to one inch from the top.

3. Screw lid on and set in cabinet, out of sunlight and heat.

4. Shake the jar once a week. After 6 weeks, strain off the liquid and put it in a tincture bottle. Label the tincture.

Be careful: horsetail can increase estrogen levels. I only take one dropper once a day when my skin is feeling tight.

You can also make this into a glycerin tincture. (See page 22 for an example of how to make a glycerin tincture.)

Toothpaste
Good Enough for Grandma and Her Pearly Whites

1 tsp. baking soda

1-2 drops peppermint oil

1. Brush with this and you will have pearly whites and fresh breath!

Deodorant
Stay Clean and Toxic-Free.

¼ cup baking soda

¼ cup arrowroot powder or corn starch

5 T. coconut oil

20 drops of your favorite essential oil: lavender, rosemary, peppermint

1. Slightly warm coconut oil.

2. Combine baking soda, arrowroot powder, and essential oil in a bowl and mix into coconut oil.

3. Pour into an empty, clean deodorant stick. It will harden once it has completely cooled.

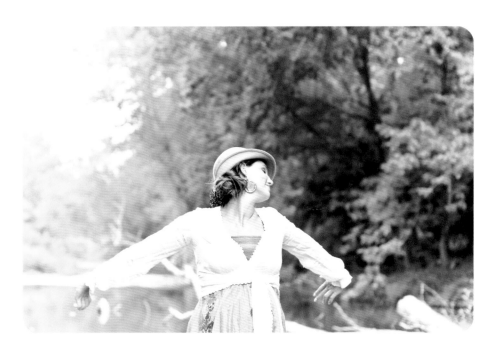

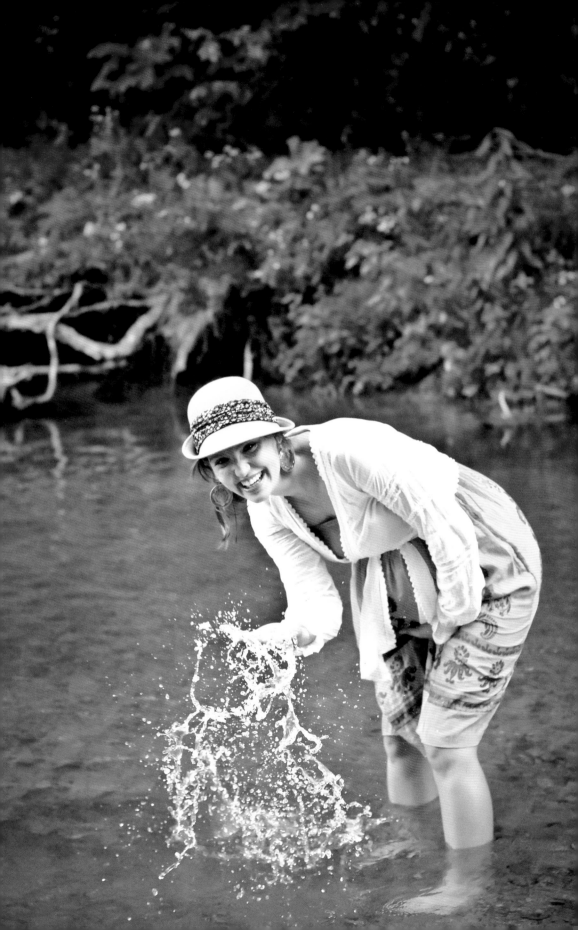

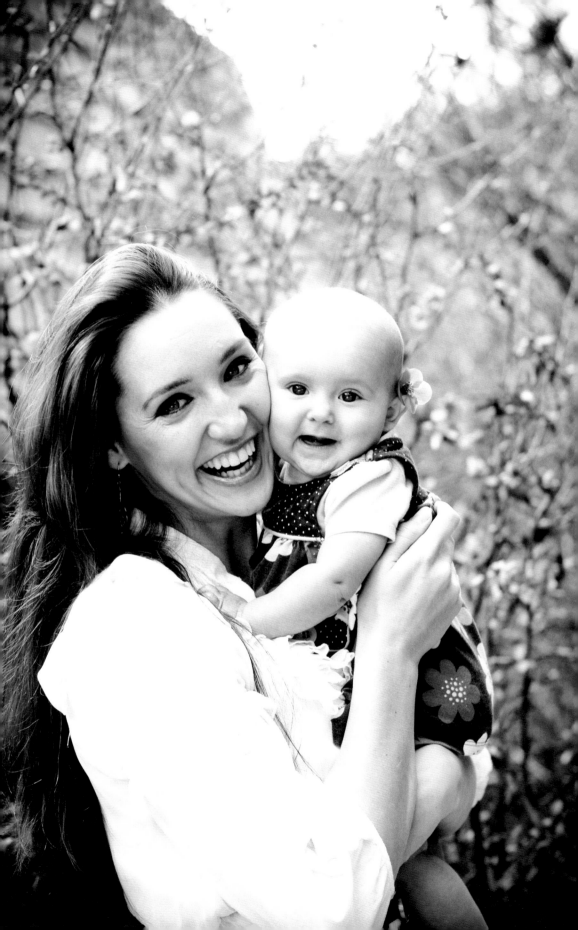

Renew Your Face

Fresh Face With Fresh Ingredients

Almond Scrub

3 T. almond flour

I T. raw honey

1. In a small bowl, mix ingredients together. With lukewarm water, wash face with gentle, upward, circular motions, using the scrub. Rinse well and pat dry.

Bentonite Clay Mask

I T. bentonite clay

I T. spring or filtered water

1. Put ingredients in the palm of one hand. Put hands together and rub, rub, rub. Apply mask to face, avoiding eye and lid areas. Relax! No talking. Let it sit for 15 to 20 minutes and wash off with lukewarm water. Rinse well and pat dry.

New Skin

I tsp. fresh aloe vera juice

1. Cut off a small piece of aloe leaf from the plant. With a knife split it open and scrape out the juice. Apply 1 teaspoon juice to face. Let it soak and dry.

2. Go to sleep and wake up with new skin.

Grandma's Remedies

Teething
What Grandma Did for Me

Method 1

1 tsp. catnip, dried or chamomile flowers

1 cup water

Method 2

4 drops clove oil

1 T. coconut oil or olive oil

Method 3

Brandy

Method 1

Steep dried catnip or chamomile flowers in 1 cup boiling water for 10 to 15 minutes, strain, and freeze in cubes or cool in refrigerator. Rub herb cube on gums or soak a piece of clean cotton gauze in the cold tea and apply directly to the child's gums. Use every two to three hours, or as needed.

Method 2

Combine clove oil with coconut or olive oil and rub directly onto the gums with a clean finger. The oil can irritate the skin and gums so try some in your mouth before giving to your baby to ensure you have diluted it enough. Repeat the treatment once every hour or as needed throughout the day.

Method 3

With a clean finger, rub a small amount of brandy on teething area. Use every two to three hours.

Grandma's Remedies

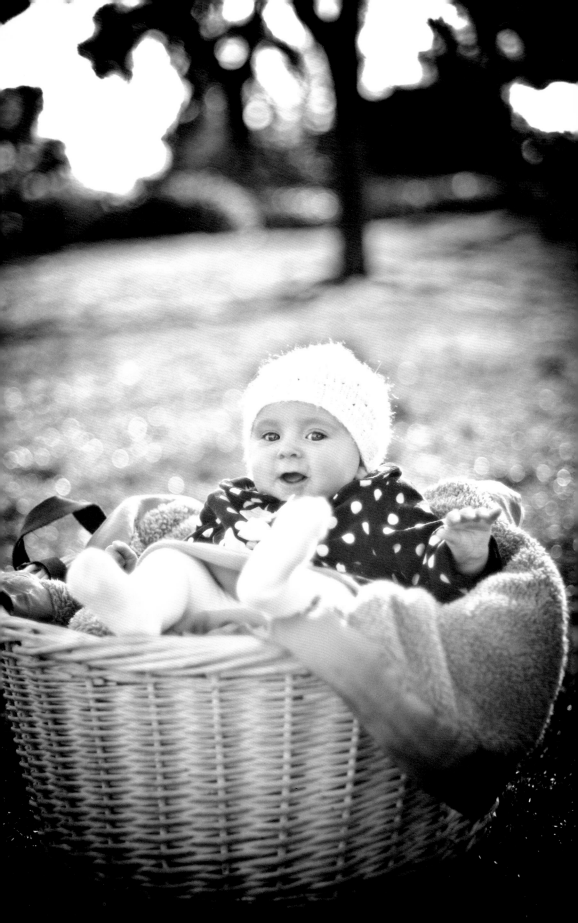

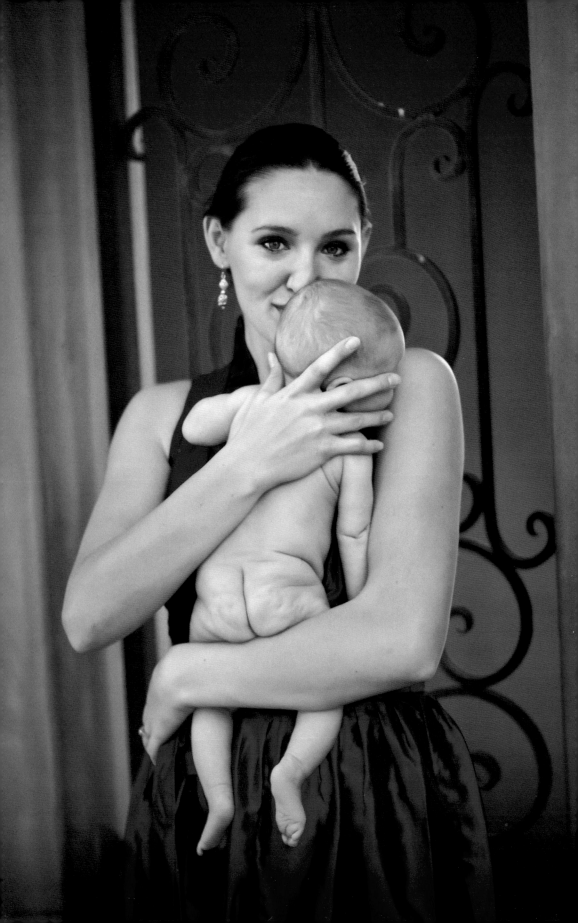

Nursing

Nursing Forms a Wonderful Bond for Life.

It is important to teach your baby to nurse correctly from the beginning. Turn baby's whole body toward you, chest to chest. Tease her with a touch of your nipple on her lips. When she opens her mouth wide, guide your breast to her. Her mouth should cover not just the nipple but as much of the areola (the darker part surrounding it) as possible.

For the first few weeks your nipples might be a little sore. If your baby is not nursing correctly, you might be in tears of pain. If that happens you might need some lanolin on your nipples. It helps sooth and heal them. Also talk to your midwife or doctor for proper latching techniques. If you have pain and cracked nipples, you are nursing incorrectly.

Healthy Butt

There Is Nothing Cuter Than a Baby's Bottom.

Calcium bentonite clay

Water

1. Mix clay and water into a paste. Apply to severe diaper rash. Reapply throughout the day as needed. The blisters should be gone within a day or two.

Fevers

Keep Your Baby Hydrated.

If your baby has a fever, make sure he is getting lots of liquid. NURSE,NURSE, NURSE!!!! Keep your baby hydrated. Lukewarm baths can also help bring the fever down.

If your baby is 6 months or older, you may be able to use garlic, lemon balm leaf, and other herbal remedies to treat the fever. If you are breastfeeding you may be advised to take the herbs and pass them on to your baby through your milk. Talk to your doctor and nutritionist.

Congestion

Breathe and Relax!

Try sitting with her in a small bathroom and let the steam of the shower or bath loosen up the mucus. You can add peppermint or a eucaliptic oil to the steam source. Mullein tea or infusion in bath to steam up the bathroom is also helpful.

Caution: Do not let yourself or your baby get overheated.

Grandma's Remedies

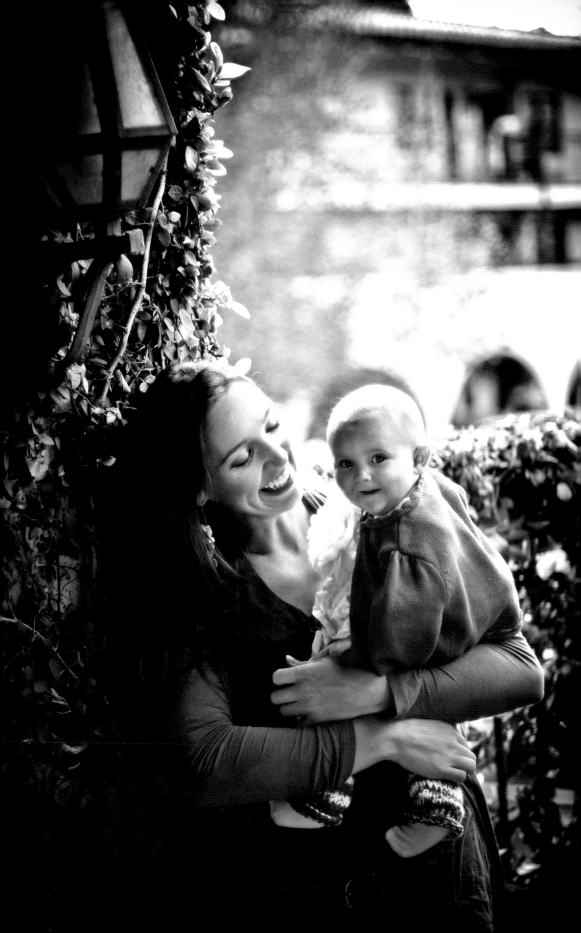

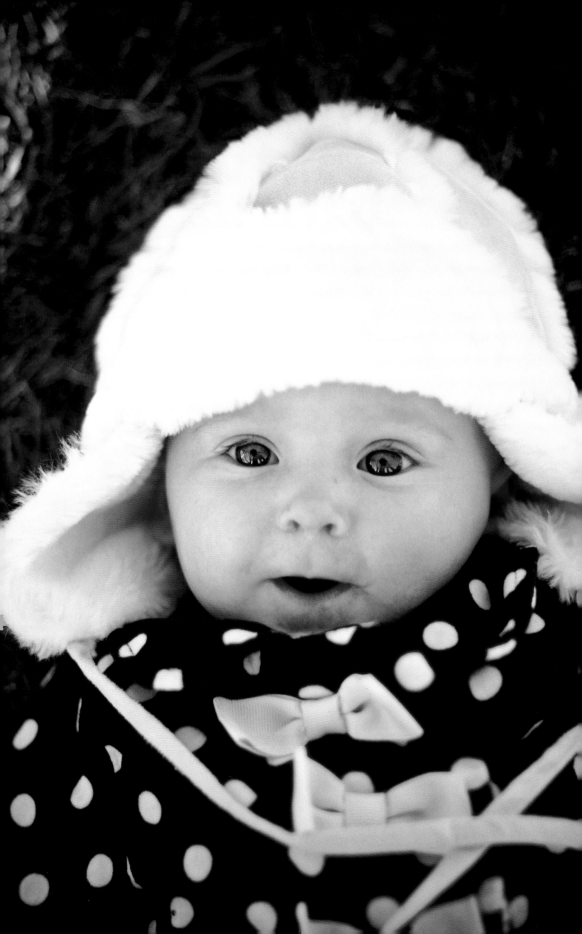

Ear Infection
This Really Helps!

1-2 T. olive oil

1 garlic clove

1. Heat olive oil until warm/hot.

2. Crush one clove garlic in oil.

3. Let sit 3 minutes, take garlic out.

4. Test the oil's temperature on your inner wrist. It needs to be warm but not hot.

5. Tilt head so that the infected ear is facing up. With a dropper or teaspoon, put 2-3 drops in the affected ear. I put a little cotton in the ear to keep the oil and heat in. It is best to stay lying down for 15-20 minutes. Use three times a day until pain is gone.

Do not use this remedy if your ear drum is already burst.

Washing Fruits and Veggies
Keep It Clean!

1 cup water

1 T. vinegar

1 T. lemon juice

1. Soak berries or anything that has cracks and crevices for 2 to 3 minutes.

2. Wash and lightly scrub firm things, then wipe dry.

3. Wash everything before you peel it. Chemicals are everywhere. Wash them off!

Grandma's Remedies

Household Cleaners
Give Your Baby a Healthy Start.

Oven Cleaner

Baking soda

Water

Liquid soap

1. Make a thick paste with baking soda and a little water. Scrub! If the oven is greasy, add a small amount of liquid soap.

All-Purpose Cleaner

1 quart vinegar of your choice

Peels from 3 oranges and one lemon

1. In a glass jar add vinegar and citrus. Screw lid on and set in a cabinet for two weeks.

2. Pour off peels. Use liquid concentrate or dilute. Pour into a spray bottle.

   Do not use on grout, because the vinegar will eat away at it.

Glass Cleaner

1 quart warm water

¼ cup white vinegar or 2 tablespoons lemon juice

1. Mix ingredients and store in a spray bottle.

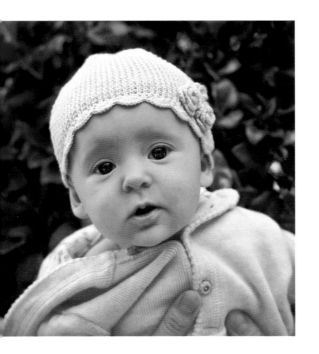

Sweet Aroma
Refresh Your Surroundings!

You can have a sweet-smelling house without all the chemicals and toxins.

8 cups water

1 cup dried herbs, your choice: lavender, rose, eucalyptus, rosemary, cloves, cinnamon, lemon peel, peppermint.

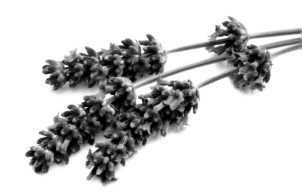

1. Simmer on stove top to purify and fill the air with a refreshing aroma.

Smells
Goodbye Smell!

Method 1

1 T. white vinegar

1 cup water

Method 2

Baking soda

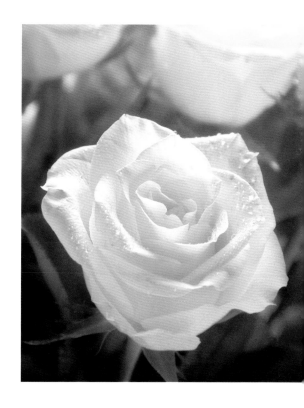

Method 1

1. Set out a dish of vinegar, or boil 1 tablespoon white vinegar in 1 cup of water to eliminate cooking odors.

Method 2

1. Use baking soda in refrigerators, closets, and other enclosed areas to absorb odors.

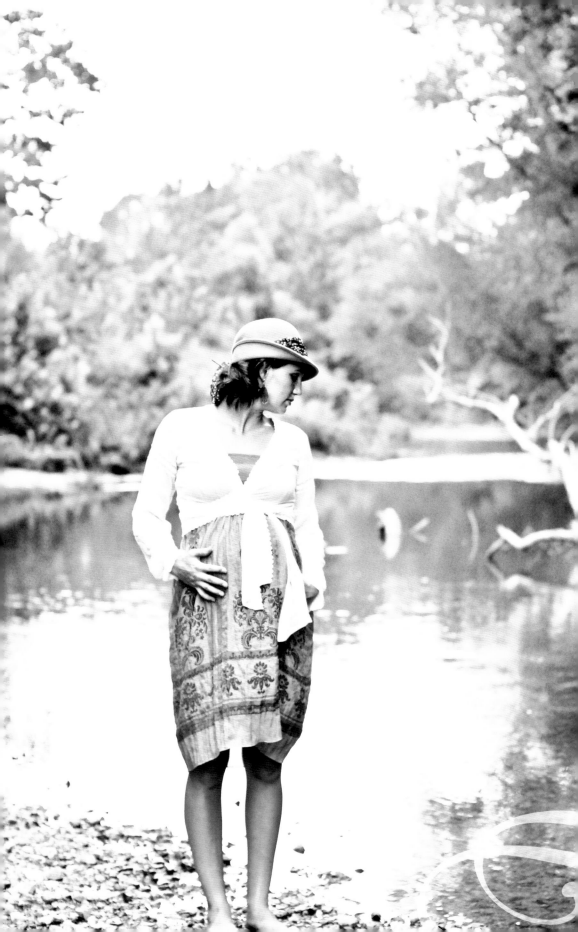

making babies

Baby Diary

Mama: _____

Daddy: _____

Baby's Due Date: _____

Sex: _____

Baby's Name: _____

Baby Diary
1st Month

This month, do something you have never done before but have always wanted to do.

A spectacular event occurs when sperm meets egg and makes a life inside of you. As small as a chia seed, your baby is starting to develop organs. Hundreds of cells are multiplying madly, forming your baby. Your body has built a house for your baby called an amniotic sac. You are a mama!

1 month and counting...

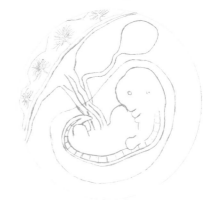

Take a picture every month to see
how your baby is growing and
changing your body.

Tape your photo or use photo tabs.

Date: _____

Weeks pregnant: _____

_____

_____

_____

Take B vitamins – especially folic acid.
They are very important. Eat raw
almonds. They are high in folate which
is the natural source of folic acid.

Where I was when I took my first pregnancy test:

How I told your daddy:

Who we told first:

My Checkup

Date: _____

Iron: _____

Weight: _____

Baby's heart beat: _____

Belly measurement: _____

Blood pressure: _____

Notes: _____

_____

_____

I need to work on: _____

_____

_____

There is love like no other love and it is
here between you and me.

Baby Diary
2nd Month

date

This month you need to dress up and go on a hot date with your man!

Your baby is about the size of a jelly bean, but he is growing so fast that in the next few weeks, he will be the size of an apricot. He is already kicking and stretching; and even though you cannot feel him, he is full of life.

2 months and counting...

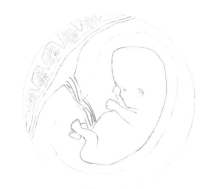

Take a picture every month to see
how your baby is growing and
changing your body.

Tape your photo or use photo tabs.

Date: _____

Weeks pregnant: _____

_____

_____

_____

Eat iron! Spinach, kale, chia seed, turnip greens, and red meat are all good sources. You and your baby need it.

Dear Baby, _____

_____

_____

_____

Love, Mama

Foods I have been craving: _____

_____

Foods I have been eating a lot of: _____

_____

My energy level has been: _____

My Checkup

Date: _____

Iron: _____

Weight: _____

Baby's heart beat: _____

Belly measurement: _____

Blood pressure: _____

Notes: _____

_____

_____

I need to work on: _____

_____

_____

A reflection of my love comes from you.

Baby Diary
3rd Month

date

This month buy some plain onesies and fabric paints. Invite some friends over and design your baby's first fashion statement.

Your baby might be sucking her thumb right now. Her brain has developed, giving her a new world. She can make faces, and even pee. She is about the size of a lemon, but she is growing so fast that in a few weeks she will be the size of an avocado.

3 months and counting...

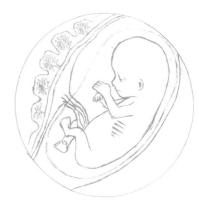

Take a picture every month to see
how your baby is growing and
changing your body.

Tape your photo or use photo tabs.

Date: _____

Weeks pregnant: _____

_____

_____

_____

Take omega fish oil – brain food for you and your baby. Eat some fish, raw nuts, and coconut oil.

Dear Baby, _____

_____

_____

_____

Love, Mama

People ask if you are a boy or a girl. I think:

_____

My sizes are changing. I am wearing: _____

_____

I have been feeling: _____

_____

My Checkup

Date: _____

Iron: _____

Weight: _____

Baby's heart beat: _____

Belly measurement: _____

Blood pressure: _____

Notes: _____

_____

_____

I need to work on: _____

_____

_____

You are the perfect distraction.

Baby Diary
4th Month

_____

_____

_____

_____

_____

_____

_____

_____

_____

_____

_____

_____

_____   *This month read <u>Bradley Birth the</u>*
                                  <u>Natural Way</u>, and start preggo
                                  exercises.

Your baby measures about 4½ inches long, crown to rump. She is about the size of a mango and weighs about 2½ ounces. She has developed fingerprints on her tiny fingertips. If you are having a girl, she has more than 2 million eggs in her ovaries. She is developing an ultra-fine covering of hair, called lanugo, all over her body, which later she will lose.

4 months and counting...

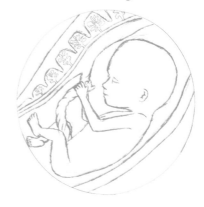

Take a picture every month to see
how your baby is growing and
changing your body.

Tape your photo or use photo tabs.

Date: _____

Weeks pregnant: _____

_____

_____

_____

Keep taking those Bs. They are very important. If you are having morning sickness, you might want to take an extra dose of B6.

Dear Baby, _____

_____

_____

_____

Love, Mama

When I heard your heartbeat for the first time:

_____

When I felt you move for the first time:

_____

My favorite maternity outfit is:

_____

Date: _____

Iron: _____

Weight: _____

Baby's heart beat: _____

Belly measurement: _____

Blood pressure: _____

Notes: _____

_____

_____

I need to work on: _____

_____

_____

Life inside life. Soul inside soul.
Baby inside mama.

Baby Diary
5th Month

_____

_____

_____

_____

_____

_____

_____

_____

_____

_____

_____

_____

This month cook something you have never cooked before. Eat it with one of your favorite people.

Your baby weighs about 11½ ounces and is about 11 inches from head to heel. His heart is now pumping about 25 quarts of blood each day, and this amount will continue to increase as your baby continues to develop. His brain is growing fast and is very active, developing smell, taste, hearing, vision, and touch.

5 months and counting...

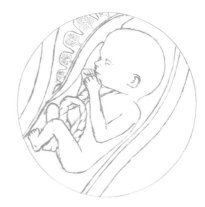

Take a picture every month to see
how your baby is growing and
changing your body.

Tape your photo or use photo tabs.

Date: _____

Weeks pregnant: _____

_____

_____

_____

Make sure you eat lots of greens. You need whole food iron.

Dear Baby, _____

_____

_____

_____

Love, Mama

Names we love and might name you:

_____   _____

_____   _____

_____   _____

Date: _____

Iron: _____

Weight: _____

Baby's heart beat: _____

Belly measurement: _____

Blood pressure: _____

Notes: _____

_____

_____

I need to work on: _____

_____

_____

God's art. Man, woman, making
babies, BABIES.

Baby Diary
6th Month

_____

_____

_____

_____

_____

_____

_____

_____

_____

_____

_____

This month get a movie, make some Cracker Jack, and have a home date with your man.

Your baby weighs about a pound and a half and is 14 inches. She is growing faster than ever now. She can feel you dance and hear you sing. She recognizes your voice. She has developed lips, eyelids, eyebrows, and tiny tooth buds beneath her gums. As you get to know her as she flips around, you might even notice her schedule.

6 months and counting...

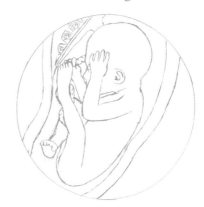

Take a picture every month to see
how your baby is growing and
changing your body.

Tape your photo or use photo tabs.

Date: _____

Weeks pregnant: _____

_____

_____

_____

Calcium is a must. Your baby's bones are needing lots as they harden.

Dear Baby, _____

_____

_____

_____

Love, Mama

The weirdest food craving I have had:

The times you move around the most:

What triggers your movement:

My Checkup

Date: _____

Iron: _____

Weight: _____

Baby's heart beat: _____

Belly measurement: _____

Blood pressure: _____

Notes: _____

_____

_____

I need to work on: _____

_____

_____

Time goes by quickly if you sing,
slowly if you sigh.

Baby Diary
7th Month

This month buy yourself something that fits and looks fabulous.

Your baby weighs 3½ pounds and is about 16 inches long. He can turn his head from side to side. Your baby will gain a third to half of his birth weight during the next 7 weeks as he fattens up. You will be feeling a lot of movement as your baby gets stronger and ready for the world.

7 months and counting...

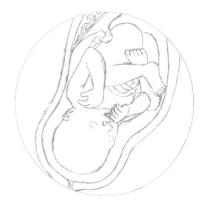

Take a picture every month to see
how your baby is growing and
changing your body.

Tape your photo or use photo tabs.

Date: _____

Weeks pregnant: _____

_____

_____

_____

Nutritional demands are growing. You'll need plenty of protein, vitamin C, folic acid, iron, and calcium.

Dear Baby, _____

_____

_____

_____

Love, Mama

The first time I felt you hiccup:

_____

Can you pee anymore? I pee:

_____

I talk to you about:

_____

Date: _____

Iron: _____

Weight: _____

Baby's heart beat: _____

Belly measurement: _____

Blood pressure: _____

Notes: _____

_____

_____

I need to work on: _____

_____

_____

Mama's eyes, daddy's hair, grandpa's
wisdom, and grandma's heart;
making babies!

Baby Diary
8th Month

_____
date

_____

_____

_____

_____

_____

_____

_____

_____

_____

_____

_____   *This month go out with the girls.*

_____   *Get a " small" dress for after you*

have your baby.

Your baby is about 6 pounds and gains around an ounce a day. She is more than 18½ inches long. She's shedding the fine hair that covered her body. Her kidneys are fully developed now, and her liver can process some waste products. She needs to put on some more fat and soon she will be arriving!

8 months and counting...

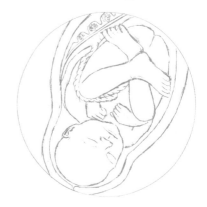

Take a picture every month to see
how your baby is growing and
changing your body.

Tape your photo or use photo tabs.

Date: _____

Weeks pregnant: _____

_____

_____

_____

Take plenty of omega fatty acids, and eat small amounts of protein throughout the day.

_____

_____

_____

_____

The first time a stranger put her hands on my belly:

_____

The first time I noticed a stranger being nice because I'm pregnant: _____

The first time I saw my belly move from your acrobatics: _____

My Checkup

Date: _____

Iron: _____

Weight: _____

Baby's heart beat: _____

Belly measurement: _____

Blood pressure: _____

Notes: _____

_____

_____

I need to work on: _____

_____

_____

You are on my mind all the time. I
love you, sweet baby of mine!

Baby Diary
9th Month

date

This month enjoy the quiet moments with your man. Spend as much quality time with him as you can.

Your baby will probably weigh anywhere from 7 to 10 lbs. The average newborn weighs about 7½ pounds and is about 20 inches long. His skull bones are not yet fused, allowing them to overlap as he passes through the birth canal during labor. He is still working hard building up fat to live in this world.

9 months and counting...

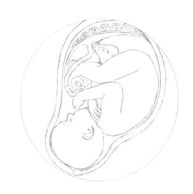

Take a picture every month to see
how your baby is growing and
changing your body.

Tape your photo or use photo tabs.

Date: _____

Weeks pregnant: _____

_____

_____

_____

Keep taking all your vitamins and drink lots of water.

Dear Baby, _____

_____

_____

_____

Love, Mama

Getting sleep is: _____

I cannot believe how much my body has: _____

The music I play you most is: _____

My Checkup

Date: _____

Iron: _____

Weight: _____

Baby's heart beat: _____

Belly measurement: _____

Blood pressure: _____

Notes: _____

_____

_____

I need to work on: _____

_____

Perfect, precious, priceless, and part
of me, my baby!

We love you,

_____ !

Baby's Name

Take a photo of your newborn baby.

Tape your photo or use photo tabs.

Date of birth: _____

Your Birth

Where I was when my water broke: _____

_____

I was in labor with you for _____ hours.

You arrived at: _____ : _____ AM / PM

You were born in _____ , _____ .
                        City   State

I gave birth to you in _____
                              (my bed, bathtub, etc.)

at _____ .
              (home, hospital name, etc.)

You were delivered by : _____

Who was at your birth:

_____   _____

_____   _____

_____   _____

_____ cut the umbilical cord.

How it felt the first time I saw you:

_____

_____

Dear Baby, _____

_____

_____

_____

_____

_____

_____

_____

_____

_____

_____

_____

_____

_____

_____

Love, Mama

Music plays, summer haze, loving you always. Hold my hand. You have my heart. You are God's form of ART.

Left Hand

Right Hand

Left Foot

Right Foot

Mother's name: _____
Date of birth

Father's name: _____
Date of birth

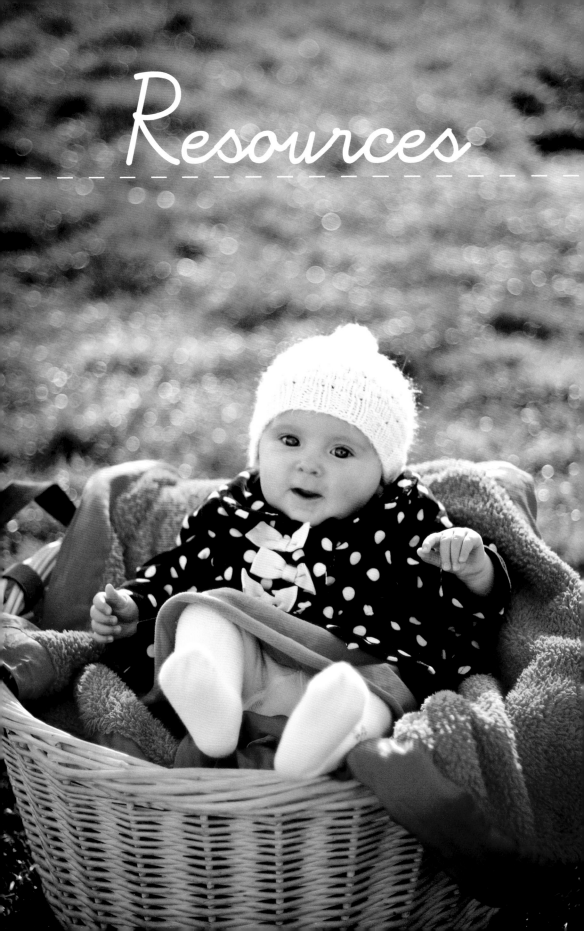

Resources

Books

The ABC Herbal For Children's Health
Steven H. Horne
Whitman Books, Inc. (1992)
Available at Bulk Herb Store

Fresh Food From Small Spaces
By R. J. Ruppenthal
Chelsea Green Publishing Company (2008)
Available at Bulk Herb Store

The Herbal Body Book: A Natural Approach to Healthier Hair, Skin, and Nails
By Stephanie Tourles
Storey Publishing (1994)

Herbal Remedies for Children's Health
By Rosemary Gladstar
Storey Publishing (1999)
Available at Bulk Herb Store

How to Grow Fresh Air
By B. C. Wolverton
Penguin (1997)
Available at Bulk Herb Store

Husband Coached Childbirth: The Bradley Method of Natural Childbirth
By Robert A. Bradley, M.D.
Bantam Books (2008)
Available at Bulk Herb Store

Living Clay
By Perry A~
LivingClayCo.com
Available at Bulk Herb Store

Natural Baby and Childcare
By Lauren Feder, M.D.
Hatherleigh Press (2006)

Natural Baby Care: Pure and Soothing Recipes and Techniques for Mothers and Babies
By Colleen K. Dodt
Storey Publishing (1997)
Available at Bulk Herb Store

Natural Childbirth the Bradley Way
By Susan McCutcheon
The Penguin Group (1996)
Available at Bulk Herb Store

Naturally Healthy Pregnancy: 4th Edition
By Shonda Parker
Loyal Publishing (2008)
Available at Bulk Herb Store

Naturally Healthy Skin: Tips and Techniques for a Lifetime of Radiant Skin
By Stephanie Tourles
Storey Publishing (1999)
Available at Bulk Herb Store

The Natural Soap Book: Making Herbal and Vegetable-Based Soaps
By Susan Miller Cavitch
Storey Publishing (1995)
Available at Bulk Herb Store

The Nontoxic Baby: Reducing Harmful Chemicals from Your Baby's Life
By Natural Choices
Lotus Light Publications (1991)
Available at Bulk Herb Store

The One-Minute Cleaner Plain & Simple: 500 Tips for Cleaning Smarter, Not Harder
By Donna Smallin
Storey Publishing (2007)
Available at Bulk Herb Store

Organic Body Care Recipes: 175 Homemade Herbal Formulas for Glowing Skin & a Vibrant Self
By Stephanie Tourles
Storey Publishing (2007)
Available at Bulk Herb Store

The Perfect Pregnancy Cookbook
By Patrick Holford, Fiona McDonald Joyce and Susannah Lawson
Storey Publishing (2010)
Available at Bulk Herb Store

Prescription for Nutritional Healing: 5th Edition — A Practical A-to-Z Reference to Drug-Free Remedies Using Vitamins, Minerals, Herbs & Food Supplements
By Phyllis A. Balch, CNC
Penguin Group (2010)
Available at Bulk Herb Store

Put 'em Up
By Sherri Brooks Vinton
Storey Publishing (2010)
Available at Bulk Herb Store

Raw Energy: Raw Food Recipes for Energy Bars, Smoothies, and Other Snacks to Supercharge Your Body
By Stephanie Tourles
Storey Publishing (2009)
Available at Bulk Herb Store

Salt Your Way to Health: 2nd Edition
By David Brownstein, M.D.
Medical Alternatives Press (2010)
Available at Bulk Herb Store

Smart Medicine for a Healthier Child: 2nd Edition - A Practical A-to-Z Reference to Natural and Conventional Treatments for Infants & Children
By Janet Zand, N.D., L.Ac., Robert Rountree, M.D., Rachael Walton, MSN, CRNP
Penguin Group (2003)

The Vaccine Book
By Robert W. Sears, M.D., F.A.A.P.
Hachette Book Group (2007)

Websites

American Association of Birth Centers
www.birthcenters.org

Birthing centers all over the country.

Baby Center
www.babycenter.com

When I was pregnant with my first child, I signed up on this website to receive weekly e-mails about the growth and development of my baby. I loved them! I looked forward to reading them every week. The e-mail also covers what pregnant mama is going through.

Baby Earth
www.babyearth.com

Lots of organic products.

Bulk Herb Store
James and Shoshanna Easling's family business

877-278-4257

26 West 6th Ave
Lobelville, TN 37097
www.bulkherbstore.com

We not only sell quality herbs at great prices, we teach you what they're good for and how to use them. We are family-owned and work hard to give you the service you deserve.

Cutie Poops
www.cutiepoops.com

Cute, custom-made diapers.

Diapers.com
www.diapers.com

Diapers and wipes at a good price.

DONA International
www.dona.org

If you want a doula to coach you through your birth, here is a website to find one. A doula is a birthing coach that talks you through labor and delivery, rubs what hurts, and is just there for you.

Natural Eco Organics
www.naturaleco.com

Great products from herbal remedies to organic clothes.

Nurturebaby
www.nurturebaby.com

This is a cute website full of great ideas and recipes for baby food.

Panano
www.panano.com

Organic clothes, toys, and bedding.

100% Pure New Zealand Colostrum
www.nextag.com/sedona-labs-colostrum-powder

I love this stuff! It works great and is the cheapest I've found.

Glossary

Alfalfa is a medicinal plant. It is extremely rich in vitamins and minerals. It has 8 essential amino acids and the highest chlorophyll content of any plant. Available at Bulk Herb Store.

Almond butter is made from almonds that are ground into a butter. Almonds are a good source of healthy fats, protein, vitamins, and minerals.

Apple cider vinegar with the mother is raw, unfiltered, and unpasteurized vinegar and is a powerful cleansing and healing elixir and a naturally occurring antibiotic and antiseptic that fights germs and bacteria.

Arrowroot powder is a medicinal, nutritious root. It is an easily digested food and an excellent thickening agent in recipes. Available at Bulk Herb Store.

Avocado is a fruit high in enzymes and healthy fats. It is great for your skin and digestive system.

Berry Herbal Brew is a mix of Indian gooseberry, bilberry fruit, bilberry leaf, pomegranate, fig leaf, and grape leaf. It is a unique blend of specially formulated ingredients that combine during the fermentation process to release their healthful benefits, including antiviral, antimicrobial, and very high antioxidant properties. Only available at Bulk Herb Store.

Beet root (Beta vulgaris) is a vegetable that contains high levels of important vitamins, minerals, and micronutrients. It is very good for you! Available at Bulk Herb Store.

Bentonite clay is an effective and powerful healing clay used to treat both internal and external maladies. Its greatest power lies in its ability to absorb toxins, impurities, heavy metals, and other internal contaminants. Available at Bulk Herb Store.

Blackstrap molasses (sulfur-free) is made from leftovers of sugarcane and is filled with minerals and vitamins. It has a high iron content and is used to holistically overcome anemia.

Blanched almond flour is simply ground, blanched almonds. You can make almond flour in a blender or food processor.

Blessed thistle is a medicinal plant that is high in potassium and sodium. It is most commonly used to enrich and increase milk in nursing mothers and to help balance females. There have been warnings to avoid internal use during pregnancy. Available at Bulk Herb Store.

Bragg's Liquid Aminos is an all-purpose seasoning. It is made from non-GMO soy that has been fermented. Most of the time I say run from soy, but because this is non-GMO and fermented, it is good for you.

Buckwheat is not related to wheat. It is a fruit and is gluten-free unless it is contaminated with cross-pollination. It is high in digestive protein and contains all eight essential amino acids.

Burdock is a medicinal plant that is a strong blood purifier and cleanser. Burdock root has been used to neutralize and eliminate toxins in the system. Available at Bulk Herb Store.

Casein is found in milk. Many people are sensitive to it in cow's milk and do not eat dairy products. Sometimes people are even sensitive to it in goat's milk.

Catnip is a medicinal plant that is used to sooth the belly and prompt sleep. It is full of vitamins and is used often in the treatment of children's ailments. Available at Bulk Herb Store.

Cayenne is a pepper and is one of the most powerful herbs for stimulating the body's energies for healing. Available at Bulk Herb Store.

Chamomile has medicinal flowers that are known to settle the stomach and calm the nerves. It is probably one of the very best nervine herbs for children. Available at Bulk Herb Store.

Coriander is the seed of cilantro, a wonderful herb. Coriander seed is used a lot in Indian food. It is full of vitamins and minerals.

Coconut flour is derived from the meat of a mature coconut. It is a gluten-free option when baking and is very nutritious and wonderful for you.

Coconut milk is derived from the meat of a mature coconut. Coconuts have antibacterial and antiviral substances that help protect your body from viruses and diseases.

Coconut oil is extracted from the kernel or meat of a matured coconut. Coconut oil is great for your skin and has many wonderful health benefits.

Coconut water is the juice that comes out of a young coconut. Full of electrolytes and soooo good for you. Coconuts have antibacterial and antiviral substances that help protect your body from viruses and diseases.

Cumin is a medicinal seed that has a nutty, peppery flavor. It is used a lot in Middle Eastern and Mexican cooking. Cumin is an excellent source of iron. Available at Bulk Herb Store.

Curry powder is a mixture of widely varying herb spices from Asia. The combinations of herbs are blood-purifying and anti-aging.

Dandelion is a medicinal plant. It might look like just a weed with a puffy ball and yellow flower that grows in your yard, but it is not a weed at all. It is a wonderful herb, high in iron, and one of the best blood purifiers and builders available. Available at Bulk Herb Store.

Double-E Immune Booster is a combination of nettle leaf, peppermint leaf, echinacea root, echinacea tops, whole elderberries, eleuthero root, and rosehips. It is highly nutritious and a great immune booster. Only available at Bulk Herb Store.

Doula is a person trained to help the birthing mother cope with the pain. She helps give the mother the best birth experience she can have. If you are having a hospital birth, you want a doula. She will help you have a natural birth and deal with the hospital tug-of-war.

Eden Salve is an organic mix of herbs and oils used to numb pain, as well as heal and soothe. It acts as an astringent to draw out infection and poisonous bites. It is an antiseptic and fights bacteria. Only available at Bulk Herb Store.

Eleuthero root, commonly known as Siberian ginseng, is a medicinal root. This herb has been shown to enhance mental acuity and physical endurance. Available at Bulk Herb Store.

Epsom salts are made up of a naturally occurring mineral that is found in water. It is easily obtained at any drug store or supermarket. From easing stress to improving oxygen, epsom salt is very beneficial.

Essential oils are concentrated liquids containing volatile aroma compounds from plants. They are used medicinally and fragrantly.

Fenugreek is a medicinal seed. It is a very nutritious herb that promotes a healthy digestive system and helps to dissolve cholesterol and fatty substances. Available at Bulk Herb Store.

Fennel is a medicinal plant. The seed is used commonly for spice. It has a nice flavor that children love. It is marvelous for colic in small babies or for stomach aches in people of all ages. The fennel bulb is used in cooking like a vegetable. Available at Bulk Herb Store.

Fish sauce is a condiment that is derived from fermented fish. It is an essential ingredient in many curries and sauces. It is very high in omega-3s.

Flax is a seed that is highly beneficial to your health. It is high in omega fatty acids, B vitamins, and so many other vitamins and minerals. Available at Bulk Herb Store.

Folic acid is simply vitamin B9, folacin, and folate.

Garlic is a wonderful herb known to be a natural antibiotic. It is a blood purifier, antibacterial, antifungal, and more. Garlic powder is available at Bulk Herb Store.

Ginger root is a medicinal root used to treat nausea and indigestion, colic, irritable bowel, loss of appetite, chills, cold, flu, poor circulation, menstrual cramps, and so much more. Available at Bulk Herb Store.

Ginkgo leaf comes from a medicinal tree. It is used to treat poor circulation. Studies have shown it to be effective in increasing peripheral blood flow. It is also great for the brain. Available at Bulk Herb Store.

Gluten is a protein found in wheat. It is said that due to the increasing genetic alterations in wheat, more and more people are showing signs of wheat allergies. A gluten-free diet is one that excludes foods with gluten. Gluten is in almost everything you buy with a label.

Glycerine (food grade) is a nontoxic, natural food substance derived from palm or coconut. It is sweet to taste but does not cause blood sugar problems. Great for making an herbal concoction. Available at Bulk Herb Store.

Hawthorn berries are medicinal berries. They regulate high and low blood pressure, arrhythmic heartbeat and irregular pulse, and help with all-around strengthening of the heart. Available at Bulk Herb Store.

Hibiscus is a medicinal flower that is colorful and tasty. It has a tart, fruity taste and a rich, red color. Hibiscus has been used as a nutritious relaxant. Available at Bulk Herb Store.

Horsetail/shavegrass is a medicinal plant. It is known for its silica and is a great herb that gives your skin elasticity. Available at Bulk Herb Store.

Infusions are like very strong teas. They are made similarly to tea, but by increasing herbs 10 to 15 times and letting stand until cool.

Jojoba oil is produced in the seed of the jojoba plant. It is one of the closest oils to our skin's oil, which makes it so wonderful. It is anti-aging and great for hair and skin.

Lavender is a medicinal flower. It has a relaxing effect on the mind and body and makes a good remedy for anxiety and nervousness. Lavender is an aromatic herb with countless benefits. Available at Bulk Herb Store.

Leeks are vegetables. They are full of vitamins and minerals. Leeks look and taste similar to a big green onion.

Lemon balm is a medicinal plant. It has been a favorite with herbalists for a long time. It is good for the nervous system and digestive system, and strengthens the brain and memory. Available at Bulk Herb Store.

Lemon grass is a medicinal plant. It is a mild sedative, promoting sleep and health throughout the body. It can be made into a tasty tea that the whole family can enjoy. Available at Bulk Herb Store.

Lentils are grown and cooked like beans, but they are seeds. They are highly nutritious and very beneficial for everything from conception to everyday life. Lentils are a superfood!

Mama's Red Raspberry Brew is a mix of red raspberry, alfalfa, nettle, and peppermint. This combination of herbs is highly nutritious, delicious, and great for the uterus. Some sources caution you to wait until 14 weeks into your pregnancy to use red raspberry. Only available at Bulk Herb Store.

Mama's Milk Tea is a mixture of red raspberry leaf, fennel seed, nettle leaf, fenugreek seed, dandelion leaf, and blessed thistle. This combination was made by a nursing mama who needed to increase her milk supply and the nutritional value of her milk. IT WORKED for her and many others. Only available at Bulk Herb Store.

Masa is corn that has been soaked in slaked lime or ash and water, removing the hull and making hominy, then rinsed, dried, and powdered. It is used for making tortillas, tamales, and many other Latin American dishes.

Mineral rocks/salt rocks are all-natural mineral salts. The salt rock keeps bacteria from building up and creating a smell, keeping you fresh without adding chemicals to your body.

Mullein is considered the herb of choice for respiratory problems. It helps loosen mucus and expel it from the body. Available at Bulk Herb Store.

Mustard is a medicinal seed that is a very good source of omega-3 fatty acids and a good source of iron, calcium, zinc, manganese, magnesium, and more. Available at Bulk Herb Store.

Nettle is a medicinal plant. This herb is packed with vitamins and minerals and is used as a diuretic, relieving joint pain, and more. Available at Bulk Herb Store.

Oatstraw is a medicinal plant. It is a great filler herb and an excellent source of the major minerals used in the structure of the body, including magnesium and calcium. Available at Bulk Herb Store.

Omega fatty acids are essential, unsaturated fatty acids. They are found in fish and nuts, and they promote heart, skin, and overall health.

Passion flower is a medicinal plant. It is used to treat pain, insomnia, the nervous system, tension, stress headaches, and smooth muscle spasms. Available at Bulk Herb Store.

Portobello mushrooms are flavorful, meaty mushrooms ranging from button-size to pancake-size. They are high in vitamin C and packed with other vitamins and minerals.

Potato flour is a flour which is produced from cooked potatoes, which are then dried and ground.

Potato starch is starch extracted from potatoes. The starch is then washed out and dried to powder.

Psyllium is a medicinal seed. It has been called a "colon broom," because it scrubs the colon. When mixed with a liquid, it creates bulk and pulls putre-factive toxins from the sides of the intestines. Available at Bulk Herb Store.

Quinoa is an edible seed. It has a mild, lightly nutty flavor. It is great to use in the place of rice or mashed potatoes. It is rich in protein, amino acids, fiber, and more.

Raw honey has not been pasteurized or refined. It is honey in its raw state. Honey is best in its purest form, straight from the beehive, full of bee pollen, propolis, antioxidants, and more. Available at Bulk Herb Store.

Raw sugar (turbinado) is unrefined sugar that still contains minerals and nu-trients that are stripped from refined white sugar and regular brown sugar.

Red raspberry leaf is a medicinal leaf. It is a wonder herb for the uterus. This king of women's herbs promotes healthy and strong female functions. Some sources caution you to wait until 14 weeks into your pregnancy to use red raspberry. Available at Bulk Herb Store.

Rhubarb stock is red and looks a bit like large celery pieces. It is a vegetable that is used more as a fruit. Rhubarb is a superfood and great for fertility.

Rise and Shine Tea is a mixture of bilberry leaf, ginkgo, green tea, peppermint, cloves, and ginger root. It is a wonderful burst of flavor and a punch of energy. Only available at Bulk Herb Store.

Rooibos is a medicinal leaf, rich in antioxidants, a sweet and slightly nutty flavor. It is naturally non-caffeinated and contains high levels of copper, iron, potassium, calcium, fluoride, zinc, and more. It is a wonderful tea that both pregnant and nursing mothers can enjoy. Available at Bulk Herb Store.

Rose hips are medicinal and come from the dried fruit of roses. They are full of vitamin C and great for fighting stress and infections. Available at Bulk Herb Store.

Sea salt is unrefined and unprocessed salt, free of chemicals that are very harmful. Sea salt is full of minerals and helps to level the sodium and potassium in your body. Available at Bulk Herb Store.

Sleep Tight Tea is a mixture of catnip, chamomile, lemon balm, and passion flower. It is a sweet-tasting tea that is full of nutrition. It relaxes the muscles and promotes good sleep. Only available at Bulk Herb Store.

Sorghum flour is made from the grains on top of the sorghum cane. It is a gluten-free alternative to wheat and is best used when mixed with other flours and starches to give a wheat-like texture.

Sparkling water (also called mineral water, carbonated water, club soda, soda water, seltzer, or fizzy water) is water with carbonation, resulting from dissolving carbon dioxide in water. In certain places, it even comes out of the ground that way.

Spearmint is a plant that can be made into a medicinal tea. With a refreshing taste, it increases the production of digestive fluids and enzymes, relieves smooth muscle spasms, and more. Available at Bulk Herb Store.

Stevia is an herb that tastes sweet but does not change your sugar levels. A small pinch of stevia leaves can sweeten up a glass of tea.

Sucanat is sugar cane that is not refined or processed like white or brown sugar. It is essentially pure, dried sugar cane juice, retaining its molasses content.

Tapioca flour is a starch extracted from the root of the plant species of yuca. It helps to give gluten-free flours consistency.

Tahini is a paste made from ground sesame seeds, used in cooking. Tahini is made with hulled, lightly roasted seeds.

Thai chili peppers are about an inch long and very hot. The red ones are ripe, and the green ones are not, but you can eat either one and mix them together for color.

Tinctures are medicinal extracts in a liquid such as alcohol, glycerin, vinegar, or honey. In a tincture, an herb is broken down into the liquid by heat, alcohol, or fermentation.

Vegenaise is a healthy alternative to mayo. It tastes better and is much better for you. Available at most health food stores.

Very Berry Tea is a mixture of bilberry fruit, bilberry leaf, elderberry fruit, red raspberry leaf, and orange peel. It is a delightful tea that is anti-aging and full of vitamin C. Only available at Bulk Herb Store.

Xanthan gum is derived from the bacterial coating of Xanthomonas campestris. It is processed, but it is said to possibly promote gut health. There is so little used in cooking that it is unlikely to do much healthwise, one way or the other. It really makes a positive difference in textures when preparing gluten-free meals.

Yarrow is a medicinal plant. It helps soothe the skin, heal bruises, and stop bleeding. It is also used to treat colds, flu, and fevers. Available at Bulk Herb Store.

Yellow dock is a medicinal herb. It is known as "the herb for anemia." It is a wonderful blood cleanser, purifier, and builder. Available at Bulk Herb Store.

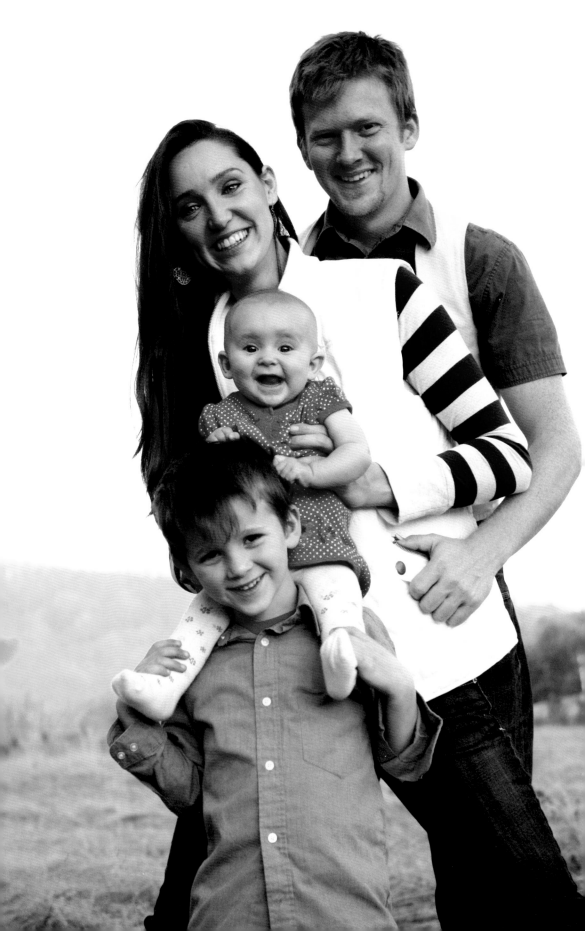

Learn and Live Well

Six years ago my husband and I moved into a rental. We did not know it at the time, but the walls and floor of the house were full of black mold. Within a short time we both had gotten sick. Two months later, I ended up in the emergency room with heart pain. I had developed a mitral valve proplapse, heart arrhythmia, and 3 calcified lumps in my lungs and glands. I could not walk 10 feet without blacking out. My husband was testing the house for everything under the sun when he found the mold. We moved out and I began researching, trying to get our health back. For over a year, I was so sick I could not even research much, but little by little I did. Research led me from one thing to another. I could not handle doing cleanses I found, because they would set off my heart. That is when I started making my own cleanses: DetoxPlus, Liver Cleanser, Herb-a-Smoothie, bentonite clay baths, and more. I made them to strengthen my body while detoxing it. It was a long road to recovery and even now, I am still working on fixing my mitral valve prolapse. It is much better already and I think I will have completely healed it within a few years. It has not been easy. From that one moldy house, my family has been through a lot of illness, but with illness, we have found health and been able to help others.

Six years later I have a beautiful, healthy, 1-year-old baby girl. She is the talk of the town, because she is so smart, cute, bossy, and sweet. I am blessed! I am truly blessed! I want this to be an encouragement to all of you who are sick or have been sick. Don't give up. Get your blood tested, research, learn, and talk to your doctor and nutritionist. Step by step, you can do it. You can LEARN AND LIVE WELL!!

Index

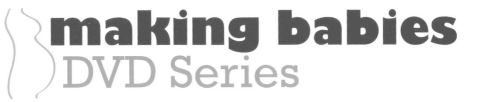

making babies
DVD Series

The *Making Babies* DVD series follows Shoshanna through her pregnancy, birth, and 6 months postpartum. Watch her stay healthy and strong as she builds a baby! This DVD series is full of delicious recipes, herbal remedies, tips, and more. Watch her peaceful labor and delivery as she teaches you how she does it. This is 7 hours and 5 minutes of pure fun, packed with information. It also features Johan C. Dinklemann, DC, Nancy A. Armetta, MD, Elaine M. Wakeland, CNM, and Jay Gordon, MD, FAAP. You will learn so much in this wonderful *Making Babies* DVD series. Available at Bulk Herb Store - www.BulkHerbStore.com

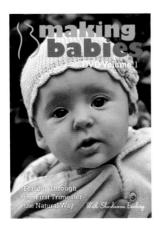
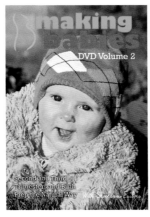
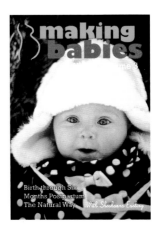

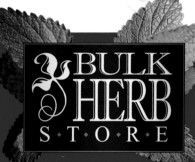

Bulk Herb Store

At the Bulk Herb Store, we provide homemade concoctions, our experience, and the tested wisdom of others. We want to do more than sell quality herbs at great prices. We want to inspire you to learn and research. Sign up for our free weekly e-blast, containing a fun and informative article, a YouTube video, and coupons. Learn and live well!

Making Herbs SIMPLE

DVDs Volumes 1 and 2

Making Herbs Simple volumes 1 and 2 are just that. They show you the simplicity of using herbs. Join Shoshanna as she teaches you how to find herbs in the wild. Learn what they are good for and how to use them in these captivating, educational DVDs. Check them out at BulkHerbStore.com.

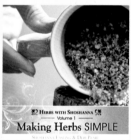
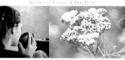
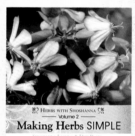
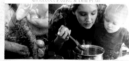

with Shoshanna Easling

 Get it at BulkHerbStore.com

Eden Salve
formulated by Shoshanna

This salve was formulated using an effective blend of herbs and natural ingredients to numb pain, as well as heal and soothe. It acts as an astringent to draw out infection and poisonous bites. It is an antiseptic and fights bacteria. When you and your family need it, nature's healing touch is here for you!

"Hi I just wanted to tell you how much I love your salve! I basically use it on everything! It does wonders on a tiny little baby bottom all the way to a sore 96-year-old grandma's skin. I always feel really confident when I use it because I know there is nothing unsafe about it! I keep it in my purse and am always pulling it out when friends need it. Thanks so much!"

-Carlene

Get it at BulkHerbStore.com

Health Begins with
Good Water

Filter your water with a Berkey water filter

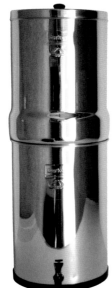

Healthy living begins with good drinking water. The water you drink is flushing your body and giving you health. Taste the difference of filtering out the heavy metals, E. coli, parasites, detergents, foul odors, herbicides, pesticides, and much more. You can taste and feel the difference in your health by drinking GOOD WATER. Up your energy! Up your health!

 Get it at BulkHerbStore.com

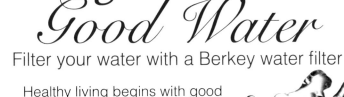

Thank You

A special thanks to: Audrey Madill for a wonderful design, Laura Newman for her fun and artistic photography of my family, and also Patricia Cohen, Lauren Brandt, Nate Crouch, Clint Cearly, Alicia Easling, Hanna Stoll, and Erin Harrison for wonderful photography. Shalom Brand for being there and helping me with anything I needed. Michael and Debi Pearl who raised me with confidence, love, and compassion, teaching and guiding me, making me the woman I am today.

Photo Credits

Laura Newman Photography: Cover, 2-4, 7, 8, 11, 14, 16, 54, 57, 62, 66, 78 (bottom left), 120-122, 123 (top), 124, 128 (bottom left), 144, 163, 167, 175, 176, 179, 186, 187, 191, 193, 200, 201, 214, 217, 234, 235, 242, 249, 251, 258-260, 270, 271, 277, 279, 283, 284, 287, 293, 299, 300, 305, 307, 308, 312-315, 321, 323, 325, 342, 344, 348, 350-352, 355, 356, 359, 360, 363, 364, 367, 371, 372, 376, 379, 380, 383, 384, 386, 389, 390, 393, 394, 396-398, 401, 402, 405, 406, 408, 410, 452, Back Cover

Patricia Cohen: 39, 50, 51 (bottom 4), 74 (bottom right), 131, 180, 183, 184, 185, 188, 192, 195, 196, 203, 204, 208, 212, 215, 216, 223, 224, 228, 231, 232, 236, 239, 240, 243, 244, 247, 250, 253, 254, 257, 261, 262, 265, 266, 269, 273, 274, 278, 281, 282, 285, 286, 289, 290, 294, 295, 297, 298, 301, 302, 306, 309, 310, 316, 317, 318, 322, 326, 329, 330, 333, 334, 337, 338, 341

Lauren Brandt: 65, 69 (top), 70 (top), 73, 74 (top), 77, 78 (top), 81, 82, 85 (top and bottom right), 86 (top), 89, 90, 91, 93, 94, 97, 98, 102, 115, 118, 139, 142, 143, 147, 152, 155, 159, 164, 173, 211

Nate Crouch Photography: 151, 207, 220, 227, 241, 335, 368, 375

Clint Cearly: 35 (bottom left and bottom right), 68, 86 (bottom right), 99 (bottom right), 127, 128 (right center), 168 (bottom right)

Alicia Easling: 12, 15, 19, 23, 35 (top), 36, 37, 42, 43, 44, 46, 47, 48, 49, 53

Hannah Stoll: 28, 31, 32, 40

Erin Harrison: 52 (top 3), 140, 466

Shoshanna Easling: 35 (bottom center), 86 (bottom left and center), 99 (top and bottom left), 101, 219